Healing Earths:
The Third Leg of Medicine

A History of Minerals in Medicine with rare illustrations from 300 to 1000 years ago

W. Rudolph Reinbacher

With a foreword by

William C. Mahaney

York University, Toronto, Canada

ISBN: 1-4033-5095-7 (e-book)
ISBN: 1-4033-5096-5 (Paperback)

This book is printed on acid free paper.

1stBooks – rev. 02/24/03

In Memoriam

Robert H. S. Robertson
1911-1999

Erudite classicist, tireless researcher

into earth's resources,

Friend and advisor to many,

And a true Scotsman.

…He spat on the ground, and made clay of the spittle, and he anointed the eyes of the blind man with the clay, and said unto him, "go and wash in the pool of Siloam". He went his way therefore, and washed, and came seeing.

New Testament, Gospel according to St. John, Verse 9, King James Translation.

Terra in carne est	Our flesh is from earth,
aer in halitu	Our breath is from air,
humor in sanguine	Our blood is from moisture,
ignis in calore vitali	Our life's warmth is from fire.

St. Isidor, Bishop of Seville
~600 AD

El Santuario de Chimayo (New Mexico)
in the year 2002:
Pilgrims to this little adobe church
still visit a small room to obtain
an earth believed to cure
bleeding scratches and skin itches.

Preface and Acknowledgements

The concept for this history of minerals in medicine developed out of my previous research into moonmilk, a cave sediment used for external and internal healing. Moonmilk was first described in detail in a monograph [then called a dissertation for teaching purposes] by the Kiel, Germany, professor of medicine Johann Daniel Major (1634-1693). Historians of medicine unfamiliar with moonmilk in geological context never took his "Dissertatio medica de lacte lunae" seriously. It is an introduction, in 90 pages of baroque Latin, to the subject of minerals in medical use.

The use of minerals in medicine is spread wide over time (over 5,000 years) and space (the entire world except Antarctica). The knowledge about this topic is scattered throughout many erudite volumes and papers, more often in ethnology and natural history than in medicine.

Intentionally or unintentionally, few histories of medicine contain any reference to minerals used for healing, and none mentions the actors of the past 150 years who proved the efficacy of clay: Addinell Hewson in the United States, Sebastian Kneipp, Pastor Emmanuel Felke, and Julius Stumpf in Germany. Histories of pharmacy (for example, Cowan & Dawson, 1988) often list only the traditional ancient writers, and they at best speculate on how many medications might have been based on plant material, how many on zoological material, and how many on mostly unidentified mineral substances.

I would like to express my sincere gratitude for the use of the facilities and collections of the Lane Medical Library of the Stanford University Medical School, and of Green Library of Stanford University including the Department of Rare Books and Special Collections. The Special Collections Department of the Public Library in St. Louis permitted access to one of the last copies in the world of a 1720 publication in their Benjamin Franklin Shumard Collection.

The accessibility on the internet of the Library of the Wellcome Institute for the History of Medicine in London proved a boon by allowing me to check roughly 5000 publications for possible content relating to earths in medicine. During my visit to London in February of 2001, the Wellcome Institute Library went out of its way to have almost 60 books on my wish list prepared on a library cart for quick and easy perusal. From Germany the granddaughter of our hero Julius Stumpf provided photographs and personal data about Julius and then helped to find information on Silesia.

Other libraries provided access to a few very rare special references, such as the German National Museum in Nürnberg. The Rare Books Department of the Library of the University of Erlangen let me hold and study a manuscript from 1100 AD; the Museum of Pharmacy in Heidelberg helped with copies of old journal articles. Würzburg University and the city archives provided records on the life of Julius Stumpf. Altogether libraries on three continents gave me access to more than 300 mostly rare books and publications.

No author can survive without critical review of facts and of style. I am indebted to geologist Dr. George W. Moore of Oregon State University for meticulous and at times painful instruction in subject and style, to speleologist Dr. Trevor R. Shaw, OBE, of Bath, England and of the Karst Research Institute at Ljubljana, Republic of Slovenia, for his knowledgeable comments, and to Don Eisenhour, Director of Research, American Colloid Company who is intimately familiar with the earths to be discussed and shared special knowledge with me.

Many thanks for the unperturbable patience of Chris Reinbacher who, after searching for her husband for five years in the 17th century while he wrote a biography of a professor of medicine, this time had to locate him somewhere within five millennia. Her proofreading is evidence of her dedication to this project. She participated in the ardors of field reseach travel and carried more than her share of work in the libraries we visited. And yes, she understood why at times I needed to dig into our savings to visit libraries for the study of books that have rested quietly in special collections for a hundred, 500 years, one even for eight hundred years.

All of them helped me in the unimaginably exciting journey through the world of rare and old books.

I offer special thanks for permission to reproduce illustrations from one of their rare holdings to

THE WELLCOME INSTITUTE LIBRARY, LONDON, for permission to reproduce many of the earth coin illustrations of C. G. Ludwig, 1748, "Terrae musei regni…"

THE PIERPOINT MORGAN LIBRARY, NEW YORK, for permission to reproduce four drawings from a 12th century incunabulum "Circa Instans" by Matthaeus Platearius,

THE OTT VERLAG UND DRUCKEREI, THUN,(SWITZERLAND) for allowing the reproduction of illustrations from the 1509 Hortus Sanitatis from their book by Hans Lüschen, "Die Namen der Steine", 1969.

<u>Foreword</u>

Minerals in medicine, or medications derived from natural earths, is a topic of long standing in human memory. It probably has traces extending well into the Paleolithic, with a history evolving over many hundreds of generations of humankind. Searching sources in ethnology, ethology, medical and natural history, W. Rudolph Reinbacher rekindles interest in the important use of clay and other minerals in medical treatment. Beginning with the very root of pharmacognosy—recognition of healing substances of nature—ancient peoples learned to enhance and protect life using organic and inorganic substances that became more varied as humans spread across the globe invading different habitats and encountering new diseases. The evolution of healing substances has had a long and complex history among different peoples, and no doubt evolved earlier amongst various groups in the animal kingdom. Indeed, as Reinbacher points out, ancient peoples may have learned about natural earths as medicants by observing the animals ingesting soil, a behavior known as geophagy.

Healing earths in the corpus of medical knowledge has never been totally erased from human memory. It would take two or three generations to obliterate totally all reference to healing earths. As pointed out by Reinbacher, ailments of one kind or another have ravaged human societies, and healing earths were used to combat many of them. First medical research into internal use of clay medicants was reported about 100 years ago in Germany, where it produced astounding results and proved great curative power in the treatment of vomiting and diarrhea and other gastrointestinal upsets. The slow evolution in the use of healing earths, from gypsum, kaolin, and alum in the ancient world of the Mediterranean has been all but eclipsed by the development of modern drugs. Medical doctors and researchers alike would do well to acquaint themselves with the healing earths and the experiments carried out by the physicians in the 19th and 20th centuries, all described in *The Third Leg of Medicine*.

Geophagy has been considered by many physicians (who frequently call it pica, the craving by pregnant women for odd foods, including earths) to be totally without value in the treatment of various malaises. As Reinbacher points out, this may be all well and good where antibiotics and inoculations can be had, but in regions of the Third World the use of clay medicants can be helpful in the treatment of diarrhea and dysentery, as well as cure for infectious wounds. Even cholera can be held at bay by ingesting small quantities of kaolin clay materials. The full story of kaolin and associated clay minerals, as well as carbonates and sulfates useful in the treatment of stomach ailments and associated gastrointestinal upsets, is told with verve and attention to detail. For those with an interest in alternative medicine and its historical roots in the natural world, this is an important work, one that should attract considerable attention.

Prof. Dr. William C. Mahaney
York University
Toronto (Canada)

Table of Contents

A Puzzle for the skeptical Reader:

Where would you look for these medicinal earths today?

1. Magnesium and aluminum hydroxide?

2. Bismuth subsalicylate?

3. Attapulgite, a clay?

4. Calcium carbonate?

5. Magnesium hydroxide?

6. Aluminum sulfate?

4) Mylanta®, Tums®

1) Maalox®

3) Kao-Pectate® liquid

5) Phillips "Milk of Magnesia"®

2) Pepto-Bismol®

6) Nick-Fix® styptic pencil

Answer: All are in your local pharmacy/drugstore

Chapter One: Introduction to a History

Throughout history, medical treatment was supported on three legs:
The first leg consisted of herbal selections, the second of animal products.
The third leg was the use of minerals such as healing earths.

Tribal needs for medications

Long, long before humankind had developed social speech as a communal tool and as yet had no pictorial, ideograph or alphabet writing, our omnivorous ancestors were mostly concerned with food and the health they needed to sustain life and surviving nature's adversity. No matter how isolated in time or geography, our human ancestors everywhere found the same or similar life benefit through animal, vegetable, and mineral medications. This recognition of healing substances by experience (*pharmacognosy*) migrated with them as they spread over the globe. It adapted to conditions in local regions. Because herbal, animal, and mineral medications did not always suffice, the fourth access to succor was magic or religious belief. In at least one language, that of the Mano of Liberia, "nye" connotes both magic and medicine (Cowen & Helfand, 1988, p.18).

Peoples' medical needs were threefold: Immediate attention was required for external injuries by animals, fights, or accidents. Sprains, fractures, sores, and swellings had to be treated then and there. Second, they needed to cure recurring internal complaints that kept them from fulfilling their tribal duties, diarrhea being a major debilitating one. Third, they needed relief from illnesses that did not respond to their medications. Since they could not comprehend the cause of such evil, they turned to beliefs, taboos, and spiritual practices to please the gods. This applied to "tribal illnesses" as well, that is: to changes in the condition of their natural environment that affected the tribe's survivability.

Impersonal or group evil

Such tribal evil could be an inexplicable non-seasonal long-term change of climate such as the drying up of the Chilean highlands, when the Ice Age mountain caps of frozen water had mostly melted, and the Atacama region became waterless and reverted to rainless desert. In their fear, the Atacameños placed elaborate geoglyphs on hillsides[1] as supplication to their gods, frequently related to the increasing impossibility to use llamas[2] to transport and trade salt from the ocean over the Andes, their major livelihood. Their priests prayed to the gods on top of the mountains and offered sacrifices to atone for their sins, which surely must have been the cause of the disruption of their lives.

In other parts of the world, the evil could have been the disappearance of the people's favorite hunt animal such as the buffalo or the eland. Then the people painted such animals in their caves and rock shelters. Elsewhere the evil could have been volcanic fire and brimstone so frequent that it made the afflicted societies move from healthy highlands to safer, but less salubrious lowlands. Wherever they lived, they needed help from gods above or below the earth to beg relief from such humanly insurmountable problems.

Medicinal uses of earths

Afflictions that our ancestors could understand were those for which they witnessed successful cures by observing tribal associates or animals in their environment. Their healing efforts then were not steeped in magic, but were based on the acquired knowledge of plants, animals, and minerals in their local environment. Very close to them and widely used as remedies were the earths they walked on, clay and mud.

Here my major topics are the use of medicinal earths and the afflictions cured by or with them. Unfortunately, in the history of medicine, reports of the use of earth during the last 5,000 years are sparse and not always easy to interpret from ancient languages. Frequently they are tinged with superstition, influenced by religious belief, and hampered by lack of knowledge as well as by crudest quacksalvery and quicksilvery. The nadir was the *Dreckapotheke* or filth dispensatory of the Early Modern Age, which experimented with useless, dangerous, and even poisonous medicines.

Medicinal use of clay, chalk, alum, gypsum and other earths is as old as mankind. It has been known since earliest recorded history. It has been reported continuously on all but one continent, in all kinds of writing, in manuscripts, incunabula, and in printed pharmacopoeias after printing was invented. But since even "healing earths" do not heal every illness, and because quack doctors and quick doctors misused minerals along with their other ludicrous concoctions of herbal and animal origin, there was at least one prominent medicine man in every century who thought he knew everything better, who declared that the use of earth or clay in medicine is only an ancient fable, of no use whatsoever, now or ever.

The perennial deprecators

Toward the end of the 20th century one such agnostic was Claus Priesner who dispatched earths as medicines with few words (Priesner, 1999). In the 19th century it was Albert Wiegand (1879) who said: "The majority of physicians considers the whole mineral scene at present as medically without value," and in the 18th century it was Nils Rosen (1739). In addition, many prominent histories of medicine totally ignore earths and especially clays as medicaments, but they mention unicorn horn, bezoar, smoked toads, mashed baby swallows, and other medical oddities.

Priesner's deprecatory statement appeared in print almost exactly one hundred years after a German physician consistently healed wounds, dried wetting ulcers, and successfully cured dysentery and Asiatic cholera with a fine white clay. Around one hundred books and journal articles recited scientifically acceptable proof of that. Chapters Four to Six are about that.

In his textbook on pharmacognosy Wiegand (1879) made his derogatory statement ten years after an American surgeon had used clay in a surgical ward of an East Coast hospital and wrote a book with over 50 case histories and sound reasoning for why clay heals wounds. Possibly Wiegand had not heard of him nor had read of the successful clay treatments of Sebastian Kneipp and the clay pastor Immanuel Felke in Germany toward the end of the 19th century. They, too, had enviable records of success with clay, which is a mineral and used to be called "an earth."

Nils Rosen (1739) at least had the excuse that he denounced mainly "perverse" uses of adsorbing medications such as clay. Truly, fantastic exaggerations by the incredible multitude of medical writers between 1500 and 1800 trying to make clay or earths and evil minerals into panaceas for all of mankind's ills, always with an exculpatory "so God will", have thrown suspicion on all uses of clays. No, clay did not cure bubonic plague then nor cures AIDS today. It cured cholera then and can cure it now. No, it did not cure tuberculosis, but it cured infected putrid wounds then and can do so now. It did not cure smallpox, but it cured dysentery then and does so now. It got rid of putrid organic smells then and can do so now.

Evidence that clay healing is efficacious is that it was the preferred treatment in general medicine for more than a quarter century before arrival of antibiotics and reliable vaccinations. As medicine is turning to a new millennium, physicians need not know any more about clay as a still useful medicine, unless they work in far away regions in countries where antibiotics and inoculations as well as doctors and pharmacists are few.

Earth medicines: healing examples

Other medications also cure cholera now, and thus clay is not the most modern remedy. The continual vast increase in medical knowledge since about 1850 makes the therapeutics of any generation seem absurd to the second succeeding generation, but clay can still heal.

There are two noteworthy points to make here: According to the World Health Organization's predictions, almost 2.5 million humans, mostly children, will die of diarrheal diseases per year even unto the year 2020 (Murray, 1992). The second point is that today, worldwide (purchased by me in the US and in Germany) is a prominent antidiarrheal tablet, marketed by a major pharmaceutical company, consisting of 75% clay, in the USA containing a clay called *attapulgite* or *palygorskite* (essentially aluminum silicates) and in Germany a clay called *kaolin*, the white fine Chinese porcelain earth also known as *Bolus alba*.[3] These tablets are available on every drug store shelf nowhere near alternative medicines, and in Germany you can still purchase *Bolus alba* and have prescription of clay suspended in acetic acid (*essigsaure Tonerde*) prepared for you to alleviate sprains. You can purchase the white earth *Bolus alba* and use it to brush teeth and gums deeply and cleanly. Hence clay is available today and not a faraway promise of biogenetic engineering. In my youth, the vinegar and clay mixture was a staple at home. Today I brush teeth and gums once a week with a relative of *Bolus alba—Bentonite or sodium montmorillonite* to polish stains and to reach and clean deep gum pockets.

Another "earth"

It was made prominent in the 17th century as *moonmilk*, natural cave calcium carbonate from Switzerland, and was used as an antacid and a remedy for an upset stomach caused by overindulgence in food and drink. Today calcium carbonate is still a 50% ingredient in a diarrheal over-the-counter medication for adults as well as for children. 400 years ago it was shipped by the cartload from its Swiss cave to consumers throughout Europe. Today calcium carbonate is still a fifty percent ingredient in a diarrheal over-the-counter medication for adults as well as for children while the name moonmilk has receded into glossaries of geology.

Three thousand years ago, clay and calcium carbonate cured the same afflictions (Holland, 1977). They did not then and do not now cure any of the avid and spurious claims promoted for them. Nowadays physicians consider clay, calcium carbonate, and gypsum with disdain if they know about their medical usefulness at all.

Doctors consider dirt on wounds as anathema, but we must distance ourselves from the notion that sand, clay, mud and other earths must be dirty. There is nothing inherently dirty about minerals that unwashed vegetables or meats do not exhibit either. And using dirt internally? Forget the notion that minerals are dirty just because digging in earth makes our hands "dirty." Earths, as other medications, must be cleaned, sifted, and sterilized. Almost all staple antidiarrhea medicines fall into the category of "earths."

In 1667, 1869 and 1898, so medical literature informs us, treatment with a mineral cured deep, old, suppurating, and evil smelling ulcers of the tibia (generally the shinbone, the inner and larger of the two bones of the lower leg) within 2 weeks with bandages of medicinal earth. Each was publicized in print as prominent in the development of medical practice of its time. In 1667 it was calcium carbonate, in 1869 it was a yellow clay, in 1898 it was a white clay.

In the 4th, 17th, and the early 20th century, the newest invention was to blow powdered clay into noses and other body orifices to stop bleeding or evil smelling secretions. The Roman physician Priscianus (Meyer, Th., 1909) did it in the late 4th century, Johann Daniel Major (Major, 1667) did it in the 17th, Trumpp (1909) reported it early in the 20th.

In the 16th century 2 separate tests were made at two separate noble houses with *terra sigillata* as anti-poison for mercury sublimate (a test on a human) and for three vegetable poisons (test on 6 dogs). The success of these tests (the human survived, the three dogs also receiving the antidote survived) had been verified at two German state archives (see Chapter eighteen).

Earth alone is not dirt

One would not choose to eat earth covered with feces nor would one eat vegetables like that, yet there was a time in pharmaceutical history when prescriptions included feces, urine, scraped body sweat, expectorations, and nose phlegm. Earwax and even fat rend from drowned women[4] were touted as remedies. There were few doctors, most practiced far away from little towns and villages, where people continued to eat clayey earth for some of their illnesses and do so now in yet to be developed countries, either because the people have no access to modern medicines or cannot afford them. In 1998 I needed a refill of electrolytes to counteract some stomach distress in Madagascar. The pharmacist had packaged clay powders but warned me that they are expensive. I bought three packets at the equivalent of

US$0.30 each, that is, for the same amount as local people pay for enough rice for supper for the family. To them, that is expensive.

Earth is always where the patient is when the patient is ill, which cannot be said for all medicinal plants or for animal remedies or even for itinerant quacksalvers. Only earths and gods were always available. Clay does not run away. Clay may crack, but does not die in droughts like plants do. Clay was there before doctors, during few doctors, and even during many doctors. Clay is where you need it when you need it, because it covers 95% of the land area of our earth.

Throughout the history of medicine before 1800, most "doctors of physick" were trained in ancient misconceptions, often sworn by their universities to support unproven procedures. They garnered their income mostly from treating the nobility and the rich who could afford many personal physicians in the hope that one would be able to cure what befell them. But the "common people" could not afford doctors and pharmacies, even if they were in their vicinity. The burden of healing remained with the family, usually with its senior women, even into the 20th century. Clay was always one of their staples.

In May 2000 a visit to the Greek island of Lemnos brought forth a medicine consisting of clay and grape juice boiled to a syrupy consistency called *Mustachoma*, for minor stomach illnesses and sore throats. The local pharmacy decried the use of *Mustachoma*, usually prepared by the grandmother in the family. Instead the pharmacy suggested the use of Kao-Pectate® which contains a higher percentage of clay than Mustachoma and commands a much higher price.

In February of 2001 during a visit to Mali in West Africa I found two clay medicines sold in the local market by special pharmacies concentrating on old remedies that the people trust and can afford. One is a cigar shaped clay stick of Niger River mud to wet and roll over insect bites or sprains. The other clay sample is sold as an anti-diarrheal medication.

As late as 1950, it was not uncommon for doctors to make house calls when the patient was immobilized by illness. When pharmacies were not ubiquitous, many household remedies had to be in store at home. So, fine clay was stored in the house, and it was recommended by physicians for medical emergencies such as the many injuries by farm equipment.

Clay as deodorant

Besides relieving symptoms of diarrhea, clay has another very desirable property: It is a powerful deodorant for the foul odors of defecations and also for the penetrant odor of suppurating wounds.

Animals with odiferous feces instinctively try to cover their discharge with earth, which deodorizes and dries it. Domesticated cats still pay paw service to this deodorization, long forgotten is the time in the wild when enemies would trail bounty by its smell. Some animals still cover their kills with earth to keep trespassers away. Kitty litter is clay (nowadays in the US mostly bentonite, a sodium montmorillonite). Clay absorbs several times its weight in moisture. In the right consistency and quantity clay is inert and non-irritating to skin and stomach. Though humans cannot smell as well as most animals can, when hospitals had large halls as wards, the stink of decay from a single suppurating ulcerous wound could be intolerable to all the other patients.

Possibly we do not need clay or other minerals as medicine anymore, even though Robert Robertson (1996) showed that many people in African upheavals died from cholera due to a lack of medicine when they might have been saved by clay. Just because our medical arsenal, if available, is much more powerful nowadays, the basic value of clay treatment has not vanished. It was there before pharmacology, and it will also survive the current emphasis on undocumented herbal cures. The most telling reason for the survival of earths as medicines, in contrast to all the weird medicines of earlier millennia, is that the earths were always useful and effective in healing.

Comments and Explanations

[1] Geoglyphs are pictorial designs made with stones on hillsides. Several of the thousands of geoglyphs along the length of Chile may be the only Western Hemisphere here record of the Supernova of 1054, now the Crab Nebula which is generally believed not to have been observed in the sky except in China. For some reason it was not observed in Europe, even though it was bright enough to be seen in the daytime cloudless sky for almost 3 weeks.

[2] Llamas are limited in the weight they can carry (about 25 kg) and, in contrast to camels, the distance they can go between watering spots is only about 50 km. The great majority of geoglyphs are recognizable representations of llamas. They are outlines made with stones on bare hills or as bare spaces on fields filled with stones, thus in essence allowing "positive and negative" stone pictures in dry hillsides, visible from quite far if the daily winds do not obscure them with blowing dust and sand (see also glossary).

[3] In the US Kao-Pectate ®, in Germany Kao-Prompt ®, in Greece Kao-Pectate ®, all made by Farmacia Corporation. Liquid Kao-Pectate® actually names *attapulgite*, an aluminosilicate, the all-inclusive name of clay.

[4] Unwed mothers accused of suffocating a child they could not feed, were subjected to a test to elicit the truth. They were bound and thrown into deep water. If they came up alive, they were guilty (from Malleus Malificarum—the Witches' Hammer—a detailed, legal and theological document of incredible brutality and callousness, written by the Jesuits Johann Sprenger and Heinrich Krämer; 28 editions were printed between 1486 and 1600 and adopted by both Catholics and Protestants).

Chapter Two: A Roadmap to Earths and Cures

Five thousand years ago, an earth was an earth was an earth. Forty-five hundred years later the consensus was that a mineral is any substance obtained by mining, including earths. In 1600 AD this was refined to say that a mineral is any natural substance that is neither vegetable nor animal. By 1730 it was accepted that a mineral is either a poison or a medicine. Since 1813 a mineral is considered any inorganic substance that is naturally part of our Earth having a consistent and distinctive set of physical properties and a composition that can be expressed by a chemical formula, except that from ancient use the term "mineral" has also been grandfathered in to be applicable to some mineral-appearing substances of organic origin, such as petroleum and coal.

The meaning of "earth"

So, what is earth? If we want to investigate ancient "healing earths", it is essential that we define the term "earth". First of all, we have the meaning of "the Earth", the member of our celestial neighborhood. Both the English word *earth* and the German word *Erde* can be traced to an early common linguistic root. For the same definition, romance languages use another common word derivation: in Latin the word is *terra* and in French it is *la terre.*

Another meaning of earth is that of the firm earth beneath our feet and beneath our homes. It is soil for our plants, a partner with the air for our birds and the water for our fish. In English and German the word is *land*. In Latin, again, the word is *terra*, the dry hard stuff as opposed to ocean and atmosphere.

Most romance languages do not have the earth-land split. The meaning of the word terra must be implied from the context in which it is used. English and German have also adopted some terra-associated words, but they clearly appear as imports. "Terrain" is familiar in both languages (sometimes "terrane" in English). The basic meaning of "Terrine" is the same, even if in English it is a clay bowl for stew, in German a clay bowl to serve soup, in French a clay pot to hold comestibles such as liver paté. Peanut is an English term referring to a nut which grows underground and its relation to the pea family of plants; in French and German it is "earth nut" (French: *terre-noix*, in German *Erdnuß*) suggesting the "nut in the earth", the peanut (which botanically is a legume, not a nut at all).

The lowest floor of a multistory building in America is generally designated the first floor, in England and in France it is the ground floor, par-terre in French, Parterr (or *Erdgeschoß* = earth level floor) in German. Yet when Americans want to participate in a promising enterprise or venture like an IPO[1], they want to get in on the ground floor, not the first floor. When Italians refer to *rimanere a terra* they remain on land, but the meaning is that they missed the boat. When the French want to express that a wine from a specific growing area tastes like it is supposed to, they call it *goût de terre* which does not mean a wine with an earthy taste. A terrier is an earth dog trained to dig into earth burrows of fox and badger.

With the Latin "terra" we are by no means on terra firma. About the only thing it does not mean is air and water, but it can mean anything you walk, slip or climb on from mud[2] to silt to clay to hardened lumps of loam to rocks and minerals. For the inquiry into healing earths, the Latin term always has an adjective or defining noun such as *terra arenosa* (sandy soil), *terra rubrica* (red earth), *terra alba* (white earth). The latter can include white clay, calcite, gypsum, borax, chalk, or sedimentary rock. The term comprises *terra viridis* (green earth), *terra bituminosa* (pitch), or *terra ampelita* (vinestock earth to protect plants from insect attack, *terrage* in French). Most often though the secondary name of terra is the name of its provenance, a geologic "type locality" such as *terra melitensa* (Maltese earth) or *terra saxonia miraculosa* (Saxon wonder earth). While we acknowledge the existence of the term "terrae medicinales", medical or healing earths, no individual earth is so called; it is a group designation. In the following, earths that are mentioned are always "medicinal earths", those used for some curative purpose unless clearly defined otherwise[3]. Very often the seal contained the words terra sigillata as sort of a quality implying "seal of good clay keeping".

Terra sigillata and bolus

Throughout the history of healing earths, we encounter two particular terms: *Terra sigillata* and *bolus*. Among medicinal earths the term *Terra sigillata* means a flat disk or compressed ball of clay, which is branded or stamped (minted or coined) with a seal, trademark, or logo denoting its origin to an often very specific site. The first well known sealed or sigillated earth was the *terra sigillata* from the Greek island of Lemnos in the Thrakian Gulf of the Aegean Sea. The simple use of generic term "terra sigillata" means any earth considered equal in its physical appearance and its healing properties to the original from Lemnos. Seals on disks of 28-30mm diameter earth coins, when healing earths became better known, were a form of advertising and promotion, such as "Earth of the Holy Mary" or "St. Paul's Earth". The seal implied—as it does with a sealed letter—that somehow a sealed earth is more valuable than an unsealed one, an impression the vendor hopes for and fosters.

A word of caution and explanation

The term *sigillata* comes from sigillum, a small figure which is imprinted or impressed on seals by signet rings on sealing wax, corporate seals on paper, and a decoration on leather parts. The term *terra sigillata* has also been used for pottery decorative design relief made by impressions in pottery molds and is prominent in the 1st through 3rd century in Roman pottery. In this book, the ceramics or pottery meaning of the term *terra sigillata* has not been used or meant at all. The healing earth has been named *terra sigillata* because it, too, involved an engraved stamp or seal which appears in relief on the face of earth disks used for medication. Henceforth I will call them "earth coins".

Bolus, originally a large pill for large animals, later the size of a smaller pill or troche (a round to oval medallion), is a form of healing earth also often flattened by a seal at which the imaginary distinction between *terra sigillata* and *bolus* is totally lost. A pill is easier to swallow than loose dry clay powder (though the proper way to ingest clay is to wet the pill and make a paste or creamy drink). Because languages do change, bolus became a synonym for healing earth, often used interchangeably with terra, so eventually there were the terms terra armena and bolus armenus both denoting the same reddish clay from Armenia[4]. In contrast to terra, the term bolus always connotes a medication pill, but then so does *terra sigillata* whether you start out with bolus (that, anyhow, is a terra) or with terra. Don't look for any distinction between the two. Yes, some writers have used *bolus sigillatus*. As we said in the beginning, an earth is an earth is an earth. To really confuse the student, some earths are known as bolaric earths (*terrae bolaricae*).

Because we are concerned with only a few medicinal earths though they may come from different locations, we need to discover those minerals that are believed to have healing properties. Basically those are variations of aluminosilicate clays (Al_2O_3+SiO_2) with or without minor percentages of iron, calcium or magnesium that account for colors in clay. Clays are chemical weathering products of crystalline rocks of an extremely fine grain size of 4 micrometers or less[5]. The extreme fineness of the particles seems to be the key to efficacious healing earth such as fine calcium carbonate, sodium or calcium montmorillonite clay, and gypsum.

Loess distinguished

A mineral material known but not promoted as a medicine until after 1925 was actually the one for which the term "healing earth" was coined originally. It is a postglacial wind-borne dust called loess, forming vast deposits in many areas of the world where the winds left them. These particles are commonly covered with a fine skin of quartz[6]. Both clay and loess are good absorbers, but loess never became popular in first-line earth medicine despite claims that the medical clay could possibly produce coproliths[7] and loess wouldn't (Peyer & Röpke, 1927). For such a problem of gut blockage you would have to eat a glob of dry clay, and that could be as uncomfortable and dangerous as swallowing dry rice, beans, or lentils, but there were no recognizable case histories of coproliths due to clay, rather this claim was more a marketing strategy for the loess. Even today rumors tell of gut explosions from eating dry earth.

There are a few references to what probably was diatomaceous earth in classic times, but more often it was used as a filler for bread dough in times of famine. Other healing earths were calcium from chalk, egg shells, coral, and similar calcitic substances to quell stomach aches and "heartburn"[8].

Cures by earth

A basic question arising from our inquiry is "what did the healing earths cure?" The only firm answer is "what was known and documented as afflictions cured", by which is meant that the question predates the answers that medical research found early in the 20th century, namely, diarrheal illnesses such as dysentery and cholera, nasal infections, diphtheria, white vaginal discharge, eczemas, parasitic worms, and eye infections. Modern earth treatments by physical therapy practitioners involve mud baths, fango (originally heated volcanic mud) packs and cataplasms or poultices to reduce swellings, ameliorate sprains, and relieve arthritic pain. These clay treatments are often quite effective due to the slow release of relatively high heat in a fango pack or mud bath, and patients can tolerate a higher temperature in mud than they can in water.

To extrapolate from known procedures dating back only to 1889 (Stumpf's successful external application of clay), respectively to 1905 (Stumpf's successful internal application of clay) to ancient illnesses is very complicated and uncertain. Earths may (and certainly seem to) have been used in desperation or ignorance for afflictions that clay has never proved to cure. Illnesses described in antiquity, the Middle Ages, and even in the early part of modern medicine may not be what they are called now. Descriptions of the symptoms may allow multiple choices of sufferings. Typical is the word "pestis" or "pestilentia" which could mean anything from an epidemic or pandemic to today's meaning of bubonic plague and as often as not encompassing small pox, scurvy, cholera, typhoid fever, and even starvation. St. Anthony's Fire, a poisoning with ergot-infested rye flour resulting in terrible skin lesions, could also have been erysipelas, gangrene, or syphilis. An example of an indeterminate disease is the epidemic of 430 BC reported by Thucydides during the Peloponnesian wars. Thucydides called it pestilence, but Ackerknecht (1965, p. 9) does not believe it was bubonic plague[9]. Where the epidemic indeed was bubonic plague, it is not surprising that in desperate hope to cure their patients, doctors prescribed healing earth compounded with wondrous medicines useless against the Black Death. Pest is a plague and it is today still prominent as an illness of cattle, cattle-plague or *Rinderpest* which is a virulent infectious disease affecting ruminants, especially oxen, with fever, dysentery and inflammation of mucous membranes.

When a locality was in the grip of a real bubonic plague epidemic, it was a catastrophe. In the 14th century two-thirds to three fourths of the European population died. In London 1664/5 70,000 people died. There was no therapeutic approach to the "pest" (Cabanés 1899, p. 764), often doctors were the first to flee: "En plusieurs endroits, lorsque la peste arrive, apoticaires et chirurgiens deslogent le premier"[10].

Scrutinizing meaningful literature, I have restricted myself to actual mentions of earths, even if their nomenclature is not quite clear as to the type of earth or whether it meant a purposeful or coincidental mixture of earth with other compounds (ammoniac in earth from beneath latrines, for example,) or a more esoteric ill-defined connotation such as "soil from under the bed of a widow".

Regarding illnesses healed

A fully acceptable cross-check was to look at both what the earth has been known to heal since 1850 and to guess at what this illness might have been in antiquity. A survey of the diseases, injuries, and surgery in early populations (Brothwell et al., 1967) contains the following illnesses which in my judgment are purely based on possible similarity of 20th century cures with ethnologic determinations (see Chapter Seven), such as famine, loose gums, intestinal parasites, Baghdad boil, eye infections from flies, ear infections, vomiting during childbirth (anemia?), typhoid (if bowels empty), diphtheria, snake bites, eczemas, bloody and mucous discharge (Ruhr), dysentery with fever (Asiatic cholera), nasal discharge, insect bites, itching, tonsillitis (fêng kho), influenza and catarrhs, ringworm, psoriasis, ulcers of the lower legs, skin lesions, total failure of digestion (cholera?). Problems associated with pregnancy would have been considered to be within the province of healing earth application, it has been reported often enough in ethnological reports and by personal accounts from older societies. What speaks eloquently for the use of healing earth within the medical arsenal is the fact that its use has never been forgotten long enough to depart totally from the pool of medical knowledge. It would have taken not much more than two generations to forget about healing earths had the illnesses ceased or cures failed, had modern medicine devised treatments of equal presence and potency. Thus a healing continuity is different from certain arts, such as the making of damascene blades (Verhoeven, 2001), which for lack of proper materials and practice disappeared completely within two or three generations. Illnesses were present at all times in all locations, and so were healing earths and healing practitioners.

Except in the rarest cases the nature and cause of an illness was purely speculative. Human excretions or discharges (rheumes, distillations, murrs and lyentery) were recognizable and effective treatment of such repetitive illnesses were the strength of the family or tribal knowledge of the three legs of medicine. Diarrheal perturbations, nausea and vomiting (especially by pregnant women), and bloody discharges occurred often enough that a body of experience was built up.

"Doctors of Physick", never having been apprentices in internal medicine, were steeped in the ancient medicine of Galen of Pergamum and the herbal and mineral cures of Dioscorides, wrote books which every other doctor lauded and ignored. They invented and patented medicines and there is no correlation between the medicine of one doctor and the medicine of another doctor for the very same illness. Some created compound medicines with 40 ingredients (an important Arabic number) or with 69 ingredients, where 69 became the "lying 8", symbol of infinity. Almost as old as earth medications were the mysterious compound medicines called theriak or Mithridate, the latter referring to Mithridatus IV of Pontus, whose wild ingestion of poisons was said to have given him resistance against being poisoned himself.

Comments and Explanations

[1] Initial public offering of a company's stock, usually an opportunity to make a sizeable profit if allowed to participate although usually reserved for private and large investors.

[2] Mud and silt and clay: Clay is soil of extremely fine particles (0.002 mm or less) and for the purpose of this history consists mostly of silicon dioxide and aluminum oxide with various percentages of other minerals. The term mud refers to a shiny or slippery mixture of water and silt, which may contain larger particles including sand, but for medical use particles of larger size are not considered benefical.

[3] Because most rules have to have exceptions, there are "terrae" that are actually plants. For example, we will encounter *terra japonica*, which is a tree but was once thought to be an earth. *Terra censualis* is the income derived from leasing land.

[4] Note that *lapis armenus*, Armenian stone, is something different entirely, from its description possibly a copper vitriol $CuSO_4$. In old English terms Armenia and ammoniac have been distorted to "armoniac".

[5] Particle sizes go from coarse to medium to fine to very fine silt, then to coarse clay to medium clay to fine clay. Clay and fine particles range between 2 one- thousands and one half thousands of an inch in diameter.

[6] Quartz is crystalline, but the silicone dioxide clay component is often an amorphous structure. Loess contains between 60 and 70% quartz, composed largely of silt-sized (0.02-0.05mm) grains loosely cemented with calcium carbonate. It has high porosity and adsorbing capacity. When taken dry or almost dry, loess will grate between the teeth, clay will not.

[7] Coproliths are hard intestinal obstructions. When dry goods are swallowed dry when they still can adsorb moisture, they can grow big enough to burst the gut. Coproliths were never reported with clay, however, because it was adminstered as a soft slurry which does not cause obstructions.

[8] A major source of calcium was the lens or flat pill (see *oculi cancri* in the glossary) produced by the riverine cray fish *Astacus astacus* and stored near his belly until it is needed to replace its exoskeleton.

[9] Pestilence could be any virulent and usually contagious disease of any animal of plant judged to be a threat to people and their interests (Encyclopedia Britannica). It could be anything fatal to public peace that plagues in any way, a pestilential vapor, mist, or hot exhalation (Oxford Unabridged Dictionary). Zedler (Universal Lexicon) says bubonic plague was first reported in Egypt, passed through Syria and Asia Minor to Constatinople, reached Italy in 543 AD.

[10] "In many places, when the pest arrived, apothercaries and surgeons were the first to flee."

Chapter Three: The Hero who Conquered Cholera:
Prof. Dr. med. Julius Stumpf (1856-1932)

Julius Stumpf is the main actor and the hero in the next three chapters dealing with the use of clay as healing earth. This brief look at his life is presented to form subsequent chapters into a cohesive unit on the medical use of clay in modern times and to lay a technical foundation for much of the earlier history of clay as medicine. Rarely do we have the opportunity to look back into historical facts and present them in modern scientific terms on which to base logical deductions for earlier times. The key to the scientific basis of clay use in medicine is Dr. Julius Stumpf, the hero who conquered cholera and gangrene a century ago.

Julius Stumpf was born on June 30, 1856. His parents were Johann Jakob Stumpf (1815-1887) and his spouse Barbara née Hitter (1825-1914). They owned and operated the family's land holdings[1] in Bavaria. Julius was the sixth child of ten, the fourth of five boys.

University schooling

After finishing the local primary school (age 6-10), Julius attended the Gymnasium[2] in Münnerstadt. Based on a normal upper school graduation at age 18, Julius Stumpf was admitted to the University of Würzburg am Main about 1874. Records show that he studied from 1874 through the summer semester 1879. Medical studies then averaged four semesters of preclinical medicine and no less than eight semesters of clinical medicine, a total of about six years. On July 18, 1879 he received his degree of "doctor of medicine, surgery, and the art of obstetrics" based on his inaugural dissertation about diagnosis and treatment of diafragmatic hernia. He obtained his license to practice medicine[3] (*Approbation)* either at the same time or in February of 1880, according to Herwart Fischer, Stumpf's successor as county medical officer, who wrote the obituary of Stumpf in the German journal of legal medicine (Fischer, 1932). It appears unlikely that Stumpf would have wasted eight months at this point in his life doing nothing.

Anyhow, either late 1879 or early 1880 Stumpf opened a general practice in the hamlet of Bütthart and practiced medicine until he was called for his obligatory six-month tour of duty in the Bamberg Ulan[4] Regiment. After this interruption he returned to his practice and prepared for and passed the *Physikat* test. This was a state examination required of graduate physicians who desired to enter government service. The test encompassed subjects in which the government might have peremptory interests, such as forensic medicine, administrative medical inquiries, public hygiene and epidemic control, venereal disease control, pursuit of illegal abortions, executions, and similar legal-medical subjects.

Marriage and family

In 1881 Julius married Anna Schmitt, daughter of a Bavarian Supreme Court justice. They had two boys, Gottfried and Paul, with two girls between them. The boys, in time, pursued careers in upper level government service. One of the girls died of diphtheria at age 4; the other became a nun in a London convent. Stumpf's wife Anna died in 1902 and Julius

Stumpf would not remarry for almost 20 years, when he was 65 years old. His son Gottfried had three children.

Gottfried's younger daughter Irmgard, currently resides in Munich. She established contact with me when a friend apprised her of a Würzburg newspaper article about an American author doing research on Prof. Dr. Julius Stumpf at the university and the city archives. She took it upon herself to poll her relatives for any photographs, newspaper clipping, records and memories of their ancestor and to obtain their permission for publication in my book. Thus she is my source of much of the history we have of the Stumpf family in general and Julius specifically. For instance, the oldest boy of Johann Jakob Stumpf, Thomas, became a physician and died early. Johann, the second child, had only daughters who could not or would not take over the estate and it was sold. Julius had elected to study medicine as had Thomas.

Government medicine

Julius Stumpf was appointed to his first government post in 1899 as deputy county physician and also as physician for the state railway[5] in the town of Werneck, a post he held until 1925. Also in 1899 he was appointed associate professor of forensic medicine at Würzburg. The King of Bavaria (Luitpold, prince regent of Bavaria 1886-1912) appointed him over the objections of the Würzburg university senate, probably because Stumpf had a better track record as government medical officer. Stumpf was granted a full professorship in 1924. During his tenure he taught courses and held practice laboratory sessions with regularity every semester. His lectures were popular with students and the public beyond the university's medical school limits[6]. Field trips included government medical installations, notably the jail and the guillotine. Stumpf would explain that there was a small room with a table and chairs on the ground floor, the cell of the condemned person on the next floor, and the guillotine under the mansard roof. After sentencing, a plea for mercy would be dispatched to the king. On the day it came back in a sealed envelope, the judges and the prisoner would meet in the office on the ground floor. The prisoner witnessed the opening of the envelope, which usually contained affirmation of the judgment. Then, within 24 hours, the prisoner had to be executed. Of note is that, between executions, the frame of the guillotine remained in the attic, the blade was moved to a secret second location, the block and tackle to raise the blade and the trip mechanism were stored in a secret third location, to prevent the unauthorized use of the guillotine in case of a riot or revolution (crowned heads in Europe had not yet forgotten the French revolution about a hundred years earlier.)

Stumpf had to attend most executions. Being questioned once why the sawdust filled sack at the head end seemed to have rips or tears, Stumpf indicated that the teeth of the dead man could still snap at the sackcloth. The visit to the execution chamber appears to have been the best attended field trip of his course.

His experimental and developmental work with clay in external and internal medicine is described in the following three chapters. His work curing Asiatic cholera peaked in 1914, about the beginning of World War I., when there was much cholera in the eastern European regions. He continued his university lectures until he was near the age of 70. Thereafter he was ailing for a long time and died in his 76th year on April 12, 1932. Records of his life are imbedded in university files[7] and in the memory of his granddaughter Irmgard. His career as a successful government employee and university professor was augmented by private practice and by applying the rediscovered methods of the use of clay in medicine to cure three scourges of mankind: Asiatic cholera, gangrene, and diphtheria.

Comments and Explanations

[1] Definition of Gutshof: A prominent farm or agricultural holding, a well-to-do agricultural entity.

[2] An eight to nine year high school leading to university admission qualification providing mandatory classical language lessons, Latin or Greek or both, distinct from the curriculum of the non-classical *Oberschule* or high school. Students not wishing to go to university could either complete four more years of the basic elementary school and then be apprenticed to a master craftsman (and until 1914 they all were men), or they could go from the basic elementary school to four years of *Oberschule* and gain entry to middle management careers.

Completing highschool with the "Abitur"-exam (graduation exam) gave acces to study at university in any of the five faculties—medicine, law, natural sciences, economic sciences, and philosophy. The faculty of natural sciences was the last to be added, the faculty of law used to be the school of "both laws", civil and ecclesiastic.

[3] Personnel records of Würzburg University and of the State of Bavaria (then a kingdom), also obituary of the local paper "*Würzburger General-Anzeiger*" April 12, 1932. In Germany, then and now, an MD is not a "professional doctorate" but earned similar to a PhD now in the US. Though not frequent, one could be licensed to practice medicine without an MD and law without a JD.

[4] Historical term for a regiment of lancers, a prestigious cavalry unit of the armed forces.

[5] Railroads then and now were state-owned enterprises providing government physicians to verify illnesses and accidents and thus controlling access to government insurance and pensions.

[6] Personal information from Irmgard Stumpf in Munich, granddaughter of Julius. She also contributed an article copy from the *Main Post* newspaper dated June 6, 1953, entitled "Würzburg um die Jahrhundertwende."

[7] Such records as "File 214" of the university personnel department as well as documents from the City Archives of Würzburg where I was given access and permission to copy. A seldom found document is Julius Stumpf's 62-page book with the major title (translated) "About a realiable curing regimen in case of Asiatic cholera as well as in cases of severe infections, vomiting, and diarrhea" and the minor title "about the relevance of Bolus (Kaolin) in the treatment of certain bacterial illnesses". Stumpf in 1906 foresaw the benefit of bolus in other occasions of poisoning, namely the poisoning by canned goods by bacterial spoiling (actually at home more "glass goods" for home canning). Careless sterilization, also by commercial producers, led to bacterial invasions of the food (usually meat products) and thus to the increasing frequency of poisonings.

Chapter Four: Clay for External Medical Application

Old ineffective treatment of wounds

Before investigating clay for treatment of festering wounds we need to ask the question "what was used before clay?" By the 19th century open wounds were covered with muslin[1] bandages, bran boxes[2], cotton balls, jute[3], or sphagnum moss[4]. Excelsior[5] bandages were in use during the later 19th century. Use of bran boxes was still mentioned by Dr. Addinnell Hewson in 1872 and was found awkward and unsatisfactory. Muslin bandages were used mainly to hold cotton balls, sphagnum moss, and wood-wool (excelsior) in place over wounds. All these materials absorbed fair amounts of blood and fluids, but offered only modest protection against infections, and rotted quickly.

The major desired property

The capacity to absorb blood, wound secretions, and pus was wanted primarily. Not far behind was the desire for a material that would not be corrupted by rotting too quickly. Mielck and Leisrink (1882) found a moss constituent of peat that, once dried, does not tend to absorb water quickly and thus works as a barrier to wound infection. Similarly, the application of black peat earth resulted in healing of wounds without heavy pus formation. Sphagnum, due to its open cells, will absorb moisture through its capillaries into its hollow areas, different from cotton, jute, and gauze which only absorb along their fibrous interstices. Mielck noted that peat moss need not be doused with antibacterial chemicals then in use, such as Jodoform® or carbolic acid. Leisrink stated that bandages with peat moss were aseptic, remained sterile and generally absorbed the odiferous exudations of wounds. Peat moss is soft enough that it can be bandaged with uniform pressure on the area of the wound. Kronacher (1890) concluded that a combination of cotton and sphagnum worked better than either material alone and also better than excelsior.

To begin the history of healing earth with its proved successes at the end of the 19th and the beginning of the 20th century allows a basis for judging and interpreting earlier applications of healing earths. It appears preferable to begin with the physician who reinvented (or rather revitalized) the serious use of clay in medicine and his astounding successes with it.

Altering traditional historic medicine, Stumpf was among the first to destroy the millennia old concept of "laudable pus", the Greek physician Galen's indicator of a healing wound. He was the first to banish single-handedly the centuries old scourge of cholera prior to the invention of sera and antibiotics. As government employee he had to support the government's regulation for medical treatments, but he did experimental research on his own while also teaching forensic medicine at a then sleepy little university in a then sleepy little town on the river Main[6].

What a dead body can teach

The concepts Stumpf developed for wound treatment and for treatment of intestinal ills, are based on a fortuitous happening in 1882: Stumpf was asked to attend an exhumation at which he first encountered clay in a medical context. In his recollections he wrote of this experience (Stumpf, 1906, pp. 3-4):

> "My first work regarding this question [the bactericidal effect of clay] took place on 23 September 1882, when, as a young county practitioner, I had the opportunity to observe a judicial exhumation of a body buried 37 months earlier. It was a case of a 25-year-old female who had died eight days after giving birth. A suspicion had arisen that her husband had poisoned her with arsenic, but the suspicion was not borne out. [Stumpf inserts a footnote here that because the suspect's second wife had died of arsenic poisoning, there was prosecutorial reason for an order to exhume the first wife].
>
> The appearance of the body at the exhumation created a long lasting impression on me, because the body was extraordinarily well preserved: For instance the abdominal walls were still completely closed and the intestines could be removed in one piece. The dried liver showed a certain greenish color (gall bladder) and the enlarged puerperal uterus showed a noticeable bloody spot (seat of the placenta").

Stumpf then described the earth in the cemetery as clay for the entire depth of burial. Next to the cemetery was a large pit with a clay depth of several meters. He thought for years about this preserved body and the clay pit and formed an opinion that in the clearly homogenous clay all organic life must be minimal if not completely absent. He contemplated that clay might have a property of resisting decomposition, which might help heal ichorous (infectious and wetting) wounds.

The prestigious *Münchener Medizinische Wochenschrift* accepted his paper on clay bandages as a healing medium (Stumpf, 1898b). He wrote about the experience with the exhumation and included a case history of a festering and evil smelling ulcer of the tibia that he had treated.

The first case history of clay on wounds

The patient had been an elderly, very poor man who lived with his family in a remote mill building. He had a badly neglected ulcer of the tibia (shinbone). The bedridden patient spread a terribly fetid odor throughout the building and even into its surroundings. The ulcer was several years old, quite extensive and quite deep, baring the tibia in two places. Stumpf was convinced he would have to amputate below the knee, but the patient refused the amputation.

Stumpf instructed the relatives of the patient to get rid of the filthy rag used to cover the ulcer and to douse the wound instead with dried and finely sifted powdered clay. This impulsive decision resulted in an immediate cessation of the fetid odor. With repetition of the clay treatment, the ulcer healed completely within weeks, "better than anyone could have hoped for" (Stumpf's words.)

From then on he kept a supply of powdered clay in his office for similar applications. He had serendipitously discovered that a suitably dried and powdered white clay was available in pharmacies under the name *Bolus alba officinalis* or *Argilla officinalis*, which we know to be a kaolin, porcelain, or Meissen earth, an odorless, inert, and very cheap clay powder used as a pill constituent. (I could still order a 5-kilo bag in a pharmacy in a small town in Germany in 1998, a hundred years later. Pharmacists of an American supermarket chain, however, did not even know what I was talking about.)

More uses of clay

Stumpf began to use *Bolus alba* for the [then] frequent head eczemas. Cleanliness was still a problem in the countryside at a time when sanitation had barely arrived in the cities. He used bolus for various pus-forming wounds, for pemphigus, a nasty water blister type infection in small children, and for poorly granulating wounds from injuries so frequent in agricultural work. Stumpf was pleased with the healing and drying effect of the clay. His book (1906) continues with a 1896 case history of the explosion of a rifle that tore a young farmer's left hand apart.

At first Stumpf tried to save some of the fingers, but that led to septic phlegmones of the forearm[7]. Five days after the accident it became necessary to amputate the hand at the wrist. Several days later he lanced the phlegmones and ten days after that he applied white clay to the badly festering and odiferous amputation wound[8]. Two days later, skin had formed in thick folds over the wound and no trace of pus was observed. Complete healing followed incredibly fast (Stumpf's term.)

Stumpf followed this with another case history in June of 1898. A 54-year-old farmer arose from his bed one morning and, grabbing for his slippers under the bed, was badly bitten in the right hand by his medium size bulldog. The animal had bitten so hard into the hand that the dog had to be dragged from under the bed by the bitten hand, only then could the dog's mouth be disengaged from the hand. Though bitten deeply into the ball of the thumb, there had been little bleeding. The farmer, rather than call a physician, placed a cold compress on the hand. The ensuing evening severe pain caused the farmer to visit the doctor's office after all. The entire hand was badly swollen, red, shiny, and very painful when touched. The multiple lacerations near the root of the little finger showed some pus formation. The patient's temperature was elevated at 38.7° C.

Treating highly septic wounds

What to do with these highly septic wounds? After due consideration Stumpf decided to forego any disinfection of the wounds. He covered the entire hand all around with a layer of about 5 cm thickness of bolus and wrapped this with a bandage. Wanting to see the patient again early the next morning, what Stumpf hadn't dared to hope for, had occurred. When the patient approached his office the next morning, he joyously waved the injured hand and showed the mobility of the fingers under the bandage. The redness and sensitivity to pain had ceased completely, the swelling had become peculiarly soft and doughy, a significant improvement. Though the patient now had a temperature of 39.3° C, Stumpf surmised correctly that it had been higher during the night and that it was now subsiding. Indeed, the following night it was normal. The bolus treatment was repeated twice a day and the hand healed completely in a few days.

Stumpf treated two more major hand injuries the same way in 1899. One was a hand shattered by a pistol bullet; the other was a severe laceration by an agricultural implement. The former was placed into a bag full of bolus and that led to rapid healing and recovery. The latter, after the nearly separated fingers had been pushed back into place under anesthesia were also placed into bolus. The injury healed rapidly. After some months the hand had regained almost the whole range of mobility of the torn digits.

Now Stumpf extended treatments even to fresh wounds, especially suture punctures, with a cover of white clay [alternately referred to as *Bolus alba* or *Argilla*, both are synonyms for the white clay] under a gauze bandage. The way he expresses himself in his book still reflects the marvel of the discovery and excitement of the search for the reason for the healing effect of clay.

What makes clay do that?

Basically, Stumpf surmised that the dry powder absorbs secretions and deodorizes offensive smells. The latter he proved in a severe case of infection of the mucous membranes in the sinus cavities (ozaena) by blowing dry powder into the nose. The patient had suffered for weeks from sanious, stinky secretions from the nose, to the point where she had been ostracized in church and at social affairs. She even was shunned by her relatives who thought the smell unbearable. After a few weeks of standard (ineffective) treatments, Stumpf changed to blowing powdered clay into the nose with an amazingly good result regarding the discharge and odor, yet it took clay treatments for a whole year to cure the ailment fully.

Curious about the drying effectiveness of powdered clay, he experimented with imbedding samples of calves' liver in a box of clay. They dried to a leathery consistency after 48 hours in the clay. He repeated his experiment with 30 grams of beef buried in clay powder. After two days the weight was reduced to 23 grams. In ten days the piece was hard enough to be broken by hand. Another test was to roll cotton into filbert size balls, drench them in either water or defibered pigs' blood and then roll them in dry clay. The clay-covered balls grew as long as free moisture from inside was available, but after 15-20 minutes growth ceased. If a ball was then fractured, the cotton fell out like a nut from a shell, completely dry, and the clay was wet with water or blood.

Stumpf's first conclusion was that clay adsorbs moisture and dries out wounds which then heal because there cannot be bacterial activity where there is no moisture. Where there is no bacterial activity, there cannot be an infectious reaction. In reading up about clay he encountered the classic earth *Terra sigillata* or *Terra lemnia* that had been used for wound treatment in antiquity and still in early modern medicine. Stumpf hoped his colleagues would begin to spread his rediscovery of the bolus treatment and bring it into mainstream medicine.

Peer comments and tests

The colleagues did. Langemak (1899) reported four months later from a Kaiserswerth hospital that they had begun to use white clay, argilla, for wound treatment as soon as Stumpf's paper had been read. Two months of application showed that (1) it was very inexpensive; (2) it was not toxic; (3) it had inordinate power of adsorption, thus reducing the need for frequent changes of bandages, very important where the physician cannot make extended daily patient house calls and where the often none too bright relatives of patients cannot be left to change the bandage themselves; (4) the clay had no odor by itself, but instead effectively deodorized putrid wounds; (5) it did not irritate the wound nor the adjacent area (no infections or eczemas); and (6) the drying-out effect helped to rebuild the skin over purulent amputation ends.

Langemak was not entirely pleased, however. In some instances he found that the healing of a wound treated with clay was delayed by scab formation and he finally used an ointment or wet clay bandage. The scabbing caused Langemak to dispute Stumpf's statement "that wounds heal especially rapidly", yet he conceded that he could not say that healing with *argilla* is slower than with other bandages. For some applications such as eczemas on the head, and superficial lacerations, Langemak's hospital used a mixture of bolus with 12.5% glycerin and 25% Vaseline, claiming that it reduced scabbing without delaying the healing process.

Further, Langemak suggested heating the clay to 150°C to improve pulverization and to sterilize the clay, even though the latter is not deemed critical with wounds that are suppurating anyhow. For the physician or nurse applying the clay, Langemak suggested using a spoon rather than a shaker, because the ultra fine particles can get into the air and dry out the nose, even cause fits of coughing.

Testing for desiccation

Not long after Stumpf's seminal article, the hygienist Buchner, a former teacher of Stumpf's, instructed his assistant, Dr. Megele, to undertake tests on the desiccation achieved by clay (Stumpf, 1906, p. 11). Among various drying media, Megele tested white clay as well as red clay, sawdust, dried moss (sphagnum), wood shavings (excelsior), flour, and bandage gauze. Megele first placed 10 gram pieces of calf liver into test tubes with these drying media (Megele 1899). Every three days he weighed the test pieces for a total of 15 days.

The weight reduction was generally 65% for red bolus, 58% for white, 43% for sawdust, 63% for dried moss, 60% for wood shavings, and 55% for flour. Tests with gauze were stopped and weighing was discontinued after six days, when the meat smelled rotten.

The physical appearance of the test pieces at the end of the tests was basically the same for meat in bolus and excelsior, that is: odorless, completely dry, leathery. Moss and wood shavings resulted in dried pieces with a light to strong putrid smell. They were generally dry outside, but soft inside.

To cross-check his results, Megele repeated his experiments by hanging up cloth bags in air with the samples in drying media. The weight loss results were slightly but not significantly higher. Another series at 37°C showed little difference between drying in ambient or heated air.

Megele then undertook a series of tests on hard-boiled eggs (shell removed) and on unbroken raw eggs in the same media except in gauze. After 38 days the weight loss of boiled eggs was similar to that of the beef pieces. Eggs dried in bolus were odorless and hard as stone; those in sawdust were odorless but "elastically hard". Those from excelsior and moss smelled badly and were slimy on the outside. Raw eggs in the shell lost less moisture in all the tests. The bolus media showed the highest (15%) weight loss versus sawdust (4.2%) and air (3.1%). The lower values compared to boiled eggs must be attributed to the required drying action through the shell of the raw egg.

Megele assigned the higher values for red versus white bolus to a finer particle size of the clay. This could account for better moisture absorption with the red clay, but there is no reason for an inherently smaller particle size of red versus white clay if the two types are not chemically different other than that red clay contains a few percent of iron oxide. Megele did not test the basic composition of either clay. A substantial percentage of magnesium or calcium oxide could vary the absorption performance of the clay, but neither of these would be recognizable simply by the color of the clay.

These tests allow us a glimpse of some of the problems with the wound treatment materials that were in use prior to *Bolus alba*. Megele had selected these older materials for the comparison tests because they then were the only media used in medicine to try to prevent or reduce the infection of wounds. The tests indeed showed the superiority of clay. However, as will be seen, these absorption tests lost part of their meaning, when it became doubtful that the dryness of the clay was the sole key to the healing of wounds. That did not deny that clay was by far the best wound coverage material because it offered a reliable protection against infection, and there were as yet no other real defenses against wound infections if they did occur post-operatively. Certainly it was well known that surgery should be done aseptically, it was by no means assured that a hundred years ago even best adherence to asepsis procedures could avoid all infections in all hospitals after every surgery. Pus formation at suture perforations was still very common.

Comments and Explanations

[1] French: Mousselin, a plain light cotton fabric first made in Iraq.

[2] The dried and sifted husk of grains, separated from the flour after thrashing. A box was built around the wound and filled with bran to absorb pus and body fluids.

[3] Jute is a bast fiber of *Tileacea* from India. By retting (watering and steeping) the fibers are separated and resident bacteria are removed from the plant.

[4] Sphagnum is the light moss in the upper stratum of dry bogs, also called moss-peat.

[5] Excelsior was the name for fine spiral wood shavings as package filler to reduce breakage.

[6] The University's most famous alumnus was Wilhelm Roentgen, discoverer of X-rays in 1895.
[7] Stumpf had previously published a paper on acetic acid poisoning in this journal.
[8] Phlegmones: Inflammations of connective tissue, cause of ulceration and abscesses.

Chapter Five: Use of Clay in Internal Medicine

Occasionally, such as for the clay treatment of finger injuries or even amputations, Dr. med. Julius Stumpf was forced to use the clay not as a dry powder, but as a thick paste applied like a cap over a finger tip or like a plaster cast around a joint. This application of moist clay was just as successful as that of the dry clay powder. It shook Stumpf's confidence in the theory that the sole healing modus of clay was the moisture absorption it provided.

Fast action by dry or wet clay

Another realization was that the extinction of odor from large putrid wounds following coverage with dry or with wet clay powder was almost instantaneous. The moment the clay was applied, the offensive odor ceased. Such fast action, Stumpf reasoned, could not possibly have anything to do with clay's removal of moisture from bacterial growth and cessation of septic activity (Stumpf, 1906, p.17). He concluded that either dry or moist clay must influence the bacterial activity in the sense of curtailing the bacterial propagation wherever the clay reached bacteria of the wound. This theory was reinforced by the fact that a covering of clay would not eliminate the odor of non-putrid fluids (chloroform, spirit of ammonia), but only the odor of decomposing urine and other organic matter. Further, any other substance that is normally considered a good absorbent, such as boric acid, beech-wood ashes, magnesium oxide, wheat flour, and confectionary sugar could not eliminate the organic decomposition odor caused by bacterial activity. Therefore, thought Stumpf, the clay must stop the bacterial activity, and it would do this regardless of whether the clay was wet or dry. From this reasoning, it was not far to consider that clay might be useful in safely treating intestinal complaints (Stumpf, 1906, p. 17):

> "This theory requires the conclusion that powdered bolus, introduced in some manner into the intestinal canal, would have to exhibit the same antibacterial activity as it did with septic suppurating wounds. If this unvarying inorganic substance, the bolus, restricted bacterial growth and its destructive activity, it would do this whether a sufficient quantity of bolus were placed on wound surfaces or on mucous membranes of the intestinal tract."

Stumpf's considerations were reinforced by his reading about geophagy (Chapter Seven), especially the famous report by Alexander von Humboldt on the clay eating of the Ottomake natives of the Orinoco (Humboldt, 1859, pp. 248-254). Thinking that the clay eating of indigenous peoples must be an instinctive disinfection of the digestive system, Stumpf began self-tests by eating small quantities of clay powder wrapped in oblates[1]. When he felt quite comfortable with the consumption of clay, he increased the daily portions and decided to try this treatment the next time he encountered a case of diarrhea with vomiting (*Brechdurchfall*).

Stumpf's mother: The first case history

The first opportunity came on 3 June 1900. Of all people, the patient was his own 81-year-old mother. She had begun suffering from diarrhea and vomiting at midnight. The increasing severity of the attacks had the family call Stumpf in the morning.

It was a typical condition: repeated violent vomiting, severe diarrhea with painful cramps. Since a collapse of the patient did not appear imminent, Stumpf gave her as much bolus powder as he could wrap in six oblates and he allowed the patient a swallow of water with each. To his surprise all vomiting and colic was soon much reduced. Repeating the dose half an hour later further reduced vomiting and the diarrhea was only a trace of the previous condition. The treatment was repeated again in the evening. By the following morning the elderly lady could be considered cured.

Barely a few days afterward, when Stumpf was substituting for a fellow physician, he was called to treat a cavalry officer's spouse for the same affliction. He prescribed 30 grams of bolus in oblates to be taken as rapidly as possible. This was in the morning. By evening rounds, the lady told Stumpf: "Listen, this is an unusual powder! I am completely cured. I took the first portion of clay in the oblates, then ate it pure like tooth powder."

Within a few weeks, another case of diarrhea with vomiting was presented. The patient was a 50-year-old prison inmate, a physically run-down homeless person. He suffered from severe and frequent vomiting, and his diarrhea had turned to rice-water stool combined with violent cramps. Stumpf, as a prison official, first had to adhere to the approved official medical procedure of opiates and diet, which, as usual, did not help.

During the afternoon visit the patient was in extremis. He was covered with a sticky sweat, he groaned incessantly, his voice was barely audible, the diarrhea extremely violent. The underarm temperature was 39.5° C. Stumpf ordered the prison guard to bring the box of *Bolus alba* from the prison dispensary and then cajoled the patient to take as much bolus in oblates as he possibly could, probably near 30 grams. That was at 5:15 p.m. When Stumpf had to leave briefly, the condition of the patient appeared hopeless to him. The clay would have to do its job quickly. Stumpf returned at 6 PM and

> "See, I came too late. Who could describe my surprise? The patient, bathed in perspiration was lying quietly. The previously cold extremities had warmed; the hardly detectable pulse had firmed. When I asked him how he was feeling he did not say 'well', but 'who took my pain away?' It indicated how severe the cramps must have been. The rectal temperature was 38.5° C. It reminded me of the crisis of a severe pneumatic[2]."

Stumpf ordered a repeat dose of bolus. The next morning the patient could be considered cured of what had been an inordinately severe case of *Cholera nostra* (bilious cholera). Bolus should be equally promising for *Cholera asiatica* (Cholera of the small intestine), even though different bacteria where involved in each.

Although today's physician may never see a case of cholera[3] except in foreign countries, and most likely no citizen of developed countries will have seen a case except on the evening TV news, this debilitating, highly infectious and always deadly disease was a frightening scourge just as pestilence was.[4] Where it struck, human suffering was intense. There was no protection, no way to guard oneself. The German satirist Saphir (1795-1858) described the manifold useless attempts in his "Preservative Man" story: "Wear gum elastic over the skin, over it a plaster of pitch, above this a body wrap of 6 ells (~20 ft) of flannel, over the heart cavity a copper plate, on the chest a bag of warm sand, around the neck a double shawl filled with juniper berries and peppercorns, in the ears two pieces of cotton drenched in camphor, in front of the nose a smelling bottle with a sharp vinegar, and in front of the mouth a twig of calamus… (this being less than ¼ of the suggested protective measures[5])… which will guarantee you to be the first in your neighborhood with cholera (Meige, 1899, pp. 79-80)."

Professor Martin Hahn in Munich expressed it more bitterly (Hahn, 1906, p.1097): "…and yet, any thinking physician at the bedside of a patient ill with cholera will clearly perceive the total helplessness of our medical arsenal against this illness and will be convinced of the unsatisfactory avail of our knowledge." Hahn must have missed Stumpf's first publication in September of the previous year (Stumpf, 1905).

Stumpf wondered how the physical character of the bolus powder provided its inherent healing proficiency. Apparently the particle size of properly pulverized clay was very small, smaller than the bacteria. The idea that clay particles could be as small as or smaller than the then known "comma bacterium" led him away from just saying "the clay particles are very small" and made him assign a specific size, such as no more than the size of the bacterium. One hundred years later he was proven right[6].

Stumpf then concluded that if it were just that clay particles needed to be small, one could grind bricks to dust and cure cholera. Indeed, unbeknownst to him, brick dust had been used in internal medicine for thousands of years (Chapter Eight).

The attack on Asiatic cholera

Asiatic cholera broke out in the northeastern part of Germany in 1904. Stumpf was called to Berlin. From there he was sent to the cholera area of Nakel (now Poland). A 53-year-old female had been diagnosed with Asiatic cholera. As Stumpf was interviewing the patient, she suddenly sat up and vomited a quarter of a liter of a greenish liquid, typical for Asiatic cholera. Stumpf tried immediately to get the patient to swallow an oblate with bolus, but she explosively vomited again. Trying to get her to swallow two teaspoons of powder stirred into a glass of water, she immediately ejected the mixture of clay and water with the greenish liquid. Stumpf admitted to becoming quite concerned, but asked the patient to drink some more of the clay suspension. The substantially weakened woman took the glass and forced herself to take several sizeable swallows. Then it happened (Stumpf, 1906, p. 29-31):

> "Now comes the moment I shall never forget. The patient remained quiet for several moments and then whispered, obviously astonished: "I don't have to vomit anymore". Her cyanotic color faded and her face coloring became normal. She was able to sleep for hours without vomiting. Ten hours later she could be considered cured. The senior government medical officers present insisted that Stumpf immediately write a treatment prescription for distribution to all physicians in the entire area of the cholera epidemic". [The proud day was September 4, 1905, nine months before Hahn had written his desperate plea].

Hardly had Stumpf returned to Würzburg when further eastern cases of cholera made his return visit advisable. Stumpf traveled via Berlin to Gnesen to find that the local physicians had begun treating nine cases with *Bolus alba*, and all were doing well. Stumpf himself treated three more and was successful. He returned home to find the message that "regrettably" no new cases of cholera had occurred that might require Stumpf's presence.

Treatment specifications

Stumpf published a preliminary paper on his experience with Asiatic cholera (Stumpf, 1905, pp. 1199 ff.). He emphasized that the clay treatment must begin with an empty stomach, but that is anyway one of the symptoms of Asiatic cholera due to the repeated vomiting and diarrhea. If then an adult patient receive 70-100 grams of bolus, children 30 grams, nursing babies 10-15 grams, the following result may be expected: The nausea ceases immediately (at worst there is one more vomiting), then to great relief the patient is given to breaking wind and no more diarrhea. The patient's temperature will drop within half an hour with attendant perspiration. The clearest result of imminent healing is the sudden strong desire to sleep. Patients fell asleep so quickly that they had to be roused to continue taking their doses of clay that should not be delayed beyond 20-30 minutes. Besides an empty stomach, an absolute requirement is the avoidance of any food and alcohol during the first 48 hours of treatment with bolus.

Even in an advanced stage of the illness the clay treatment is still effective. The clay is suspended in water, stirred frequently, and drunk in small portions. Infants appear to love to drink the mixture from a bottle, but if they refuse to drink, they must be force-fed. The principle of the treatment is the drenching of the bacteria with a surfeit of clay of the finest particle size. Bacteria will stop propagating and toxin production will cease[7].

Stumpf, upon being queried, said that he knew very well that Asiatic cholera and diarrhea with vomiting (bilious cholera) are two different things caused by different bacteria, but the same clay material can be used to combat both. Cholera was now curable.

Between 1906 and 1910 there was no cholera in Germany. Stumpf therefore assisted in the treatment of epidemics in bordering countries, especially in Serbia (Stumpf 1914a, pp. 759-763). This time Stumpf wanted to make sure that neither local authority nor local physicians would limit the application of bolus since there had been many cases where insufficient amounts of bolus were given the patients.

Drigalski (1943, pp. 405-6) reminisces about cholera in Serbia where he was cholera commissioner when cholera was rampant among the military and civilians there. He became fully convinced of the value of *Bolus alba* and later, during WW I, carried bags of it into the field. In a curious aside he even mentions *Bolus alba* as the healing agent for the badly beaten Candide in Voltaire's work of the same name, but copies of the text in three languages do not suggest this to be probable[8].

Success in Serbia

In Nisch (now Niš) in Serbia, Stumpf faced thirty cholera cases in a large ward attended by several international physicians from Switzerland and Russia. With the help of a German-speaking nurse Stumpf prepared his bolus and water mixture and began to dispense it. Several of the less debilitated patients left their beds to ask for the "white drink," which had first been given to the very ill who were too weak to hold the beakers with the solution.

The next day in the ward Stumpf treated several patients whose prospects for recovery seemed practically nil. One, a huge man, was brought in supported by two guards. After trying for 2 ½ hours to get the patient to keep some of the bolus mixture down, he suddenly reached for the beaker, "Hey, I'm feeling better," and took a sizeable swallow. Shortly thereafter the patient's pulse was noticeable again and the following day the patient was cured. For two more days no patient died of cholera. Altogether Stumpf had treated 31 cases in a few days and lost only the one who had been already near death the night before Stumpf had arrived. The ward at Niš was then closed for lack of new patients.

From Niš Stumpf went to Belgrade and treated 20 female patients in the local hospital. Three were hopelessly moribund by the time Stumpf got there, but 17 recovered within 24 hours. Stumpf's efforts and successful introduction of the bolus therapy were rewarded with a high Serbian decoration. The chemical company Merck had provided Stumpf with 300 packets of their *Bolus alba officinalis* of 200 grams each (60 kilograms) free of charge.

In Germany, the chief at a children's polyclinic, Prof. Dr. Seitz, had agreed to do some bolus tests with infants suffering from the then typical "summer diarrhea". 20 babies between 14 days and 9 months of age were treated, nine recuperated, three were improved and five were not cured. Stumpf later concluded that, as was done too often, the doses given were inadequate.

Diphtheria next

About 1908 Stumpf had turned his attention to curing diphtheria (a very serious contagious throat infection often requiring months of isolation) with bolus (Stumpf, 1908, pp. 1181-2; Levy, 1908, p. 32). He reminded his readers about successes of bolus therapy in cases of diarrhea and vomiting, of Asiatic cholera, and of fish and vegetable poisoning. Then he introduced throat diphtheria into the realm of bolus therapy. The treatment was simple for all ages: Give the patient a teaspoon of 1:2 bolus suspension in water to swallow every five minutes. The frequency is the most important aspect for success. After a very short time the evil mouth odor disappears, within two hours pulse and temperature decrease. The swelling is reduced surprisingly quickly. Within 10 hours the diphtheria coating breaks up into insular pockets, showing again healthy red mucous membrane. The mechanism seems to be a scouring of the throat by the bolus particles with removal of the toxins to the stomach. Stumpf cites 15 case histories, a lot really, considering he was not a full-time practicing physician. His cases arose from treating occasional patients in and around Würzburg, whom Stumpf met when he went deer hunting in the surrounding area[9].

Levy adds that Stumpf also recommended bolus for nose diphtheria of older children via a method of gargling with bolus suspension. Since Stumpf's paper, the hospital where Levy was engaged[10] used bolus exclusively for diphtheria, because the then available serum was not reliably effective. Levy agrees that the function was a mechanical one. The treatment failed in cases where patients came to the hospital too late, suffering already from the toxin's effects such as heart complications or nephritis.

Laboratory tests with a variety of suspensions of bolus, magnesia, sulfur, talc, and plant and animal carbon proved that diphtheria toxin was absorbed by bolus. The toxin was transported to the intestinal tract where the toxin became ineffective (See Chapter Sixteen). The coagulation necrosis (dead cells) of the epithelium coverings is a nutrient for the bacteria and its removal is critical to the success of treatment. Levy points to an article by Dr.Trumpp on diphtheria in a handbook of child healing: "Even if only part of the toxins are removed or made ineffective, the growth on the membranes on the mucous side is slowed or ceases, and the leucocytes, chemically alerted by the infection process, will melt away the [diphtheria] layer." Levy further found that the physician need not face a dilemma of choices between bolus or antidiphtheria serum, because both can safely be used side by side.

Stumpf nowhere claimed to be the inventor of the bolus treatment, indeed, his research showed a historical background through the ages. But Stumpf did resurrect an ancient healing method and rescued it from the mangling it received from some Middle Ages and Early Modern Age medical practitioners. In the process he saved many lives.

---

[1] Oblates: Flexible, paper-thin pastry wrappings baked usually of wheat, used for religious observances or as pan release when baking (before Teflon® coated bake ware).

[2] Stumpf must be referring to the pneumonia crisis (prior to antibiotics), when the fever either broke on the 21st day or the patient expired.

[3] For definition only: <u>Cholera morbus</u> – noninfectious diarrhea and cramps, usually caused by contaminated foods. <u>Cholera infantum</u> – "summer complaint" of children in the warm season, with pain, vomiting, diarrhea, fever, and prostration. <u>Cholera asiatica</u> – infectious, usually fatal, violent diarrhea and vomiting, muscular cramps, and collapse. <u>Cholera nostra</u> – bilious cholera. <u>Dysentery</u> – an intestinal disease, plain, amoebic or bacillary inflammation, abdominal pain, toxemia, and diarrhea with bloody discharge and mucous feces.

[4] Cholera deaths: 1869 one half million in Hungary; 1884/5 in France and Italy 50,000 each; 1885/5 Russia 800,000 (Source: Chambers, 1938).

[5] Saphir, continued: "…Over the flannel a shirt steeped in calcium chloride, over it a cotton jacket and above that a hot brick and a waistcoat with calcium chloride, flannel leg dressings, double yarn knit stockings boiled in vinegar and rubbed with camphor. Two copper flasks with hot water and galoshes over them and two water bags behind the calves. An overcoat of sheep's wool with chloride, and as outer garment a coat of waxed linen and a thick hat. In the right pocket he would carry a pound of Melissa tea and half a pound of southernwood (Artemesium) and a half a pound of sage. In the waist pocket he carries a flagon with chamomile oil and in the trouser pocket a flask with ether of camphor. In the hat he carries a terrine of Gratten* soup, in the right hand he carries a whole juniper bush and in the left an acacia tree. With a string around his waist he drags a cart with 15 ells of flannel, a steam bath machine, 10 bath brushes, 18 bricks, 2 furs, and one comfort chair (mobile earth toilet). About the face he must have a mask of mentholated dough and in his mouth a quarter pound of sedge". This article by Meige appeared in "Janus" in 1899. Saphir lived a hundred years earlier.
*Neither Saphir's French editor Meige nor I could identify the meaning of 'Gratte'.

[6] A journal article of 1987 contains an electron micrograph of bacteria immobilized by a thin film of clay.

[7] How to take clay, mixing clay and water to prepare mixture: It can be dangerous to try to take portions of dry or insufficiently moist clay because the powdered clay can be accidentally inhaled or may stick in the throat or even cause a gut blockage, because clay will increase in volume with absorption or more moisture. In a vessel always add water to clay, because the other way around dried balls or pieces of clay, when put into water, will not gently fizz but explosively disintegrate into myriads of small particles. This was first reported about 1568. When dry clay pieces were placed in a goblet of wine the clay sprang apart and hit the glass with a clang or small crackle just as if the glass or a window pane had cracked" (Georg Anton Volkmann, Silesia subterranea).

[8] Generally the German, French and English texts agree that Candide was cured of his wounds by an emollient, by an ointment, or an ameliorating medication espoused by Dioscorides. To my knowledge, Dioscorides did not use the term bolus but knew a number of white earths that could have helped Candide but would not have been described as ointments or emollients.

[9] In Germany you not only need to pass a very stringent test to obtain a (lifetime) hunting license, to hunt you must either own the land or have leased the hunting rights to it, unless more affluent friends invite you to hunt with them on their preserves.

[10] Freiburg University, Freiburg im Breisgau.

Chapter Six: Peer Acceptance of Clay in Medical Treatment

The rediscovery of the beneficial applications of fine clay found resonance in many meetings of local medical societies and in numerous articles in prominent medical journals of the day.

Langemak and Megele (both 1899) were not the only ones to take up the promotion of the new clay treatment pioneered by Stumpf (1898-99). An unusual spate of papers was published within two years, based on the seminal work on wound treatment, on dysentery and cholera (1905), on expanded treatments in between 1908 and 1910. A review by Stumpf (1914) was followed by other commentaries in 1916 and 1917. All papers appeared in the major medical journals of Germany[1]. Subjects covered can basically be grouped into concurrence, criticisms but final agreement, new treatment applications, and new clay-like materials for treatment[2]. Despite lengthy research, I was unable to find any reference to Stumpf's clay treatments in any British, French, or American publication. Possibly international communication between journals barely existed before World War I, and most likely none existed during it.

The burden of cervical catarrh

Georgii reported (1899, p. 14) on using *Bolus alba* to combat cervical catarrhs with their debilitating smelly discharge, the "cross" that women with cervical affliction had to bear. Georgii found immediate and substantial help in the odor- and secretion-reducing properties of bolus. He took past cases of *Endometritis cervicis* back for treatment. Even though the treatment with bolus had to be repeated every three days, the clay application reduced unhealthy changes of the uterus portio, eliminated the many lower abdominal pains and totally cured the feared vaginal "white flux".

Rudolf Höpfel (1899, p. 448) wrote about bandages with clay. He was disappointed with the clay in three cases of amputations or exarticulation of fingers. He had sterilized the clay powder, the operation was conducted under strict rules of asepsis. The amputation wound was covered with a thick layer of bolus and bound tightly with bandage gauze and cotton, and it was covered with multiple windings of bandage. He found that after three days pus came out of the suture holes, the edges of the wounds were stuck together, below that was even more pus. The same occurred two days later. When Höpfel dusted the wound with a 1:4 mixture of Jodoform®[3] and Dermatol®[4] and covered it with a standard antiseptic bandage, pus formation ceased, the wound healed in six days. In five cases of foot ulcers the same treatment reached the same result. Because nobody else reported these results, and since there was general surgical dissatisfaction with the above-mentioned antiseptic solutions, one tends to believe that Höpfel had used an insufficient layer of bolus and had wrapped it too tightly.

In three cases of tibia ulcers, Höpfel washed the ulcers three times daily in dilute boric acid, then sprinkled on a substantial layer of clay and added five fold muslin tampons. This avoided the scabbing; the wound dried quickly, the ulcers healed within 8-10 days. Höpfel tried the same method with various smaller wounds that did not pus, but did scab. He actually was pleased with the result, but he believed that a combination of clay with the two other medications would be even better. Finally Höpfel criticized the clay treatment because he could not use it with an occlusive bandage (which he apparently liked) and thought that other antiseptic bandages were equal to clay, an opinion not shared in the literature.

Gangrene defeated with bolus

A paralyzed patient resident in a mental institution developed gangrene of muscle and bone in both feet. Though the patient mostly was not mentally stable, Dr. Hans Fischer (1899, pp. 378-9) felt that the condition of his feet and the rapidly progressing gangrene must impact the patient's condition of mental instability. The ulcers produced ichorous smells and secretions.

A visiting professor, Dr. Klaussner, shared Fischer's opinion that it was gangrene and felt that even after amputation the gangrene would come back. The medical council decided that keeping the wounds clean was most important and authorized a clay treatment primarily to defeat the pervading odor. Dr. Fischer then spread argilla (*Bolus alba*) into the open wounds, filling them completely. Within three days the odor had disappeared. Then followed an unanticipated healing process so different from what gangrene would normally do that Fischer would have questioned the first diagnosis of the nature of the illness.

Within two months, documented by precise case history progress, the hospital reported that all three wounds were closed and scar tissue had formed. The length of time for the healing was partially blamed on a slight mishandling of the patient during regular baths, which reopened two wounds. It was concluded that clay could conquer the curse of gangrene.

Babies are happier

From a midwife (or ob-gyn nurse) school near Cologne, Germany, Dr. Horn (1899, p. 377) addressed the concern about proper treatment of umbilicus cut-off for babies. Normally when separated from blood supply, the remainder of the umbilicus must dry out and mummify. Babies were treated with Vaseline and were bathed regularly. Horn had read Stumpf's paper that where there is no moisture, there is no bacterial effect. He instructed his staff to use *Bolus alba* and to discontinue the bathing, because bathing prevents the drying out of the remnant of the umbilical cord. Danger of infection also lurks in the bathwater. Here he was in opposition to two colleagues who insisted that not bathing the babies would lead the nursing students to sloppy procedures and to excessively careless behavior. Dr. Horn started to teach the new method (he compared teaching the new method to the difficulty of teaching old dogs a new trick) and proved that the new teaching was successful, but the seldom revised old handbook for midwives was a total roadblock to progress and better methods.

New Clay Treatments developed

A gynecologist was very much concerned about the relatively frequent infections and pus formation in the suture canals after laparotomies[5] (Stoeckel, 1900, p. 593) as well as incidence of stomatites[6]. The then used "Airolpaste", a bismuth-oxy-iodide that splits off either iodine or bismuth when wetted could let airborne bacteria pass. In a series of experiments Stoeckel compared Dermatol®, Jodoform®, and kaolin. Kaolin brought none of the stomatidal problems. Especially the kaolin was so superior, that the aluminosilicate (which kaolin is), same as Stumpf's *Bolus Alba* or *Argilla*, was used exclusively henceforth, and was also used for other types of wounds.

The first decade of the 20th century brought forth a number of competing substances for wound treatment. First came Karfunkel's lake mud, Seeschlick, which was the mud remnant of an ancient lake, hidden under a layer of peat. It was wet but dried to a gray powder. Essentially it was 76% siliceous earth (SiO_2), 8% aluminum oxide (Al_2O_3), iron oxide 3%, magnesium 2.2%, alkali 2.2% and 7.6% calcium oxide, a really fairly standard healing earth mix. Cohn named it "Xeranatsbolus" and used it on about 1,500 patients. Same as other clay of similar chemical composition, it was helpful on burns; it cleaned hands, removed scaliness from the scalp, held heat, was odorless, and had no irritants.

"Boluphen" was a new wound product, a condensate of formaldehyde-phenol and clay, proposed for large surface wounds and as a means to quickly cleanse and deodorize wounds (Hayward, 1917, p. 583).

"Geox" was a fine powder of 80% diatomaceous earth, 10% clay, calcium oxide and calcium carbonate, easy to wet and thus easy to mold to wound surfaces. It seems very similar to ancient Tripoli earth. Dr. Byk (1918, p.1-2), a specialist in stomach, intestinal and metabolism problems, used it as poultice in every case, once or twice a day. He recommended it for pain relief, calming, loosening cramps, and fighting inflammation.

While Dr. Byk apparently was 'of prominence' as public health councilor *(Sanitätsrat)*, the tenor of his paper is autocratic, and the contents are of little medical specificity:

Q:"How do I use Geox?"	A: "As cataplasm."
Q: "For which hurt have I recommended it?"	A: "233 cases of abdominal pain."
Q: "How have I used this preparation?"	A: "54 times without other therapy."
Q: "Which successes have I achieved?"	A: "Relieved many cases of rheumatism of the abdominal muscles."
Q: "How does Geox work?"	A: "Primarily because it is a cataplasm".

This closes the vicious circle. Then, almost like earlier (and later) nonmedical purveyors of miracles, Byk had patients explain their joy of the success of Geox: "The treatment does me well", "The treatment does me very well", "I am very satisfied, I believe it helped me", all without any reference to a case history. This is endemic among claims for cure by alternative medicines. I would not have selected Dr. Byk's Geox article here, had it not been the only published reference to a diatomaceous earth with significant clay-like components. Apparently it had beneficial effects.

Not much more elucidating is an article about a new fango preparation, (polyfango, which means multiple mud). Prof. Karl Grube (1919, p. 1087) describes this product as a fine mud of gray color from the shores of a mountain lake in the Eifel middle mountain range in Germany. Such lake mud was also called Eifelfango. In contrast to other powders that need to be mixed with hot water, this polyfango, when mixed with cold water will shortly rise to 60° C temperature and is good for poultices. Temperature increases when dry mud is wetted have been reported often.

Three physicians expressed their thoughts of the use of clay (*Bolus alba*) to dry out body orifices by blowing powder into the afflicted areas. This had been known, but had been forgotten from 1,000 and from 400 years ago. In all cases it was the nose that was powdered partly because of ozaena (sinus inflammation) and partly to stop bleeding after a fight. Max Nassauer (1910, p. 82) reminded readers of his opinion that bolus treatment could be also expanded to other body cavities. Trumpp (1909, p. 2422) also had excellent results blowing bolus into noses, thus reaching the locus of the infection or injury.

Nassauer's contribution was the invention of a rubber squeeze-bulb-activated blower on a powder glass reservoir (not unlike a basting tool) that he primarily used in cases of the then-frequent "white flux", the white odorous vaginal discharge. In his remarks he does not want to appear overly optimistic, but the symptom of discharge ceased within 2-3 days. Internal cleansing and repeated powder application seemed to alleviate the problem for good. Adding to the effort to treat this complaint, Ernst Poppel (1914, p. 2406) reported on a new preparation that consisted of bolus with silver phosphate, silver encapsulating each grain of bolus. His experience was that conditions of gonorrhea and cervical catarrhs were cleared up with several applications unless there were severe complications such as a vicious *Bacterium coli* infection. He considered some of his results unclear, because the recurrence of gonorrhea was probably due to a reinfection by the husband.

More peer comments

Others related more benefits or discoveries about *Bolus alba*. The pharmacist Georg Hoffmann (1910, p. 234) based the success of *Bolus alba* not only on an absorption mechanism restricting bacterial growth, but also on the absorption of toxic enzymes and putrefaction gases. G. Salus (1917, p. 378) added that, in water, bolus acts as a negative colloid, so bolus primarily absorbs by cation exchange. His tests showed that staphylococcus is absorbed better than typhus bacteria. Stumpf had experimented with typhus treatment but had not considered it promising unless the alimentary system was as empty as it usually is after onset of cholera diarrhea.

Expanding bolus application to diarrhea and meteorism (flatulence), Johannes Görner (1907, p. 2383) used bolus in eight cases of acute gastroenteritis including severe fish poisoning. In all cases the first or second treatment with bolus stopped the diarrhea and led to convalescence. After the 50-100 grams of bolus suggested by Stumpf for treatment of adults, stool remained liquid, after the next treatment it became mixed with bolus and then was firm. In the case of a serious influenza pneumonia a patient experienced frequent vomiting and many mucous discharges. Oral use of bolus stopped the vomiting, 100 grams infused rectally led to normal stool within 48 hours. With hindsight, it might have been more propitious to repeat the oral doses. Stumpf did not recommend rectal treatment, at least he did not write about it.

Görner agreed with Stumpf that, in case of typhus, bolus only worked on an empty stomach and intestinal system. He was successful with three cases of typhus treatment. Dr. Gräser (1911, p. 1991) had reported six years earlier that he was successful curing different typhus-caused diarrheas due to meat (canned meat) poisoning, and diarrhea with vomiting. He emphasized that the malodorous diarrhea of typhus ceased soon and stools became normal. He also advocated that, similar to keeping bolus in the house, it should be available on shipboard.

Infections due to use of clay was an occasional subject, usually ill researched. H. Möser (1909, Pp. 249-50) preached the not unfamiliar gospel according to St. Tetanus. P. Zweifel (1910, p. 1787) communicated a hospital incident, where after 10,000 perfect cases of umbilical cord treatment suddenly 12 infections occurred that were traced to a double control failure in the sterilization of bolus. Zweifel rejected the midwives' explanation that the bolus was sterilized at 170°C to be "as likely as holding your hand into fire and not being burned". In steam of 100°C all tetanus spores were dead within two minutes; in dry heat all spores were dead after 10 minutes at 150°C. Since Zweifel's hospital insisted on three hours at 200°C, no bacteria could be alive. He was convinced that an error caused unsterilized bolus to be used on the patients.

From the pre-WW I. German colonial holding of Kiautschou in China, a German colonel in the medical corps, Prof. Dr. Martini and his apothecary (Martini & Grothe, 1910, p.900) discovered the eating of certain clay prevailing in the province of Shantung. While "eating earth" will be treated in Chapter Seven, this eating of clay to minimize intestinal catarrhs by heavy users of opium might be considered a use of bolus against (voluntary) poisonings. An analysis of the earth was very similar to bolus with a high content of silicic anhydride and aluminum oxide, a clay. Martini and Grothe in essence observed in the 20th century the use of a medicament known to history for thousands of years.

Clay and World War I

The outbreak of World War I. in 1914 led to a number of reports regarding use of bolus against trench diarrhea among infantry troops. Martin Vogel (1915, Pp.193-5), commanding a construction company field hospital of the German ground army, considered daily new minor illnesses a severe detriment to the performance of the troops. The most frequent illness was acute enteritis, especially during the first few months of the war. Many cases had to be transferred home. In Vogel's company the percentage of soldiers on sick call could be as high as 55% for enteritis. The usual opiate treatment would stop the intestinal musculature cramps but would prevent needed voiding. In 80 cases in 8 weeks Vogel first gave a strong purge to void deleterious ingesta, then followed with bolus. Fasting and 400 grams of bolus in three portions and subsequent "fletchering"[7] of foods firmed the stool after the third dose of bolus. Of the 80 cases only 11 came back a second time. Four did not come back for weeks, indicating a reinfection rather than unsuccessful treatment.

Another medical officer, Prof. Arneth (1916, pp. 935-8), addressed the problems of troops on the move. He suggested that any diarrhea immediately be treated with bolus. The troops should carry bolus premixed in a canteen with tea (shake before drinking!) and use it early to catch the illness in the initial stage. (While Arneth says water can be used too, to mix the slurry or creamy liquid with bolus, tea probably was chosen because it normally is made with boiling water and hence is safer water). A normal canteen allowed for about the equivalent of 400 grams of bolus.

Russian troops in World War I. were given 200 grams of bolus in a glass vial to carry in their packs (Wacker, 1935, pp.1279-30). Robert Robertson (1947, p. 213) says, "In the First World War, British medical officers in the Near East noticed that French troops suffered far less from dysentery than British troops. It became known that a French medical officer had ordered fullers' earth (calcium montmorillonite, a clay) to be mixed with custard and given to the men. Some years ago (prior to about 1947) when large quantities of fullers' earth were regularly exported to the Americas, sailors at Angerstein's Wharf in London used to ask for fullers' earth that had spilled from the sacks so that they could use it medically against dysentery and stomach troubles on the voyage at sea".

Other than one article (Morrison, 1916, pp. 268-272), I found no reference to advanced treatment of suppurating wounds in the UK during or after WW II. "Bibb", bismuth subnitrate, 1 oz by weight, Jodoform® 2 oz by weight, made to a paste with liquid paraffin, was the treatment published in "Lancet" as cited above. It was never mentioned again, probably because of the poisoning possibility with Jodoform®. Bismuth subnitrate had been known for years and has not been found elsewhere in the literature in connection with wound treatment. Bismuth subsilicitate is the active ingredient in today's Pepto-Bismol® antidiarrhea compound.

Now defeat of amoebic dysentery

Finally, to emphasize Stumpf's revival of internal and external bolus therapy, we look to a case history by a Swiss physician, Dr. Frei of Niederzuwil (Frei, 1910, pp. 441-4) that will give a feel for the suffering prevalent before Stumpf's discovery: The patient was a 32 year old governess employed in Egypt by the governor of Fayum, about 4 hours from Cairo. Dirt in the environment and unclean means of preparing meals caused her intestinal problems, eventually violent and frequent diarrhea. A physician prescribed a diet consisting of milk and Evian water. Then she developed a high fever. She was given some "whitish" medicine, and in 1908 she was able to travel to Europe where she was hospitalized at St. Gallen. She was given hot enemas, some food such as acorn cocoa, soft boiled eggs, and some wine. Very soon she lost basins full of blood and mucous membranes. Within weeks she lost 28 pounds. The diagnosis was "amoebic enteritis" with the prognosis "usually fatal."

Then, after having read Stumpf's monograph, her physician ordered no more food after 7 a.m. except water, and he administered a solution of 50 grams of bolus in 200 cc of water. About 10 a.m. the physician authorized cocoa, milk, bread, butter, and cheese, for lunch sweet cider, ground beef, and cooked apples. In between, he continued the bolus treatments for two months. Her bowel movements became formed, two to three times a day, pain receded, and sleep, appetite and general condition were very good. The patient was discharged as recovered. This case history, in the context of medicinal use of clay, offers several conclusions:

1) *Bolus alba* cured amoebic dysentery that heretofore was "usually fatal".
2) Had the bolus been given in Stumpf's recommended quantities in the total absence of food, the patient might have been cured in days instead of months.
3) Three thousand years ago the patient could have been cured in Egypt with the appropriate earth.

Quite possibly it is understandable that practitioners new to the concept of internal treatments with clay were impressed enough with the results to decide to try the method, but with a natural reluctance to apply it at the recommended strength and a hesitation to discard entirely other treatments and diets that had moderately served them in the past.

The most depressing part of the history of medicine is not the period when healing knowledge was not reliable or even totally lacking, I find that the period from 1600 or so on is one where new knowledge was so consistently disregarded. One can actually speak on "incubation periods" of new knowledge that variously lasted 50, 100, even 200 years, such as the time it took to believe in the harm of ingesting lead, the length of time it took to accept smallpox vaccination, the length of time it took to realize there were ways of avoiding scurvy, but the medical community was uninformed of or uninterested in cures that had come out of the seafaring population.

Reading 16th and 17th century medical books gives the impression that many doctors wrote about their thoughts or ideas, but colleagues did not read them or try their methods. Doctors also invented "patent" medicines and no two were alike or even similar for the same complaint.

Comments and Explanations

[1] Münchener Medizinische Wochenschrift, a weekly newpaper-like medical journal; Deutsche Medizinische Wochenschrift, a tabloid size, but classy weekly medical journal; Berliner Klinische Wochenschrift, a superregional weekly journal of clinical news; Zentralblatt für Chirurgie, a national central organ for surgeons and surgical procedure; Medizinische Klinik, a national weekly for internal medicine and clinical procedure.

[2] Even though it is not really a subject under our title, it should be mentioned that several medical authors (Starkenstein, 1915, referencing Wiechowsky's work in the journal Fortschritt der Medizin, Nr. 13, 1909, and Adler in Wiener Klinische Wochenschrift Nr. 21, 1912, and Skutetsky-Starkenstein in Neue Arzneimittel, Berlin 1014, p. 439; I was unable to locate the three referenced original articles) promoted animal charcoal in

¼ liter aqueous solution of saline laxatives to combat absorption mushroom poisoning (botulism toxin), heavy metal poisoning and poisoning by alkaloids such as phosphorus or arsenic, and diphtheria toxins.

This opinion is not borne out by authors like Hahn, 1906, on animal charcoal and who could not duplicate results.

[3] Jodoform® is a German trademark for an antiseptic solution or powder used as disinfectant in general surgery. It was then "the best available, but later was found to be deleterious in many cases and always dubious in antiseptic efficacy on wounds. Since Jodoform® was generally used in the solution form, it was blamed for poisonous effects.

[4] Dermatol® is a German trademark for bismuth subgallate that surpassed Jodoform® in wound sterilization in general surgery and became a general anti-inflammatory wound treatment. It was brought into commerce about 1900 to replace Jodoform® because it is insoluble and was considered not to be poisonous.

[5] Laparotomy: Incision through the top or side of the abdominal cover

[6] Stomatite: An inflammation of the mucous membranes of the mouth.

[7] Fletchering: Chewing food very finely (100 times per mouthful) to a liquid consistency before swallowing. In the hunger years in Germany after WW I, this method was promoted as emergency help to make food last longer and be more nutritious.

Chapter Seven: Eating Earth - Geophagy, Geopharma

When Julius Stumpf had his first successes curing vomiting and diarrhea with *Bolus alba,* he remembered having read about ingestion of clay by South American Indians described by Alexander von Humboldt (1859, p. 163) and thus encountered the edge of what ethnologists since have called *geophagy* (eating earth), are now calling *geopharma* (eating earth as medication) or even *geopharmacognosy* (knowing which earth to eat as medication) in all but a few cases.

Eating earth for five reasons

Geophagy is a Greek compound word meaning "eating earth". It was created around 1850 to make ethnologists sound more sophisticated than when they say dirt gobblers, mud feeders, or clay eaters. In any case, geophagy refers to the fact that almost all human societies have been eaters of some specific soil, usually clay. Not dirt, but clay. Clean clay is not dirty, but the first question is why would anyone eat clay? Did our ancestors observe animals eating clay earth to cure diarrhea? It appears so, because even today animals like deer, or gazelles, or mountain sheep can be observed licking clay (not salt!) after the fresh new grass of spring has given them a touch of diarrhea.

Geophagy subsumes the medical term "pica" which dates back to 1563. Pica is the Latin word for magpie, a bird that picks up anything it sees, not only food, but also glittering oddities as collections for nest building[1]. The medical sciences, however, have called *pica* the behavior of eating strange or unusual substances by humans and have related it mostly to some dietary behavior during pregnancy. Pica includes but is not limited to eating clay. Pica involves foodstuffs other than clay or earth. It includes foods that are considered unusual or strange to us today. We go further with the definitions by denoting geophagy as a "craving", which changes occasional pica to a compulsive obsession for unusual, even absurd foods. Ethnologists define "geomania" as an uncontrollable urge to eat earth even to the point of death. All of this is documented by research all over the world in about 300 books and articles written over four centuries since our earth was first explored by valiant sailors.

Why would humans crave earth?

M. E. Gelfand[2] said it this way: "If one remembers that it is mankind's natural instinct to inquire into or taste all that is provided by nature, one will not be surprised that earth is eaten. This is no more irrational than eating salt or pepper, or snails and frogs" [I am certain that many a gourmet will not consider snails and frogs irrational food]. It seems certain that the basic bushman or aborigine or Urmensch was quite aware of his surroundings, including the plants, the animals, and also the minerals, the only class of substance, as said above, which would not wilt in droughts or run away when hunted. This thought, however, would require that all humans are geophagists, not just many, and that is not supported by research. We have no record of an entire society given to eating clay. We also know that only some members of any society do it, however, as one might otherwise suspect, not only the poor segments of a group. Geophagy is not an indicator of social status. There is no scientific literature claiming that geophagy is a racial preference. There is literature that it is a regional preference in the tropics, but that is defeated by reports of geophagy from subtropical and even subpolar regions. Mostly, but there are exceptions, eating clay is not necessarily a continuous habit of dependency such as betel nut chewing, ingesting datura (in America called Jimsonweed), smoking tobacco, or drinking adult beverages.

The question then arises, of course, why would certain members of certain societies sometimes engage in eating clay when, at a cursory observation, it would generally be considered deleterious to health? There are several answers and theories in ethnology trying to vie for a grand unified geophagy theory.

The first reason is hunger due to a seasonally insufficient food supply. Where real foodstuffs, mostly flour, are mixed with earthy substances (clay, diatomaceous earth) to "stretch" the food supply, the reason of hunger is not irrational. Clay earth is generally safe for passage through the human digestive system, even though it cannot be considered nutritious since it has no organic components. Can it fill the stomach to give the feel of satisfaction? It has been so reported. In Germany, workers at the Kyffhäuser sandstone quarries spread "stone butter", a talc (magnesium hydrosilicate), on their lunch sandwich bread (Laufer, 1930, p. 168)[3]. C. B. Lowe reported the same for Italy and Styria in Austria (Lowe, 1920). The Swiss knew mountain flour, mountain butter, mountain cheese (Reinbacher, 1994, pp. 1-13). Scandinavian and Siberian people baked infusoria earth into bread (Halstead, 1968, pp. 1384-93). American natives mixed clay with their acorn or corn meal in times of starvation. Florida Indians ate clay mixed with ground mesquite beans. California Tatu Indians ate clay mixed with mashed acorns to make bread go further and to debitter it. The Athabasca family of Native Americans also reduced the bitter taste of wild potatoes with clay[4], Mackenzie River Tinneh Indians ingested unctuous river mud in times of famine (Sine nomen, 1895).

Other reasons

Another reason suggested for eating clay is that it is an acquired taste and an enjoyable habit. It has been considered as a substitute for salt and or pepper, but where habitual clay eating has been found, there seldom is a lack of access to salt. Where there is habitual use of betel nuts, tobacco, or other natural soul ameliorants, there is not necessarily attendant geophagy.

A third reason for eating clay is found in religion and subservience. It happens mostly in the form of lightly fired clay balls, cookies, or figures (clay figures are eaten at the temple of Tezcatlipoca), but it is more sporadic and is generally tied to specific religious events such as the annual feast of the Black Christ of Esquipulas in Guatemala, or to nonreligious events surrounding a power figure in a society, such as the eating of clay from the grave of a Madagascar tribal chief (Stahl, 1931). These reasons are not connected to a food requirement or enjoyment or religion.

The reason most often found associated with geophagy is help for specific medical complaints. This reason takes it out of the "eating earth" category and places it into the "taking earth as medicine" category, which should be distinguished as "geopharma". This grafts a time defining requirement onto the practice of eating earth, which is customary of medications. Such medical relief from eating earth should be found wherever the same complaint exists. The impressive meaning of the ethnographic reports of clay eating to achieve health is that it can also be traced to the same complaints that were treated many hundreds of years ago with clay earth. In some cases it is not clear what the underlying complaint was, but most often it is gastrointestinal (wounds were treated, too, but that is a different from geopharma, the external application of clay such as for bandages, plasters, or casts for broken bones).

An additional fifth category could be called the involuntary or unsuspecting ingestion of minerals by fraudulent addition of them into foods. It was quite a boost of income for bakers to make whiter bread by adding gypsum, white clay, chalk, ammonium carbonate (*Hirschhornsalz*), milled bones, even poisonous white lead, powdered alum, and calcium dust to flour (Paczensky et al., 1997, p. 193). This is not the same as the addition of clay to flour for medical reasons in the Aegean islands, or the filtering of wine with clay as far back as the age of Nippur, or for making clay medication palatable by boiling it with wine into syrup.

While the literature about geophagy encompasses hundreds of reports from ethnologists, physicians, and naturalists, good summaries are few in number. Two fall into Stumpf's time, but only one into Stumpf's continent. Two other major survey works on geophagy date from the 1930s, again one each from America and one from Europe.

Full credit to Berthold Laufer and Günther Stahl

The major American work on geophagy is that of Berthold Laufer, then curator of the Department of Anthropology at the Field Museum of Natural History in Chicago (Laufer, 1930). Just a year later Günther Stahl published "Die Geophagie" in Germany, a very detailed review (Stahl, 1931). In the 1890s, available to Julius Stumpf, R. Lasch (1898, p. 214) in Vienna wrote about geophagy. The magazine Scientific American had a staff article without designated author about clay eating in 1895 that most likely nobody in Germany saw, because it is nowhere cited (Sine nomen, 1895).

For a more detailed analysis of "geopharma" it is beneficial first to select examples that have been reported from early explorations and then have been confirmed by later observations. On January 1, 1938 researchers Alexander Lawson and H. P. Moon observed that Indians of the Bolivian Altiplano near Puno existed on a vegetable diet largely consisting of potatoes. After boiling and just before consumption, the potatoes are dipped into an aqueous suspension of kaolin type clay to prevent "souring of the stomach" In 1975, traveling on the Altiplano, I stopped at villages with potato fields and was told that eating potatoes that were still a little bit green under the skin when harvested, caused stomach grief. This was also reported by R. H. S. Robertson (Robertson, 1986, chapter on geophagy), who speculated that clay may either be a protection against bacterial infection of the intestinal tract (somewhat unlikely, it would be the only example), or to adsorb solanine from green skinned varieties. It appears, though, that solanine is primarily present in the potato *Solanum dulcamara,* and in the food potato *Solanum tuberosum* only in the tubers until they have fully ripened. Solanine can cause convulsions and death, and clay may have adsorbed the poison. But many varieties of potatoes are grown on the Altiplano. Stahl (1931, p. 346 ff.) said that the Bolivians do not know the use of clay but elsewhere he says they mix it with their food. The Altiplano is wide and long and may have different localized behavior or habits than the lower regions of Bolivia.

Earth as cause or cure of hookworm disease

A widespread parasitic illness in Asia and Africa often referred to as "maladie de terre" or "maladie d'estomac" was *Ancylostomiasis duodenale,* hookworm disease[5]. Laufer (1930, p. 104) couldn't decide which came first, the clay eating or the disease. Since hookworm disease is very prevalent where people do not use specified facilities (as in China), but the fields (as in India), reinfection after medical treatment is a foregone conclusion. Ludwig Gross reported (Gross, 1927, p. 1580) that in Cameroon people infected with hookworm eat baked clay pieces as cure and succeed curing the disease. Because the clay was baked, eating it could not be the cause of the illness; rather the eating of baked clay must have rid the people of worms. In my reading of most of the available literature, there was no case of clay eating causing a parasitic disease, but cases of bacterial infections have been reported from nonsterilized clay on wounds early in the 1900s.

As an anthropologist Laufer is unique in that he critically reviews previous publications by ethnographers about geophagy. He analyzed the seminal work of the geologist C. G. Ehrenberg about reasons for geophagy and negates almost all of them except geopharma. Laufer's approach to the subject begins in China:

> "In this article is given for the first time a correct exposition of the facts concerning geophagy. For this reason China opens this investigation. The days are gone when the discussion of a problem started with the Greeks and Romans, whose importance in the history of civilization is not much greater than, and in many respects inferior, to that of Asiatic nations."

Laufer's work is not focused along lines of medical importance of earths. He does go into one question, that of ancylostomiasis, but otherwise he only reports on medical uses as they were written down during field visits. I will attempt to group the reports by the type of medical problem for which the clay was ingested.

Geophagy everywhere

Ludwig Gross (1923) reported from Cameroon that the inhabitants eat clay during pregnancy and also to improve bowel movement and to treat "some illnesses" (probably diarrhea). He speculates whether rachitic[6] children eat it unwittingly to ingest calcium, which cannot really be determined unless one knows that the clay contained calcium and even then it is medically questionable that such type of calcium is taken up by the body. A "healing earth" to be discussed later is calcium carbonate found as deposit in limestone caves that was sold all over Europe ever since the birth of Christ, mainly as an aid to lactation of nursing women. Modern lactation centers discount that ingestion of calcium improves lactation, but then again, they probably do not often see female patients as underfed and overworked as most women were 500 to 5000 years ago.

Gross also mentions that in China clay was sold in the market to help with the digestion of a diet heavy in fish and also to ease intestinal pain from excessive use of opium. There are several other reports about diarrhea from excessive eating of fish, one about Kamtchatka reported by Robertson (1947, pp. 213-215). A famous historical research travel reports cited above, that by Alexander von Humboldt (Laufer, 1930, 185 ff), states that the Ottomake Indians carefully selected a river clay and made 5-6" diameter balls and lightly fired them, but remoistened them before eating clay, lizards, small fish, and fern root, mostly during the swelling of the river in the rainy season, when fishing was hard, but they also ate great quantities of unctuous clay (up to 1 ¼ lbs a day), when the fishing was good in the dry season. Because Humboldt had spent only a part of one day with the Ottomakes he based his report on the opinion of a Franciscan friar, Ramon Bueno, who cited J. Gumilla's Historia Del Rio Orinoco (1791), who denies the Ottomakes ever ate pure clay, but mixed it with maize and crocodile fat. There are confirming reports of such clay and maize eating by Laufer citing the explorer Cortambert, and the inference can be made that when the river was running high, the Ottomakes could not successfully fish, so then they added clay and maize to their diet.

Reports worldwide

Many reports of a medical nature refer to eating clay by pregnant women for stomach relief, to stop vomiting and to stop diarrhea: Malaysia (Lasch, 1898), Virginia settlers (Stahl, 1931, p. 353), Persia (Lasch, 1898, passim), New Guinea (Meigen, 1905, p. 55), Queensland in Australia (Laufer, p. 133), and Baholoholo in the former Belgian Congo (Laufer, 1930, p. 146). Egyptians ate Nile mud with lemon juice (Wacker, 1935, p. 1279). The Ainos of Japan living on the north coast of Yesso in the valley of Tsietonai (eat-earth-valley) cooked clay with lily roots for a soup (sine nomen, citing Love). A Chinese pharmacopoeia (Li-Shi-Chen, 1997), Pen Ts'ao Kang Mu (now: Bencao), contains 61 clayish substances sold as mud pills. (See Chapter Eight).

Among unusual uses of clay we find consumption or application of white clay by Chinese women to obtain a pale complexion, as did the noble ladies of Spain. Women of the Moluccas used it in the hope to "have white children" (Laufer, 1930, p. 133). Indian women liked fine clay as cosmetic (Robertson, 1947, p. 213,). The natives of the Runjut Valley in Sikkim chewed clay to cure goiter, which also seems to stem from the Scientific American article in 1895. In India and Australia it is not unusual that women would eat pieces of termite hills to fill their need for clay (Lasch, pp. 214-222).

In line with earlier reference to calcium carbonate, there are references to a "healing earth" that appears to replenish itself. Usually the material exists in mountain caves. It has been known in Switzerland (called moonmilk), Tibet, Malta, and Jerusalem. Calcium carbonate in limestone caves has this capacity.

Eating clay was not strange to the early people. It was their third major source of relief from maladies that plagued them. While excessive consumption of earth—as that of almost any substance—can lead to health problems including death, the healing earths were an important part of medical treatment besides animals and plants.

There are a few discussions of anemia caused by continual clay eating (rather than assumptions that iron-containing earth improves the iron content of blood) and concerns that clay particles can pass through intestinal walls by "persorption" (Volkheimer, 1933). In either case, this, if at all, will rather apply to geomania, not the short-term use in geopharma for specific ailments or food problems. Contrary reports consider anemia the result of eating earth.

Julius Stumpf was much encouraged by what he read about geophagy and he continued his clay procedures with self-ingestion to determine the safety of clay in internal applications. The history of clay (minerals) within the history of medicine reinforced his conviction of the practicality of using this abundant earth material in the treatment of patients.

---

[1] This bird was characterized as the "thieving magpie" (Die diebische Elster) by Franz von Suppé, German operetta composer of the end of the 19th century.

[2] Gelfand, M.E., cited from African Medical Journal, 1945, #22. Original not found.

[3] The lunch sandwich with clay is also reported from Meissen, a German porcelain pit, in English often referred to as Dresden china, in French as Porcelain de Saxe. Common German name is Meissner Porzellan.

[4] Even without food shortages, it is necessary to de-bitter wild acorns, yams, taro, and tuberous roots. This was done in some cases by special boiling, in others by the addition of clay (Paczensky, 1997, pp 29 and 38).

[5] Hookworm is the common name for the genus *Ancylostoma* of the class of nematodes. They are parasitic in humans, dogs, and cats. *Anclyostoma duodenale*, 8-13mm long worms, exist on all continents, but mostly in warm regions. After the female lays its eggs in the host's intestine, the new generation passes out with the stool and hatches in the soil within 24-48 hours. After 2-3 days it can reinfect the host or infect a new host by penetrating the skin and thus burrowing into the host, traveling in the blood stream to the lung from where it migrates into the mouth, is swallowed and passes into the intestines. There is sucks blood and can cause inflammation and anemia. Constipation alternates with diarrhea, supposedly causing increased appetite for clay.

[6] Rachitis: Whistler in 1645 misnamed the Greek word for spine, rachitis, as "rickets" which became a medical term in the English language. This illness of retarded calcification of children's bones was later recognized as deficiency of vitamin D.

Chapter Eight: Medicinal Earths in Antiquity

When humans began to coalesce from tribes into nations, even before they began to write they began to leave physical evidence of organized, interpretable, and repeatable thought on caves walls, stones, clay tablets, papyrus, bamboo, bones, or cloth, their healing traditions included medicinal earths. Writing as we know it from its early forms onward, served to enable the administration of larger human societal entities. Recorded experience allowed to express concern with medicines and the curing of illnesses. Healing, controlling pain, and improving well being, were the most important comforts besides food and shelter, at times they were more important than either of the others. Evidence shows us that the early use of earths as medication was contemporaneous in China and India, in Australia and the Americas, as well as in the Middle Eastern "Fertile Crescent", that fruitful cradle of knowledge of Asia Minor between the Euphrates and Tigris, prior to Greco-Roman culture.

China's earths, soils, stones

In the Far East, Read and Pac (1936, p. 4) mention three ancient halberds (a style of battle axe) found at the Yin site at Honan. Tsurumatsu Dono, in the Bulletin of Chemical Society of Japan, analyzed them and showed that one sample was free of tin; another contained only 0.06%, and the third 2.29%. He concluded that the similarity between Chinese and Sumerian bronzes is noteworthy, because the introduction of low-tin bronze occurred as a transitional period that came between the Copper and Bronze Ages. This period was very short, yet it happened continents apart at the same time.

It cannot then be forbidden to compare the earliest mention of healing earth as contemporary in Sumeria, Egypt and China about 1800 BC at the latest. There is a similarity of earth appellations as well as similarities in the medical conditions treated with clay and related materials. Both regions knew the concept of "green" earths, even though the meaning is yet unclear. Both knew red and yellow clay. Sumeria and Egypt had terms for clay such as "clay from the gate", "clay from a statue", and "clay from a wall". China had terms like "soil under a pillar", "soil from above the tomb", and "soil from the east wall".

Fragments of papyri and pieces of clay tablets have been recovered, some dealing with mineral medicines. From an old Chinese dispensatory (a comprehensive list of available drugs) we know in great detail about mineral medications. This most unusual document of healing is a materia medica that has been compiled and updated continuously for about five thousand years and was last reprinted in 1977. Since before the concept of a "total China" was born, Emperor Shen Nung, who is believed to have lived between 3217 and 3077 BC, commenced a catalog with 365 medical plants, one for each day of the year (Chen and Ling, 1926). It was and is called *Pen Ts'ao Kang Mu* and now includes 1074 herbal, 433 animal and 354 mineral medicines. Of the latter, 61 are "soils" or earths. Under every emperor this *materia medica* was checked, corrected, and updated, often by a lifetime of work by a designated court official.

It was first written in ancient Chinese ideographs on pieces of bone, slats of bamboo, and on silk. It was revised 25-219 AD by the Han dynasty, and it has existed on paper since 105 AD. Again it was revised 502-556 by the Liang dynasty, 618-905 by the Tang dynasty, and it was printed in 1597 for the first time by the son of scholar Li Shih Cheng [also written Li Shih-chen] of the Ming dynasty, who worked on a new revision for 30 years. It then had 1,871 drugs altogether[1].

All of the drugs were illustrated and described, sort of a combined lapidary and herbal. Except for very few, the "soils" have never been fully[2] translated. "Minerals and Stones" was translated and analyzed in 1936 (Read and Pak, 1936). Most of the metals are the same as those known to us from post medieval European literature. Some are ancient and not far removed from magic, such as tarnished mirrors made of a 50-50 copper and tin alloy. Old coins were made of a 50-30 copper and zinc alloy. Among precious stones was powdered jade, especially blue jade as an elixir to confer immortality. Red coral is among the precious stones. Lapis lazuli and malachite were used well before Dioscorides' herbal and lapidary. Gypsum ($CaSO_4.2H_20$) is among the stones, and so are soapstone (steatite), talc ($Mg_3H_2Si_4O_{12}$), creta gallica (an argillaceous earth), and calcium carbonate.

Among the so-called "marrow stones" (*Medulla saxorum*) were five siliceous clays, prominent among them kaolin (China clay, *Bolus alba*, pipe clay, basically pure aluminum silicate), and "red bole" with a chemical composition similar to kaolin[3] plus 3-5% of iron oxides.

To the non-precious stones belonged hematite (red and brown), dolomite (carbonate of lime and magnesia), bath bricks (sand and clay), riverbed sand, and fossil shells. Pisiform clay iron ore (also nodular iron pyrite) have been assumed to be bezoar of snakes[4.] They were believed to have been disgorged during the snakes' hibernation. Trevor Shaw (1992, p. 223) reports of crushed stalactite as medication in ancient China that would be comparable to calcium carbonate from caves in Europe.

Names of the earths

The soil appellations include a number of names that do not allow us even to speculate as to their chemical nature. Few names give a specific type, they are rather tied to a specific location where they might be found: Soil underneath the shoe (308-5)[5;] sweet soil from the Northwest of China (303-1) will help when having eaten poisonous herbs or mushrooms if the soil is boiled and soup is made from it to drink. Red soil (305-3) is taken to heal burns, yellow soil (305-3) cures severe diarrhea, hot stomach cramps and bloody stool; the yellow soil should be boiled several times, be sieved and should be drunk warm against the poisons of spoiled meat or of mushrooms.

Soil above the tomb (309-1) gives hope against the plague: an urn made from this clay was placed in front of the door on the first day of the New Year. Some soils may be clay portions in bee's nests, swallow nest clay with the saliva of a swallow building the nest (309-3), and rat nests (311-1). Termite hill earth is not strange (still known in Australia and Africa) and used for swellings or boils on the head and for skin ulcers (gangrene), but soil of the snail (312-1) means actually soil eaten by the snail, so about a deciliter of snails is soaked in water, the resulting mush is dried and taken with a cordial to stop vomiting. Soil of the earthworm, actually soil eaten by the earthworm (311-2) is dried over heat, soaked in water, drained and drunk with wine against diarrhea; in children this soil, when licorice is added, will cure a swollen scrotum as poultice, but it helps also with snake bites and rabid dog bites. Soil of the eel might be clay that, as clay in Victoria (Australia) does, harbors 2 m long and 3-5 cm thick "earthworms" in a deep layer of gray clay[6]. (In the above, the numbers are pages and items in the Pen Ts'ao.)

Other uses of clay in China according to the catalog of the Pen Ts'ao Kang Mu were treatment of spleen and stomach ailments, "sour flux" (reflux?), nausea, and vomiting due to gastrointestinal complaints. Limestone milk (dissolved calcium carbonate) was used to treat diarrhea, but most chalk-like substances are listed under the section on "stones" rather than soils.

The indigenous drugs of India (Chopra, 1933) either developed unto themselves or as trade exchange. They encompass the same inorganic products found in Chinese, Sumerian, Egyptian, Greco-Roman, and Arabian medicine, and traces found in Western medicine. Prominent are alum, alumino-silicate clays, calcium products, and types of bitumen. Their use parallels that among all ancient peoples.

It was no longer sufficient to bring a patient to the market in hopes of finding someone who had a similar illness and had recuperated from it (Cumston, 1920, pp. 357-360). As Majno (1975) said twenty-five years ago: "we can try to look back in time and see when the footsteps of medicine began to emerge from the night of time". While there were very few known physicians for 2-3 millennia, the few that were there wrote often of ailments and of cures, but medical texts amount to no more than a handful of fragments for a period of 3,000 years. Almost all of the few texts, however, specify instances of the use of earths to heal, even if they addressed nonmagic medicine like common clay and only for such palpable causes as suffering from parasitic worms or wounds inflicted by human agency (Dawson, 1930a, p. 357).

Mud of Ancient Rivers

Ancient Egypt had its own sources of mud for treatment including mud of the Nile and adjacent "marsh soil" written "btj" (Thorwald, 1962, p. 85). Babylonian medicine reported the use of Euphrates Mud. Ancient Peru used argillaceous earth against diarrhea and so did the Aztecs according to the Badianus Herbal (Emmart, 1940), which had been written by a bright local divinity student before any influence or contamination by Western experts could affect the translation. It contained much clay, silicon, aluminum, and magnesium. Yemen supplied bituminous products such as asphalt or pitch as salve (Thorwald, 1962) and alum. The Land of Cush[7] provided both alum and soda.

It was to be expected that writers on this subject would vie to find "the most ancient medical text". What John Webb (1957) calls the "oldest medical document" is a Sumerian clay tablet not much younger (indeed possibly older) than the Chinese dispensatory. Guido

Majno (1973) considers the Smith Papyrus from Egypt the most ancient medical text, admitting the Sumerian tablet to be 500 years older, but the Smith Papyrus reproduces text which originated many centuries earlier. For the subject of the use of earths as medicaments, this competition is unnecessary. Five thousand years ago the first light of medicine spread across the world, and because of the similarities in many lands, it is immaterial whether the lamp was lit in China, India, Egypt, or Mesopotamia. It is readily supportable that the use of earths is not an invention like paper or gunpowder, but is a reported medical use of substances known everywhere since time immemorial, not only after writing was invented.

Sir Bhagwat Sinh Jeem (1981) expressed that the Aryan indogerman peoples' group had good chemical knowledge. They knew sulfuric, nitric, and muriatic acids, oxides of copper, iron, lead, and zinc, as well as many chlorites, sulfates, and carbonates. Mukta was powdered pearl prescribed for impotency and consumption; powdered coral was given for a cough. Their mineral knowledge embraced metals, salts, precious stones, clay, alum, calcium carbonate *(khatica)*, silicate of calcium *(kardama),* silicate of aluminum *(gopichandana),* and plain silica *(sikita).*

In his examination of history of drugs of mineral origin John Nunn (Ancient Medicine, 1996) found that malachite prevents growth of *staphylococcus aureus* and *pseudomoneas aeruginosa,* when used as a dressing for burns or to "draw out" inflammations. He reported a schedule of treatment for burns by day: Day one: black mud, day 2: excrement of small cattle (sheep), day 3: resin of acacia, day 4: wax and oil, and day 5: carob and red ochre.

He developed this table of ancient medicines and some of their specific applications:

Common names	Ancient names	chemical names
Natron (sodium)	hesmen	NaCl sodium chloride, also Na$_2$SO$_4$ sodium sulfate, also Na$_2$CO$_3$ sodium carbonate, also NaHCO$_3$ sodium bicarbonate (used under bandages to draw pus).
Alabaster	shes	Calcium sulfate, but at times confused with calcium carbonate.
Alum	Ibnu	Potassium sulfate aluminum hydroxide
Black eye paint (galena?)	mesdemet	Lead sulfide
Brick (dust)	djebet	Brick dust
Calamine (?)	hetem	Zinc oxide
Chalcedony	seheret	Silicon dioxide
Chalcopyrite	gesten	Copper-iron sulfide
Clay	Im, deben	Aluminosilicate
Copper	hemet	
Dew (for clean water?)	Iadet	
Green eye paint	wadju	Cupric carbonate or malachite
Gypsum	besen	Hydrated calcium sulfate

Hematite (blood stone)	dedi (d'd)	Iron oxide (Fe_2O_3)
Lapis lazuli	khesbedj	Sodium aluminosilicate
Naphta	merket last	Desert oil? Bitumen?
Nile mud	qah	
Ochre	sety	Hydrated iron oxide and clay
Salt of Lower Egypt	hemat*	Sodium chloride?

*warm solutions are mildly emetic, often added for taste, used as skin treatment.

Mineral drugs from the Fertile Crescent

A partial text of a 4,000-year-old Sumerian clay tablet addresses medicine. The red clay tablet, 10 by 17.5 cm, was dug out of the silt of the Euphrates. It does represent the earliest medical notation among successive nations in the Fertile Crescent. Its author lived in the third dynasty of Ur, the last efflorescence of Sumerian culture between 2350 and 2025 BC (Webb, 1957, p.2). From here on, written records about the use of earths in medical texts are few among no more than 1,000 fragments total for a period of 3,000 years. Of the few medical fragments found, even fewer were analyzed (Majno, 1973, p.36).

Hematite (bloodstone) was used in ancient Mesopotamia to treat wounds. Pitch or bitumen served for leprosy and as wound treatment, and as salve for boils (Martin, 1966, p.128 and p. 162). Babylon used Yemenite alum as mouthwash, as styptic pessary for hemorraghia, itchy scalp, gonorrhea, purulent ophthalmicia (pus-forming eye infections), and excessive secretion in dysentery (Martin, 1966, p. 165). Houri clay was very pure clay from ancient Egypt (Martin, p. 189). Nubians dug the earth from Schendi, gray-brown, soft to the touch, a specific for syphilis, if indeed it was syphilis (Lasch, 1898, pp. 214-222). The widespread deceptive adulteration of comestibles at least proved white clay mixed in flour as safe in internal consumption (Lasch, ibid). Clio Medica (Dawson and Hoeber, 1930, passim) mentions burnt ochre as pill (maybe with nurse's milk) to swallow for children's diarrhea. Earaches were treated with 'pounded' (powdered) alum inserted in the ear.

The most prominent reminders of earth use in medicine came from a variety of found papyri, notably the Papyri of Ebers, the London, and the Berlin Papyrus. The Ebers Papyri I-III were named after the German egyptologist Ebers who acquired them about 1873. This medical record dates back to 1550 BC and describes even older medicine (Bryan, 1931, pp. 10-14). It stems from a working diagnosis of illnesses or complaints from the often cryptic descriptions by the scribes. Of the 81 listed afflictions, the ones that might have been ameliorated by use of clay are diarrhea, indigestion, colic, dysentery, melæna[8], piles, inflammation of the anus, tapeworms, roundworms, guinea worms, hookworms, external tumors, scurf (and dandruff), eczema, scabies, insect stings, bite of a crocodile (?), burns, cuts, abscesses, gangrene, pustules and infections, ulcers, diseases of female genitalia, teeth irregularities, gum boils, nose and ear discharges, ulcerations of the ears, eye diseases, hemorrhages, and infections. Truly clay had found its way into the medicine of the time.

There were still tendencies to use mystical terms for some drugs, probably to widen their appeal and to exculpate the druggists, even for substances such as milk, beer, and water. The pharmacopoeia contains 811 prescriptions. Some drugs which are still in use today, and many more that are weird and wonderful substances, some in all sorts of forms:

> Beer as a vehicle was described as plain beer, sweet beer, bitter beer, cold beer, warmed beer, flat beer; yeast-of-beer, froth-of-beer, beer-which-has-been-brewed-from many ingredients; in a bright moment they bethought themselves of a swill-of-beer.
>
> Milk also afforded them some scope; it appears as: fresh milk, sour milk, spoiled milk, cooked milk, ass' milk, cow's milk, man's milk, milk-of-a-woman, milk-of-a-woman-who-has-borne-a-son, milk-of-the-sycamore, and milk-juice. As for water we find plain water, well water, spring water, salt water, water-from-the-bird-pond, water-from-the-rain-of-heaven and water-in-which-the-phallus-has-been-washed.

Mineral drugs were often described with adjectives such as alabaster, meal-of-alabaster, dust-of-alabaster[9]. When we search for clay we find clay-from-the-gate, clay-from-a-statue, clay-from-the-wall, masons' clay. Simple mineral substances were calamine, collyrium (an eye wash, also an earth from the Aegean island of Samos), hematite, soda, various salts, and various stones. A scientific dispute arose about the translation of the cuneiform symbol <d'd'>(pronounced didi) as red clay, as red ochre, or hematite. The latter won out.

The Ebers Papyri I-III

The documents found and labeled as Papyrus Ebers II (Ebbels, 1937) and Papyrus Ebers III (Joachim, 1890) are additions to the first Ebers Papyrus. In it you find "green" (fresh? untouched?) lead earth and collyrium. Masons' clay found application for backaches and to cool the head. Clay-from-the-gate gave poultices for ulcers (mixed with petroleum?). Clay-from-the-wall was mixed with wheat flour and fat from the animal "deher"(?). Extract from the plant "selede" (festuca?) and yeast of sweet beer also was an external plaster for wounds.

Two other medical papyri are those of London and of Hearst (Wreszinski, 1912). Their contents are very alike in some of the mineral medications, even if translations are not always given. Both repeatedly mention an "htjn"-earth and what appears to be a measurement "oval" and "½ oval" (spoon?). The indications can change, several cases refer to a sick toe (gout or arthritis according to the German version), others to treatment of fingers, toenails, and in general ½ oval of htnj earth mixed with 1 oval of lard, or a ½ oval of htjn earth mixed with honey to be eaten at evening.

Earth (powder) of two bricks (burnt clay) prevented interference from male and female ghosts and healed the stomach immediately. So did pulverized shards of a clay vessel. Given with clay were ingredients like types of soda, salt-of-the north[10], minium (red lead), drift sand, honey, powdered alabaster, "green earth", dates, lard of antelope, snake fat, crocodile and hippopotamus fat. Treatments were often combined with incantations against bleeding or with prescribed invocations such as: "I am one who is loved by his god and he will keep me alive."

The Ebers Papyrus I. has 875 prescriptions, 47 case studies, and 700 odd remedies suggesting highly specialized therapeutics. We need to remember, though, Fielding Garrison's exhortation (1929, p.25) that when different remedies are proposed for a disease, it usually means there was little known about treatment of that disease, and also, in reverse, when a drug is vaunted as a panacea or cure for many diseases, it means ignorance of the disease (Fielding Garrison was the dean of writers of medical history at the turn of the last century).

As late as in the 11th century AD, Arabian medicine maintained the terms tîr iblîz = Nile mud and tîn Misr = Egyptian earth. Tutijâ remained in medicine as tutia through the 17th century as ashes of zinc (zinc oxide, calamine, Hüttenrauch) (Meyerhof, 1928).

For wound treatment one took some river sediment, pounded it, kneaded it with water, then rubbed the affected part with mineral oil and added the mud as plaster. "Rivers carried the right kind of mud, and people knew what to do with it: heal and build cities. Nowhere else have men and mud done so much for each other" (Majno, 1973, p. 29).

From Syria, although not written about until after Galen, we find use of clay mixed with lemon juice to stop nosebleed "even though it be necessary to cover the whole head". We find again green (fresh? moist?) earth (khespê dhê sapâ), gypsum (ampûmâ) and hematite (shîdrûch) (Budge, 1913).

Altogether, practical and available earths were part of daily medicine throughout olden times. In contrast to pulverized stones, even precious stones prescribed for high and noble patients, the earths were available to the poorest of the poor.

---

[1] The first printed edition of the Pen Ts'ao Kang Mu of Li Shin Cheng (Li Shih Chen) consisted of several volumes totaling 2,000 pages, printed on rice paper in the 16th century (State Library of Munich in Bavaria.)

[2] Mrs. Yanfeng Sun of Beijing helped obtain some translations of the "soils" terms from specialists while she was traveling with our group in China. The ancient ideographs are not understandable to Chinese physicians to-day, as I experienced when I tried to find a local medical person able to translate this in the US.

[3] Schelenz (1909) derives the word kaolin from the Kaoli Peninsula in Korea. All other authors derive it from the name of a Chinese mountain east of King-Te-Chin (Jingdezhen). Laufer (1930) has mentioned several clay sources in China.

[4] Bezoars, the leather-like or harder concretions (not swallowed stones) in many animals, mostly found in the stomach of mountain goats, deer, gazelle, monkeys, elephants, but ocassionally in birds. China believed in snake bezoars (error). They considered bezoars medicines against magic and poison much earlier than Europeans.

[5] Thanks to Alberta Wang of the Hoover Institute of Asian studies in Palo Alto, I was able to gain some insight into meanings of the Pen Ts'ao Kang Mu: "Soil underneath the shoe" is indicated when one is uncomfortable in a new environment. Drinking a mixture of water and the soil under the traveler's shoe immediately stops anxiety.

[6] My personal observation in Korrumburra (Victoria, Australia). The then crown prince, now king, of Norway studied this 5cm diameter and 2m long "earthworm". Unfortunately my visit was during the dry season, when a 5m thick layer of hardened clay lies above the habitat of the worm, so it was not possible to look for a live one. I saw two preserved ones, one preserved in a jar of formaldehyde, one in formaldehyde in a long clear plastic tube.

[7] Today's Nubia, called Ethiopia by the Greeks, an ancient region in northeast Africa south of the first cataract of the Nile, now Sudan, extending west to Lybia, east to the Red Sea and south to what is now Karthoum and Omdurman.

[8] Melaena: A disease characterized by evacuation and vomiting of dark bloody matter.

[9] Alabaster here is said to be crystallized calcium carbonate, not gypsum (hydrous calcium sulfate).

[10] Variously erroneously identified as alabaster, nitre, ochre, or Nubian earth (alum).

Chapter Nine: The Concept of Medical Stones and Metals

Previously I have alluded to the fact that in antiquity everything in, on, and under the ground was an earth, a *terra.* Equally confusing was the concept of stone, *lapis* in Latin, *lithos* in Greek. Among the stones there were such as could be crumbled into dust, a matter not too hard for dried clay or calcium carbonate. It just was a matter of degree as to how much force was required. In the olden days, a stone could be called an earth and an earth could be called a stone (with the exception of boulders or rocks, *petra* in Greek and *saxum* in Latin).

Another problem in antiquity was that even metals could be included with "stones". Among Arab scholars we find terminology such as "the stone gold"[1]. For pre-Greco-Roman times, the source for many names and properties of metals and stones again is China's *Pen Ts'ao Kang Mu (Bencao)*. Read and Pak (1936) not only established the Chinese names, but followed the subsequent history of the metal or stone and, where available, its medical significance. The Pen Ts'ao catalog has separate sections for precious stones, two sections for ordinary stones, and four chapters for metals.

Again, China first

Jade (nephrite) powder was ingested for heartburn, asthma and thirst (diabetes?). In Europe it was used for edema and calculi (calculus: little stone, kidney and gallstones mostly) by Caspar Bartholinus of the famous professor dynasty of the Bartholini in Denmark. In 1628 powdered green jade was used for spleen, bile, and hemorrhages. Indians of Brazil mention "Amazon stones", but used them not as powder but rather as amulet against snakebite and difficult parturition. Jade also was made into an elixir to confer immortality[2].

Coral powder was given to treat hydrophobia (rabies). Hindu medicine says coral "acts on" secretions of the mucous membranes. In the 16th century, Europe used coral for the amelioration of bile problems and to increase perspiration, and to act as diuretic.

Cornelian (red agate) was used in China and India to cure eye diseases. In Egypt and Crete it was used for bites of spiders and scorpions. In Europe cornelian was reported to have been used for thirst quenching during fevers.

Sapphire was a Hindu medicine against phlegm, bile, and flatulence. Europe made potions in the 17th century of ground sapphire for scorpion bites, intestinal ulcers, eye growths, and "ruptured membranes". Beryl was said to cure quinsy (tonsillitis), swollen glands, eye disease and hiccough. Lapis lazuli in Egypt was mixed with malachite and milk for cataract treatment according to the Papyrus Ebers I. Quick burned (deflagrated) and washed (levigated) amethyst with vinegar was considered a protection against (or cure for) drunkenness.

"Stones" included soapstone and five siliceous clays similar to kaolin, terra sigillata, fullers' earth, yellow and red clay (aluminosilicates). A Chinese medical curiosity is a slice of the middle part of a stalactite, which has a hole in the center (which is really not that infrequent among stalactites). Stones in China also included red and brown hematite for inflamed eyelids, in Ethiopia and Egypt for "eyes and burns", in Africa and in Arabia for bilious disorders and burns. The prevalence of eye afflictions could have been caused by blowing wind carrying fine sand from desert regions and by the unlimited number of flies searching for moisture in a dry country. They are still caused that way today. Ground malachite was used in Assyria for eye trouble, also for cardiac pains and stomach colics.

Some Chinese soils are mixed under with "stones": There is magnetite, ochre, a series of "greens" (empty green, evergreen, "green" green, flat green, and white green (all jades?), gall stones (!), arsenic golden star (yellow orpiment?), green rock, flower milk rock (?), white sheep stone, golden tooth stone, diamond, ginger stone, white bran (brown?) stone, millstone in the water, swallow fossil, crab fossil, snake fossil, silkworm fossil, turtle fossil (all sediment stones).

Other minerals are salt-for-eating, army salt (?), bright salt, halogen (?), coagulant stone, black crystal, green salt, nitre, stone sulfur, and green vitriol. The problem with these designations is that they vary regionally in ancient Chinese script and their meanings are elusive even to learned scholars of ancient Chinese writing.

Real Greek and unreal Greek influence

Much younger, but still in antiquity is the treatise on stones (*de lapidibus*) by Theophrast of Eresos, 372-287 BC, a pupil of Aristotle (Caley and Richards 1956). According to Theophrastus, all types of earth are produced by fire. From it come stones, including precious ones, whereas metals obtained by mining come from water. Some stones can turn what is placed on them entirely to stone such as objects buried in calcium carbonate or silica, for instance at mineral springs (Reinbacher, 1998). Stones also can give birth to young stones. Theophrastus must mean geodes with a stony or clayey nucleus. In any case, the stone was considered pregnant, such as the eagle stone. It became an amulet for pregnant women to ease giving birth.

Theophrastus includes among stones asphaltic bitumen (Thrakian stone) and Lyncurium ("petrified urine of the lynx" = yellow amber). Amber has been used medically into the 17th century, bitumen or pitch much longer as wound treatment to contain possible infection.

Aristotle's name appears in the title of a later (Arabian) lapidary, the "Book of Stones", but Aristotle did not write such a text. It is rather a work variously attributed to the Syriac author Hunain ibn Ishak, the Arab writers Ibn al-Baitar, Lukas ben Serapion or Costa del Luca. Of this compendium one is a translation from Arabic into German by Julius Ruska (1912), the other one is an arabicised Spanish-Latin version described by Valentine Rose (1875) as a work of Arnoldus Saxo[3]. A comparison of items in each version indicates that they originally are from the same but not unambiguously identified source.

The curious content, other than that coral and bezoar and pearls again are among "stones", is that in Ruska's translation even metals are considered "stones". In the imaginary realm, the stones included magnets that attract gold, hair, nails, flesh, and fish.

Others are credited with occult powers, such as the stone that facilitates birth (eagle stone?), the stone that brings sleep, and the stone that keeps awake or respectively drives away sleep.

Physicians mixed pearl dust into their medications such as their eye salves. Completely dissolved into "vibrating water" it will clean off white skin spots and, sniffed up through the nose, will alleviate headaches. Johann Daniel Major of Kiel, in the 17th century, mixed powdered pearl into a "prince's tonic" (*Fürstenwasser* for his liege lord the Duke of Holstein.)

Emerald will strengthen the eyes when quietly contemplated[4] (Lüschen 1979, pp. 320-322). As amulet or as signet ring emeralds will prevent an epileptic attack, if worn before the attack. As powder, about 8 grains of barley corns by weight, when taken internally after ingestion of poison, will, with God's help, prevent death and offer succor also in case of poisonous bites and stings of creepy vermin.

Onyx when used as a signet-ring stone will bring bad dreams. Hung around a child's neck it will increase saliva flow. Used as a cup, it will prevent sleep.

The Arab influence

In other Arab sources we meet again the "bezoar stone", the name bezoar being a derivation of the Persian word origin "padzähr". We must admire the tenacity of belief in animal stones in the history of medications, because there is no proof ever—in contrast to healing earths—that bezoars have cured any affliction. The concept of poison was that it was a substance that did not cause death by heat or cold, but by its specific properties that are directed against the blood of the heart and the blood of the liver. Poison will change blood into the consistency of boiled meat, spread to the arteries, and make the blood coagulate. 12-barleycorn weight of bezoar[5] will help. Calx (lime) heals wounds when mixed with oil. Sulfur cures headaches (questionable) and eczema (probably). The "lightning stone" (barkijj) is a strong aphrodisiac for women. The Indian "water stone" absorbs water, but dries out again. As a powder it will make hair grow, in the pharmacological sense of those times we need to add "so God will".

The stone "salt" is of many varieties, evaporated from water. The Arab opinion of the minerals borax, nitre, and vitriol was that borax removes phlegm from the stomach, nitre is a cleansing agent, and vitriol is dangerous because it damages nerves and causes fevers. The stone talc is useful for ulcers, it raises the lame, and it heals broken bones. Powdered coral is useful for painful eyes, reduces mouth rot, and strengthens gums. Pumice that floats in from the sea also cleans eyes and teeth when mixed with honey.

Generally, not limited to the history of mineral remedies, the stone "gagates" most likely was a polished dense coal. Another stone was amber, the tree sap fossil (*succinus = sap*). Both gagates and amber could be burned so that smoke could give relief (at least from the myriad of insects), amber could be chemically dissolved and added to bath water. Then follow the stones with names of precious metals or rather the seven planetary metals. One of the unusual miracle stones is the white marcasite that causes laughter. Galactite, milk-stone found along the shores of the Greek river Achelos and the Egyptian Nile, was considered a stone but could also be pulverized and mixed with water either as a means to whiten cloth or as a medicated drink.

Stones and metals grow

Like humans and animals, plants, stones and metals were conceived, born, grew, and reached adulthood. They did this underground to the accompaniment of heat and gases and terrible noise—that was observed from volcanoes. But one could also notice other stones growing (such as stink stone, pearls, and coral), and since one could find stones that grew into shapes like living things or as fossils of living things, it was abundantly clear that stones grow. Miners also reported metal as growing underground, because they were familiar with underground fires and forces that were required for metals to achieve copulation, growth, and maturity.

Who had not seen stones and metals grow on the edges of springs? Especially mineral hot springs? Further, metals were believed to be deposited by other planets, such as silver by the moon, gold by the sun, iron by Mars, copper by Venus, zinc by Jupiter, lead by Saturn and quicksilver by Mercury (Reinbacher, 1998, p. 53). This was not a disavowal of God's creation, but an explanation why one saw creation continuing. To keep creation going, God engaged the help of angels and of the seven planets after his original creation. Not only coral grew, pearls did. Didn't fish and flies grow by spontaneous creation? So why not rocks and stones and metals? Only after Antoni von Leeuwenhoek reported seeing "bacteria" in his microscopes (Klaus Meyer, 1998) did belief in spontaneous creation begin to disappear.

Confusing nomenclature.

What complicates the history of stones is the significant number of changes of definitions.

Alabaster was once considered a marble; we know it as fine-grained opaque gypsum. Chalk is most confusing, because the Latin word *creta* probably did not originate from the Island of Crete (Kriti in Greek and later assimilated into Latin). Crete is a classic limestone sediment island with soft friable white to grayish sedimentary rock composed of remains of minute marine organisms and high content of calcium carbonate, which is also a definition of chalk. Rather, according to Hans Lüschen (1979 pp. 257-8), the word comes from the old Latin verb conjugated *cerno, crevi, cretum,* meaning to sieve, sift, as for instance, writing chalk is very finely sieved or sifted gypsum[6] and calcium carbonate as medicine is sifted. Ulisses Aldrovandi refers to all powdered earths in his Museum Metallicum as "creta", not as earth. The Oxford Latin Dictionary goes further than Lüschen. Its first (and oldest) definition of *creta* is usually whitish clay, 2) clay or chalk, 3) any of the following: clay for potters, clay for sealing letters, cleaning clothes, for marking. It also describes *cretula* (white sigillated earth) as a kind of clay. Thus the definition includes kaolin, calcium and sodium montmorillonite, chalk, calcium carbonate, diatomaceous earth, fullers' earth and porcelain or potters' clay—all earths of antique science, so to speak, were first creta, that is: sifted.

The carbuncle stone used to be anthrax, was changed to ruby or garnet cut "en cabochon". It has been said to grow under the forehead of the unicorn. Nitrum was a universal stone; it could either be sodium carbonate, potassium carbonate or white fumigating stone. The sodium carbonate came from Macedonian and Egyptian lakes, potassium carbonate from oak-wood ashes. But then again, nitrum could be one of many salts, baurac-borax, gypsum or, as in 1300, saltpeter (KNO_3), component of many compound medications, as well as "soda."

Eating or wearing stone?

Some of the real stones, precious, semiprecious, or common, were used by ingestion. In some cases ground precious stones and finely ground precious metals were added to prescriptions for those of high rank, who wouldn't deign to take the same medicines as the poor people. Goldwasser from Danzig (now Gdansk, Poland), a liqueur, has contained flakes of gold since hundreds of years. We have mentioned above numerous powdered stone medications. If we return to the definition at the beginning of this chapter, any stone lent itself to being crushed to a powder and become a healing substance.

More frequent and conspicuous was the wearing of stones as amulets to ward off evil spirits, protect against magic, and warn the wearer of the presence of poisons. Sapphire (Greek hyacinth, see Lüschen, 1979, p. 310) was supposed to cure "spots in the eye". Kings wore sapphire around the neck for powerful protection, because sapphire protected persons who led a virtuous life[7]. Of course, sapphire was often confused with lazurite. Fraud was neither unknown nor unsuspected. Fear of magical harm and poison was a real primary mental concern[8].

Bezoar and unicorn

Ralph Major (1954) relates the efforts of a court physician to convince his king that bezoar "stones" are worthless, no matter how much they cost. The king agreed to a test whereby a prisoner condemned to death was given a poison followed by a piece of the king's bezoar. The man died and the king was furious that somebody had sold him a fake bezoar. In the same league is the unicorn horn of fabulous value, because it will assuredly warn the sovereign of poison. About 1650, when it was suggested that the unicorn horn might be the spiral horn of the narwhal (Lachmund, 1674) the scientific conclusion was that maybe the "marine unicorn" did have a horn, too, but it was not the same as that of the land unicorn (which nobody had ever seen).

Magnesite, $MgCO_3$, what the English called carbonate of magnesia (today's milk of magnesia is magnesium hydroxide), was one of the many specifics against stomach trouble. Red coral was also one of these remedies as it had been for ages, moonmilk (calcium carbonate) another, and there were always chalk, powdered eggshells, "white earth", real and fake oculi cancri, crayfish pellets.

Fine flakes of the "heavenly" metals were added to the medications of the rich. Mercury became a fad with mercury ingestion and sweatboxes. The German poet Friedrich Schiller has one of his characters say: "I know a doctor who built his house with quicksilver"[9].

Despite the superstition involved in many of the medical applications of stones, it must be admitted that 300 or more years ago fear of the unreal, of evil magic, and of early death, were eased by remedies that we would not accept today (that is, as long as we have grown up not to read horoscopes), but giving hope is a recognized specific in medicine: the victory of hope over reason (very much like lotteries).

The amethyst supposedly protected against drunkenness by not allowing the spirits to reach the brain. A red stone helps staunch bleeding, and a gold stone chases away melancholy. The eagle stone, as we learned before, helps those pregnant. Antimony, then called stibium, was taken to cause vomiting (probably right), bitumen (pitch and tar) was used to protect wounds from infections, chrysolite chased stupidity and fostered wisdom. The previously discussed galactite (milk stone) in amulet form aided lactation (drinking it would have been better) and children, with such an amulet around their neck increased the production of saliva, but elsewhere galactite taken by mouth was thought to confuse the mind. Of course with the confusion in the early nomenclature, who knew exactly what it was?

To rejuvenate themselves, stags ate vipers, but the poison heated them up and they dashed neck deep into cold water and shed tears. One of the earliest and probably the most famous European herbal, *Hortus sanitatis*, the garden of health, of about 1510, lauded the stags' tears as medication (they were found as bright stones), as well as the standard classic earths.

Albertus Magnus and Konrad von Megenberg

Legacy of the knowledge of the past before the fall of Rome (~395 AD) are a number of encyclopedic works written between 1100 and 1300 AD. In this chapter we encounter the "great lapidaries", books on stones. In the next chapter the "great herbals" will tie in to ancient knowledge of plants. Actually, both lapidaries and herbals contain descriptions of healing earths, but no new knowledge appears to have been created much before 1500 AD. New treatments of old knowledge, yes, but truly new knowledge of healing earths did not appear until the end of the 19th and the beginning of the 20th century. If we began with Theophrastus treatise on stone, extend to Pliny's Natural History (regarding stones), the thread of knowledge after the darkest of the Middle Ages is picked up by Bishop Isidor of Seville (about 600 AD), crafted further by Albertus Magnus (about 1250) and Konrad von Megenberg (about 1350 AD).

Because of his encyclopedic knowledge of things natural, Albert of Cologne (1200-1280) was honored with the name suffix "the Great" and for his knowledge of things spiritual the Roman church made him bishop and a saint. Indeed he was one of the greatest philosophers of the 13th century. His "de mineralibus" is the part of his work dealing with stones, real stones, earth as stones, and magical stones with nigh unbelievable properties (Albertus Magnus, ed. Erwin Braun, 1983; Albertus Magnus, transl. Wyckhoff, 1967). Here an excerpt from his book on stones:

Cygolite dissolves kidney and bladder stones—for these unbelievably painful afflictions people actually submitted to bladder operations without anesthesia and with unclean hands and instruments—even though the survival rate was minimal. *Andromata* helps against rage and melancholy. *Sarcophagus* is the stone that eats the flesh of the dead in 30 days (Greek: sarkos=flesh, phago=to eat). *Ophthalmus* helps against eye disease and also prevents people from seeing things, not in the sense of blindness, but in the sense that it would make thieves invisible to them. No wonder this stone was venerated by thieves. Albertus was also aware of all the stone growing in the heads of animals: the toad stone, the rooster stone, the serpent stone and the dragon stone, as long as it was taken while the dragon was asleep[10]. The pearl "Margarita" and the lynx stone "Ligurius" are among Albert's stones as are the eagle stone and the "topasion", effective against hemorrhoids and against being moonstruck.

Another stone, in ancient medical books and alchemical writings referred to as "Ramai", appears to be the same as *Bolus armenus*. It is, in Albert's sense, a precious stone of light red color, effective against strong stomach aches, bloody dysentery (*Ruhr*) and excessive bleeding during menstruation. These are the classic cures of a classic healing earth.

150 years after Albertus Magnus, Konrad von Megenberg wrote the first "book of nature" in the German vernacular, which included some of the same stones as the list by Albert the Great. Both have hematite among curative stones, also Samian earth, and both have coral as stone, and—curiously—they both call the toadstone "borax".

If we split off stones from earths and magic from medicine, the stones will remain in the arena of magic and the earths continued as specific medications for specific ills.

Comments and Explanations

[1] Checking with experts in Arabic at both Stanford University and also the University of Munich, I did not receive information that clarifies why Ruska used "stone" for both metals and stones and did not use the word "Hajar" for stone and "Ma'dan" for mineral. Probably the original author did not use them and used a term that could mean either stone or mineral.

[2] Promoted as elixir of life to Chinese emperors, several physicians lost their lives when it turned out the emperors were still mortal.

[3] Arnold Saxo, de virtutibus lapidum, on the advantages of stones, dating to the 13th century. I used the 1875 Rose article.

[4] Reduction of eyesight acuity with age before invention of glasses was a frequent but yet unsolved medical problem.

[5] Human kidney and gall stones were called "calculi" in Latin, not considered bezoar stones.

[6] Related Latin word are "creturea", that which is sifted, and "cretula" for white sifted sigillated earth.

[7] Lüschen, under sapphire.

[8] As we know the unicorn horn's ability to detect poison.

[9] Friedrich Schiller, "Die Räuber", Act 1, Scene 2 Razmann speaks. The meaning is that the doctor became rich enough to build a house from the proceeds of selling mercury treatments.

[10] Boethius de Boodt, who copied books from the 15th and 16th century, was so enthralled by the toadstone belief, that as a boy he one sat up all night watching a toad that, sitting on a red cloth, should give up the stone in its head. It didn't, and there was one boy who never fell for the toad stone again. But magic stones supposedly were found in dragons, too, at least in the head of those dragons that flew among the Swiss mountains. Same as the unicorn that nobody had ever seen, dragons nobody could see were found in literature until the 18th century.

Note: In general, while stones were almost always in the realm of magic belief and nowadays are mostly superstitions, the medical use of earths for specific ailments was almost always in the area of practical self help. It was not until main stream medicine began to develop newer and better cures that the reliance on earths, mostly clays, receded in the learned profession. In practical terms that was not unitl well into the second quarter of the 20th century, even if mostly hidden from knowing eyes. Physicians will stoutly deny the medical efficacy of clay but will prescribe or suggest it when under a cover name.

Chapter Ten: Healing Earths in Post-Antiquity and the Middle Ages
(1,000 BC - 1,500 AD)

From China and India, from Egypt and the Fertile Crescent, the burgeoning civilizations who had learned to use clay and other earths as medicine or healing medium, spread the knowledge of and interest therein to the learned men of Greece, Rome and Arabia who practiced medicine along the borders of the Mediterranean and its tributary seas such as the Aegean.

The high point of classical literature on the medical use of earths around the "inland sea", the Mediterranean Sea, can roughly be timed between Homer (900 BC), Hippocrates (460-377 BC) and Avicenna (Ibn Sina, 980 - 1037 AD).

Western heritage of classical medicine was essentially shut down between the fall of Rome (395 AD) and the resurgence of interest in natural sciences about 1,000 AD, after the wave of the destructions of cultures by the migrations of Visigoths and Ostrogoths until they, in turn, were so effectively destroyed that even their language had disappeared except for 112 words (Jared, 2000).

Thereafter for half a millennium most of the mentions of healing earths began to be collected in the works of encyclopedists and writers of herbals, bestiaries and lapidaries who had studied the ten preceding centuries, but added nothing new:

> "Most important developments in medicine between the 7th and the 11th century took place not in underpopulated Christian Western Europe, but in the flourishing cities and the lively intellectual milieu of Muslim society. Greco-Roman medicine barely survived in Western Europe, hidden in a monastic environment" (Sirasi, 1990, p.10).

Given the choice of reviewing the history of clay respectively mineral treatment either by chronology of authors or by summary of specific earths, I have chosen the latter. Many earths were in use, but the bulk of writing about them came from but a few: Dioscorides of Anazerbos (40-90 AD), Gaius Plinius Secundus and Aulus Cornelius Celsus of Rome (1st century AD), and Galen of Pergamum[1] (2d century AD). Galen's medical writings encompassed about 2 ½ million words, about as much as the British scientist Isaac Newton wrote on alchemy and the German poet Johann Wolfgang Goethe devoted to poetry and prose. Much of the medical writing by the old authors mentioned first above was deemed original. It was acknowledged that the writings from Galen's sphere of knowledge were never doubted for centuries. Dioscorides, Pliny, and Celsus (Celsus did not write in Greek but in Latin and therefore, at least then, was not read) were the first great encyclopedists. Dioscorides' herbal was taught side-by-side with Galen's humoral theories of pathology in most of European universities well into the 18th century. In some universities such as Paris, Galen and Dioscorides were taught by professors under oath not to deviate from their texts.

The healing earths of two thousand years ago can best be grouped by locality of provenance: Armenia and Anatolia (Turkey), the Greek Aegean islands, Asia Minor, and borders of other Mediterranean cultures. We begin with the earths from the Greek Aegean Islands, and among those, begin with the one most often described and analyzed.

The story of Lemnos and its earth

The most prominent (and best remembered) of the earths from the Greek islands is the *terra lemnia* of the largest northeastern Aegean island, Lemnos (today: Limnos). It lies in the Thrakian Gulf, about 50 miles east of the south entrance to the Dardanelles Narrows (also called Hellespont) that lead to the Sea of Marmara, Istanbul and the Black Sea. Lemnos does not have spectacular cliffs or beaches (which is why it is ignored by most of the tourist trade), but it has two good harbors, water, and fertile low plains. Many war episodes denuded the island of trees[2]. Travelers in antiquity stopped there to partake of the good Lemnian bread and good wine (Welcker, 1824, p. 315), while awaiting favorable winds to enter the Dardanelles.

As a way station to and from Turkey, Lemnos has participated in a fair share of Greek mythology. Hephaistos, the God of Fire (Roman name: Vulcan), was thrown out of Heaven by Zeus and landed on Lemnos. His leg, broken in the fall, was cured by Lemnian earth. The hill Mosychlos (it was once a volcano, but not in recorded history) had an earth gas flame or fire that made the earth curative, because the fire demon lived with the earth goddess in the hill of the red clay where they had been married (Fredrich, 1906, Pp. 60-86). Since the beginning of the Bronze Age the island of Lemnos had been populated. It has neolithic sites with remnants of pottery including figures cut from sheets of clay.

Mythology of Lemnos

In one mythological occurrence the enraged women of Lemnos killed all their husbands because the men had provided themselves with captured Thrakian concubines. When Jason and the Argonauts in their search for the Golden Fleece stopped at Lemnos (for two years?) they were asked to mate with the Lemnian women so as to repopulate the island with males (Welcker, 1824, p. 301). In Euripides' (484-406 BC) tragedy Hysipyle, the daughter of Dionysus' son Thoas acceded to the throne of the kingdom of Lemnos and bore two sons to the chief argonaut Jason (not twins, so they must have rested in Lemnos about 24 months).

There are old reminiscences of the annual "renewal of fire" festival, when all fires on the island were doused for nine days, and people refrained from conjugal activity while a new fire was brought by ship from the mainland (Welcker, 1824, p. 247). This legend has been associated with the annual digging of Lemnian clay or earth. It was dug before sunrise from the hill Mosychlos[3] by the priestesses of the goddess Artemis (Roman: Diana) on a summer day every year (Fredrich, 1906, Pp. 7-8) for at least 1,000 years. Again, it needs to be indicated here, discussed later in detail, that (a) there was no hill called Mosychlos in human memory, just a crater rim type of elevation, well weathered, and (b) it is a thinking error to associate a Greek goddess (Artemis) with a very holy Christian feast day, the metamorphosis of Christ on August 6.

A cart full of earth was dug, probably less than 200 lbs. The clay was made into round troches or tablets, each of which was stamped (branded, sealed, minted) with the die of a goat, the mascot of the goddess Artemis. This made Lemnian earth the first sigillated medicinal earth and wherever in literature the term *terra sigillata* appears without a location suffix, it refers to Lemnian earth, sometimes called Lemnia sphragis which is Greek for *terra sigillata* from Lemnos. Throughout history Lemnian earth was always the revered example, at times described as red, red and white, and white, probably due to striations in the clay deposit. Since the island is strategically located to facilitate control of access to the Dardanelles, Lemnos was constantly caught in battles between Turkey (to protect their mainland) and the city-states of Genoa and Venice (to protect their trade) and later between Turkey and Greece for the same reasons.

Lemnian politics

Lemnos was under Greek control from 500 BC on. It was conquered by the Romans about 197 AD, so Galen saw it as a Roman colony. By the 2d century, Christians were the religious leaders in the island, even had a Greek orthodox archbishopric. After the fall of Rome, Lemnos came to the Eastern empire. Venetians battled the Turks and conquered the island in 1204. After later battles, even at the doors of Venice, the island was given to Turkey which by 1479 was the Ottoman empire. There must have been a reversal of this later because in 1829 Crete was given to Turkey, and in exchange for the island of Euboa near Athens. Lemnos once again became Turkish. In 1912 the Greeks conquered Lemnos back and made it a part of the Greek kingdom. Whenever the island was occupied by the Turks, the trademark seal of Artemis' goat was changed to Arabic lettering and marketing was under strict Turkish control[4].

The history of Lemnian earth goes back to 900 BC, to Homer's Odyssey, wherein Homer mentions *terra sigillata*, which cured Philoctetes of pestilence (?) at Lemnos by the earth sacred to the Temple of Asklepios. Hippocrates was silent on Lemnian earth because it was associated with religious cultism, while he acknowledged other earths: Alum, argilla, bolus rubra and alba, argilla fullorum (fullers' earth); he mentions *cancer astacus* the river crayfish that supplied the calcium carbonate pellets called *oculi cancri* later (Upman, 1847, p. 422, 423, 435).

Dioscorides

Dioscorides of Anazerbos[5] reported that the Lemnian earth comes from a certain hollow cavern in an area having a marshy place or surroundings [this is correct] and that the clay, after it had been dug, was mixed with goats' blood [this is incorrect], after which the men [not the priestesses?] made it into flat round disks and sealed it with the figure of the goat. The clay was said to have the eminent faculty as antidote against deadly poisons when drunk with wine soon after, which caused vomiting up the poison. It is good against strokes, it is good for bites of venomous beasts, and it is also good for diarrhea (Berendes 1902, p. 638). At least the last is believable today, defeating heavy metal poisoning probably is possible, resisting or defeating snake venom is a dubious claim. It would need external application same as insect bites.

There is no record that Dioscorides, the unquestioned pope of herbals for 1500 years, himself visited the island of Lemnos. Galen of Pergamum, the unquestioned pope of medicine also for 1500 years, did twice. The first time his ship had landed at Kastro (now Myrina). He was too far from the site of the clay digging (about 35 km) and the ship's captain did not want to wait for Galen traveling there and back. During the second trip, Galen's ship landed in the Gulf of Bournia and Galen was able to visit the site and at the correct time to observe the clay being dug. When he asked the priestesses about the goats' blood, the priestesses laughed: "No, there is none added". People could obtain coins made of this earth in return for a gift of wheat. Galen acquired 5,000 pieces (some sources say 20,000), but the only report on any medical use of these was that it supposedly alleviated the stomach problems of Marcus Aurelius in the field camp at Aquilega.

Pliny (c. 50 AD) in Volume 35 Chapter 14 of his Natural History essentially agrees with Dioscorides. Celsus (c. 178 AD) in his eight-volume opus about medical science lists other Aegean island earths, but not *terra lemnia* (Frieboes, 1906).

Samples and testing

Until recently, there has not been a positive analysis of the Lemnian earth. As said above opinions abounded; when we saw it at Agiochoma it was light brown on the dry surface and the clay was too hard to dig to try to determine the color underneath. Looking at it in terms of chemical analysis in the 20th century, the table below lists clay samples from 5 different sources:

(1) is a sample which has resided as *terra lemnia* in the British Museum and was presumed to date to the 16th century. This was analyzed and reported by Thompson in 1913 from a 1581 text by Andreas Berthold; (2) is a sample of Armenian bole published by Read and Pak (1936); (3) is an analysis of an earth sample collected by Tozer (1910); (4) is a sample brought back by me from Agiochoma on Lemnos; (5) is from a gift to me of clay boiled with grape juice to a syrup that is used as the local Lemnian stomach tonic "Mustachoma". The mother of my taxi driver in May 2000 was the donor of this family remedy. The samples were analyzed by Actlabs-Skyline in Tucson AZ on August 22, 2000.

	Sample 1	Sample 2	Sample 3	Sample 4	Sample 5
Silica	37.23%	43%	66%	52.24%	43.12%
Ferric oxide	4.08%	5%	6%	4.82%	2.95%
Aluminum oxide	13.51%	36%	14.50%	13.64%	7.42%
Calcium oxide	22.9%	Trace	Trace	5.69%	20.59%
Magnesia, alkali oxides	1.5%	1%	3.5%*	5.22%	3.00%
Water and CO_2	17.72%	15%	8.50%	15.94%	21.35%

* sodium

Black (1956), in his interpretation of Galen, says nothing about the goats' blood question but does state that Galen took 20,000, not 5,000 clay coins with him. This would not be much more than 20 kg in the lightest case, but could be as much as 100 kg if the thickness made the weight of the coin come out at 5 kg/1,000 coins. Secondly, as I will explain below in Chapter 17, it could have taken a week's labor to prepare, clean, dry, roll, cut, and mint 20,000 coins (Ten people 40 hrs? This is highly unlikely, as we will see later.)

Black (1956) then interprets a German account of a poison test on a human first reported by Andreas Berthold von Oschatz (Latin 1580 or 1581[6], English 1587.) as follows:" A prisoner in the realm of the Earl of Hohenlohe, Lord of Langenburg, was scheduled to be executed by hanging for several robberies. It was decided to test a sample of *terra sigillata* for its propensity to protect against poisoning. The prisoner had been promised that if he submitted to the test and survived, he would be set free. In the presence of physicians and commissioners and nobles besides the earl, the prisoner received a dram and one-half of mercury sublimate in a conserve of roses and immediately thereafter a dram of *terra sigillata* in old wine. While the prisoner was ill and extremely tormented for a while, the medication finally prevailed and the prisoner was restored to health, and thus to freedom. This is said to have happened on January 25, 1581 [Gregorian calendar]. The full translation is attached at the end as Chapter 18 Part 2.

Use of Lemnian earth declined when it became too difficult and too expensive to obtain it from the Turkish government. More than 1300 years after Galen, 1100 years after the fall of Rome, the personal physician of Sultan Muhammed II Amasiaz studied Galen's reports and suggested an expedition to Lemnos to rediscover Lemnian earth. After two expeditions they finally found the location, surrounded by a fence. Under the Turks, the earth of Lemnos was no longer free for the taking. In 2000, there was no sign of a fence or remnants of it.

Other Greek Earths

The Greek island of Samos also belongs to the northern Cyclades and lies very close to the Turkish mainland. It was known for two kinds of healing earth, the first being very white and light. It sticks to the tongue, it was said, it feels mellow [soft, juicy, rich] and is easily ground [pulverized]. These properties are now known for calcium carbonate and for almost 100% amorphous SiO_2. The notation by Dioscorides "a fine potters' clay" would indicate kaolin or porcelain clay.

The second type of "earth" of Samos is called *collyrium* (Latin: liquid eye salve). It was called "Aster" (Latin: star) and was coined with the outline of a six-pointed star. (As comparison: alum was once known as coined with an 8-pointed star). Collyrium was said to have the same powers as earth from Eretria on the island of Euboea after it is washed and roasted[7]. It reduced spitting of blood, was helpful to control female discharges. With water and rose ointment it reduced infections of testicles and breasts. With water it was said to be an antidote for bites by venomous animals[8] and for deadly poisons taken.

Collyrium had an amount of star-like glitter (mica?) that gave it its name. Dioscorides treats this as a separate item as "stone in the Samian earth" that is normally used for polishing. It is hard, white, and astringent, cooling, good for stomach ills, and for strengthening of the sensory organs. With milk it is active against fluxes and for ulcers of the eyes. It eases giving birth when worn as an amulet and it protects "the fruit of conception." Berendes[9] thinks that the earth was gypsum with amorphous SiO_2 or a clay with a $CaSO_4$ in an area where clayey earths predominate[10].

Just north of Samos lies the island of Khios (Chios). Its *terra chia* is white to ashen colored (probably mixed with fine volcanic ash or soot). In physical appearance it is layered and, when pulverized, very fine. It was said it had the same powers as Samian earth (there is little geological distance between the two islands). It can smooth facial skin as well as the skin of the entire body. In the bath it cleans like natural nitre [Na_2CO_3]. To Berendes it appeared as fine clay or marl, earths that have frequently been used as cosmetics.

Close to mainland Greece, the island of Euboea (Evvoia) was famous for the earth dug near the town of Eretria[11]. White clay is found there, but the best according to Dioscorides is the ash gray type dug further towards the hills. It must be properly washed and burnt; it is astringent, cools, softens easily, fills caverns and glues edges of bloody wounds together. According to a Berendes footnote, it may be pure clay, may contain some alum or sulfur, and since it reacts with copper, it may be gypsum. Eretria also provides alum and has sulfurous springs. Celsus (Friboes, 1906, p. 605) says that Eretrian clay must be soft and turn purple when brushed on copper.

The clay islands Milos and Kimolos

Halfway between Greece and Crete, two close islands, Milos and Kimolos, were and are still famous for their clay and alum products. The clay of Milos (*terra melia*) can act as contraceptive when placed near the mouth of the uterus and it also ejects the embryo, says Dioscorides, but Berendes (1902, p. 533) hadn't found this reported elsewhere. Celsus favors Melian alum (styptic) to stanch bleeding, to use a water and alum mixture to gargle, and use it as a wash for conjunctivitis. It also removes white spots from skin (?) and relieves eczema (probably). Milos today sells fine porcelain clay to potters. This clay is not as fatty as Samian earth and thus is also suited for painters. Today much of Milos is an open pit mining area. A pure white silica mineral is the ingredient in the pure white concrete which makes Greek island villages so startlingly white, especially when offset by very red, very blue, very green, and very yellow window frames, shutters, and doors. This white clay is also baked into bread as a stomach pacifier. (This was even done as late as the 18th century in northern Germany, but mostly to cheat the public by using less flour for bread of a given size).

The neighboring little island of Kimolos provided Cimolian earth (*terra cimolia*) of two kinds: One was white, one more purplish with a feeling of a natural pinguidity (greasy touch or unctuousness), cool to the touch. Both of these, when mixed with vinegar, reduce swelling behind the ears. Placed on burns, they both help immediately to prevent blistering.

They bring relief to inflamed testicles and other inflammations of the body. They were said to cure shingles. Celsus thought them good to stop ulcers, stop bleeding, provide cooling as poultice, and would stop diarrhea. Thanks to Robert H. S. Robertson we know today that the white Cimolian earth is fullers' earth, calcium montmorillonite as described above.

Turkey (Anatolia, Armenia, Sinopia, Cappadocia)

The Asia Minor region to the east of Greece and the Aegean sea, mainly Anatolia, Armenia and Cappadocia, were the source of several healing earths. Much of Turkish soil is red clay or clayey soil (Minnich et al, 1968, p. 78). The clay has been reported as mostly 50% SiO_2 and only 12% Al_2O_3 and a high proportion of MgO (21%), very similar to clay in Mississippi, Georgia and New Mexico. X-ray diffraction clay mineralogy showed 65-70% sepiolite and 20-25% montmorillonite. Turkish clay has a little quartz, and almost 85% of it has a particle size of <0.002 mm. Where it contained more sand (up to 18%), the percentage of 0.002 mm particles was lower (60%), in comparison the above mentioned US clays had a 40-50% silt component (0.05-0.002 mm particle size). For medicinal use, the sand has to be washed out.

Turkish clay, if at all sigillated, then with the Arabic seal, was mostly clay from the northern Cyclades whenever occupied by the Turks. Harder to find and therefore more costly was the famous earth now known as "Armenian bole". Its reputation was equal to that of Lemnian earth well into the 16th century in Europe, it then was so expensive that it was considered a gift suitable between monarchs (Kentman, 1565).

The name and the clay "Armenian bole" come from mountain caves in Cappadocia, that at an earlier time was part of Armenia, now Turkey (an annexation still violently opposed by Armenians). Armenian bole was even more specifically identified as the "veritable or oriental" bole *(vera seu orientalis)*. Whereas there was agreement as to the general provenance or type locality of Armenian bole, the classical authors have different descriptions of its characteristics. Dioscorides calls this clay a thick, liver-colored, stone-free, homogenous, easy flowing earth, and names it "Sinopian earth" because, while it was collected in the Cappadocia mountains, it was brought to Sinop, then a busy harbor on the south shore of the Black Sea. It was really Armenian bole, but it was often confused with "Sinopian red ochre" (or cinnabar) of which a deposit was worked near Sinop. The Iliad mentions Sinopian red ochre that could be either of these two red earths. Theophrastus did not believe in Sinopian red ochre, he considered it Cappadocian clay.

Galen used the Armenian bole—or its Greek equivalent—but just mentioned that it was found in caves (These caves are almost directly on the present border between Turkey and Armenia and not safely accessible). 800 years later Avicenna described it in his Canon of Medicine (Part V) as "clay earth from Ani". In the 9th to 11th century AD Ani was the capital of the Kingdom of Bagratuni in western Turkey, i.e. closer to the source of the clay in the Cappadocia mountain caves than Sinop.

Armenian bole is very dry, has a yellowish to reddish color, and its best property is that it dries moist things to the highest degree. It is useful in cases of bloody dysentery, other diarrheas, coughing of blood, uterine bleeding, catharrs and "fouling ulcers" in the mouth cavity. It promised quick relief from a "tight chest" and asthma. Some drank it mixed with a thin wine as prophylaxis against the pest (?), when it either worked or didn't in which case there was nothing else as remedy. Megele (1899, p. 376) stated that Galen gave credit for the discovery of Armenian bole to a pupil of Asklepius.

Earths from Malta and other Mediterranean locations

Another famous earth came from the Island of Malta and was much touted by Christians as "Saint Paul's Earth" in a variety of shapes, piece weights, and marketed with a great variety of coinages, of which many had the letters IHS imprinted or coined, IH being Greek abbreviations for Jesus Christ, the S being a later Latin addition of "Salvator", saviour (details are in the Chapter of Illustrations, # 17), but with these we are already in the 16th century earth coinages.

The New Testament indicates Paul was born when Christ was three years old. On his third missionary trip Paul was held prisoner in Caesarea for two years. Then, about 60 AD, while on his way to Rome, he was shipwrecked off Malta. Legend tells us that he lived and preached near a cave where there was a "self-replenishing" supply of white healing earth[13].

Other earths and stones were found and used medically all around the Mediterranean. Frequently mentioned are Selunesian earth from Sicily and a diatomaceous earth from Tripoli, which in whiteness and properties was compared to earth from Chios. A *terra hierosolymitica* or Jerusalem earth is said to have existed in a cave where Mary, Joseph and the child hid from Herod's persecution, a version not clear in the New Testament. Mary accidentally spilled some of her milk onto a cave wall, where it kept "growing" and offered succor for poor lactation of women and beasts, same as calcium carbonate later. It was highly regarded by Christians as well as Moslems. An earth from Bethlehem is also known (Hasluck 1909, p. 229) (See page 153).

Classic earths by name and type

Earths less well known but prominent in history will be grouped below by type and locality. The literary source is always Dioscorides unless otherwise explained.There cannot be but some repetition in ailments for which the earths were used, but the reliable ones (dysentery, for instance) appear to be more reliable than esoteric mentions of cures for ailments not even then understood.

Alabastros lithos (gypsum, if powdered) was also called onyx. It was taken as a medicine when heated with rosin or pitch; it dissolved "hardnesses", eased "griefs of stomach" and it "bindeth gums". Related must be Arabicus lithos that may also have been chalcedony or onyx. When applied as a powder, it dried up hemorrhoids, and when burnt was used as a dentrifice. Its color was ivory. All of these can be considered probable cures.

Aimatitos lithos (Latin: hematite, English bloodstone, Fe_2O_3) exists in huge deposits almost everywhere on Earth. Mixed with blood it was used as rock painting material for Australian aborigines 50,000 years ago. In the Greco-Roman period it was reportedly found near Sinop (or was it cinnabar or Armenian clay?) on the Black Sea and in Ethiopia (which then encompassed so much of Africa that 17th century maps of Africa still called the South Atlantic the "Ethiopian" ocean). It was found in Arabia and in Spain. Its color is dark red, as dark as cinnabar with which it was confused. For healing purposes it was considered an earth. It had the faculty of binding (astringent?), was somewhat warming, and cleared scars off the eyes. With mothers' milk it was good for lippitudes (dry eye infections), and bloodshot eyes. Mixing hematite with pomegranate juice provided a medication against spitting blood, with wine it cured dysuria (frequent urination problem). Celsus added a use for cleaning out ulcerating wounds, but the hematite should be washed and made into a powder first.

Yellow amber (Latin: succinus, German: Bernstein), even though it was recognized as a resinous "stone", it was categorized as an earth because it was found in the earth like on and in sandy beaches. Pliny, although most of his account is fable, recognized it as the "flowing marrow" of pine trees. Still in the 17th century amber was dissolved chemically and added to bath water. It could readily be confused with copal, a similar but much younger amber-like tree resin mostly found on Indian Ocean shores and islands like Madagascar.

Bitumen (tar, pitch, naphtha) came from many sources. Most prominent was bitumen judaeicum, the tar and pitch globules floating on the Dead Sea. Others, those with strong smell preferred, came from Syria and Phoenicia. Bitumen was used to disinfect or cauterize wounds of war well into early modern times. From the 17th century Thirty-Years War comes a much repeated story (always attributed to a different source) that one night a field medic ran out of tar to cauterize the day's wounded warriors and he worried all night only to find that the non-tarred wounds looked much better next morning. Dioscorides prescribed wood tar (*pix liquida*) as useful against wetting ulcers and "to ripen pus formation" (we remember Galen considered pus laudable, since it told him a wound wanted to heal).

The older Greek authors knew one type of fossil bitumen as *gagates lithos*, a dense, polishable coal. It had the faculty to soften and disperse. Fumigation in the smoke of burning *gagates* helped epileptics and hysterical (? not today's meaning) women. It was also said to drive away serpents (yes, it would). It was smeared on the skin for podagra (mostly meaning gout). The source was in Cilicia by a river near Plagiopolis, the name of the bitumen comes from Gagas, the mouth or delta of the river. Frequently petroleum seeped to the surface and deposited tar products on riverbanks. Another prominently mentioned bitumen was an earth from Selenkia in Syria, called *terra ampelitis*, grape vine earth (syn. pharmakitis). It is a black substance like coal tar and was used on grape vines at the time of new growth to protect against insects or worms on the plants, but it also gained medical favor for reducing swellings, adorning eyes, and coloring hair. It was not a coal, but an asphaltic earth.

Brick dust (ground up fired brick) was a medicament from ancient Europe to modern age. The powdered dust was efficacious for dysentery and other stomach ailments. The history of geophagy is replete with instances of pulverized or well-chewed baked clay taken as remedy. Chinese dispensaries contained it, so did Europe in the early modern age where alchemists made it into "oil of bricks". There is no discernible reason why fired clay, pulverized and sifted to the right particle size, should be less useful against diarrhea than natural clay. It certainly makes clay coins more durable during shipment.

Coral, harvested all around the Mediterranean Sea (as well as other temperate oceans), was much in demand for medicinal purposes, especially the red "male" coral. Dioscorides considered it a plant that hardens when drawn out of the water. It grew near Syracuse and Naples, in the Red Sea according to Pliny, and in the Persian Gulf. "Coral bindeth and cooleth gently, represses the excrescences and fills concavities. It is effective against spitting blood and, mixed with water, helps the spleen. It is also a good diuretic (forcing urination)" (Dioscorides).

Ochre as healing earth was quite common. Dioscorides favored the Egyptian and Carthaginian; Celsus preferred the yellower earth of Sesel (Seseli). Pliny mentioned it found in iron mines (wrong as usual) and that it turns red when annealed in fire (right). It is astringent, disperses inflammations and swellings, very much the same as umber, an ochre from the Italian region of Umbra.

Nitre, a natural soda (Na_2CO_3), not saltpeter (its later meaning), was an admixture to healing earths as softening medium. Never fully identified earths are Morochthus lithos, Galaktites lithos and Melitites lithos. Morochthus, translated as soapstone and as French chalk, was originally described by Pliny (Vol. 37 p. 173, also Robertson, p. 36) as a leek-green stone giving white liquid exudation (the white exudation or "writing" puts these minerals in the classic group of the Leucographics.) It "grows" in Egypt. Basically used to whiten cloth, it was considered helpful in cases of blood spitting, grief of the bladder and excessive menstrual bleeding. Its supposed greenish color led Johann Daniel Major (1634-1693) not to consider it "moonmilk" (calcium carbonate) described in his "Dissertatio medica de lacte lunae" (Kiel, 1667). He believed, however, that all white earths such as chalk and Maltese earth were moonmilk. Major is not sanguine about Morochthus, Galaxia, or other Leucographia being moonmilk, because they have a sweet taste, and moonmilk has no taste at all (Reinbacher, 1998, see also Agricola, 1555).

Three volcanic products were among the healing earths at the turn of the previous millennium: Stypteria or alum, pumice, and mixtures of both. Medically only the feather alum or the round alum was found useful to restrain creeping ulcers (gangrene?) to stop bloody fluxes, to close gums and, with vinegar or honey, to strengthen "wagging teeth". It was found in Macedonia, on the island of Melos (now Milos), Sardinia, Lipari and Phrygia in Armenia. Pumice was used to cleanse and scour as it is today.

Other early writers on healing earths

Very little was added to the knowledge and use of healing earths until the 16th century, much was copied into later literature. Oribasios of Pergamum (325-404 AD) copied Galen and so did Aetius of Amida (6th century AD), and Paul of Aegina (7th century AD). Theodorus Priscianus (4th-5th century AD) wrote of using Samian earth mixed with soda and oil to protect against lice; he also suggested blowing powders into the nose to stop bleeding for which he recommended Alexandrine earth with powder of a dried plant or droppings of a donkey. Use of alum for loose and rotting teeth was copied from Dioscorides, Galen, Pliny, Celsus and Oribasios. His list of healing earths included "Darkens" (a crystallized salt), alum, hematite, coral, Alexandrine earth, Cimolian, Lemnian and Samian (Aster) earth and unsalted chalk or lime. Lapis magnetis (magnet stone, sailing stone) was said to cure headaches; an enema was made of red arsenic (Sandarac, possibly realgar, a bright red sulfide of arsenic) for dysentery. Celsus believed in bituminosa (*pix liquida, pix brittia*) and in powdered mill-stone (*lapis molaris*) and powdered marble (*lapis naxius*) (Meyer, 1909, p. 89ff).

Alexander of Tralles (525-605 AD), in his twelve books on pathology and therapy printed in Arabic, Latin, and Greek in the 16th century, lists asphaltos (*bitumen judaeicum*) with the same "properties" as mentioned above. All earths (Greek: ge) not mixed with other substances will dry without irritating. Unctuous earths are suitable for all parts that require drying. Egyptian earth, made into soft mud, helps against dropsy and affectations of the spleen and moist, pulpy ulcers. Tralles also lauds Lemnian earth for drying out and mild astringency, for being effective against deadly poisons, evil ulcers and blood fluxes. It stops dysentery and he considers Sinopian red earth a cure for intestinal worms. Samian earth, which Tralles believes to be gentler than Lemnian, is sticky and unctuous and efficacious against blood spitting regardless of the cause. Selunesian and Chios earth build new flesh over ulcers and new skin in case of burns. Earth from Crete is airy and cleans the skin, Eretrian gray is astringent and does not irritate. Armenian bolus dries very hard and therefore helps in cases of dysentery, stomach fluxes, ulcers, and the like. It also, like yellow ochre, disperses swellings and rotting flesh and fills remaining cavities[12].

In line with the previously mentioned brick dust are *ostraka*, the shards from potter's ovens. When finely powdered, dry, clean and smooth, ostraka is brushed onto teeth to clean. With vinegar ostraka helps against skin itches, blisters and podagra. With wax ointment it it will disperse swellings of glands in the throat. Burnt oyster shell powder was also used as dentrifice. It also heals ulcers. Finally Tralles confirms previous writings about stypteria or alum from Melos and the Liparian islands.

In Spain, an area not often quoted in other parts of European medical history since Latin gave way to the vernacular in book printing, Saint Isidor, Bishop of Seville (556-636 AD) cites in his 20 volumes of *Etymologias o Oriens* the earths *rubrica, terra melia, ochre, Cimolian and Samian earth* (Lindsay, 1911). Isidor differentiated between stones and metals, which some Arabian writers did not, unless they used a term meaning both or either. Isidor divided earths into "de pulveribus et glebis terrae" (powdered and lumpy earths)[13], which included sulphur and volcanic ash such as *pulvis puteolanis* and into Samian and Cimolian earths, which were ground and mixed with water to a paste, as well as as galactite, coral, and *lapis margarita* (pearls).

Among the prominent Arab scholars Abu Bakr Muhammed ibn Zakaritya (Rhazes 865-923 AD) wrote extensively on healing earths (Levey, 1966). He proposed coral (p.243, item 38) for urinary trouble and to stay menses. Coral is astringent, moderately chilling and detersive. The Tamil of Sri Lanka reportedly used it for bleeding piles. Red coral was suitable for chronic and for recently decayed teeth ("worm i'the tooth"), to strengthen loose teeth [this must have been a frequent complaint] and to remove odor. As a tonic, powdered coral checks vomiting and acidity from dyspepsia and biliousness, it will also help against dysentery and spitting of blood.

For borax, realgar, bituminosa, hematite, and Yemenite alum, Rhazes follows his predecessors (Levey, items 48, 126, 128, 162, 165). Among clays he favors the very fine *houri* clay from Egypt and an unspecified red earth or clay for ulcers. He agrees on yellow amber (succinus) and on bituminosa such as liquid tar for hemorrhoids, fistulas, scrofula (tuberculosis of lymph nodes?), and abscesses. He also used it as poultice for wounds (Forbes, 1936). Rhazes dispensed the clay from Nishapur near Mashad in Iran, giving doses of 30 drams in a decoction of sweet apples to cure nausea, indigestion, grave choleric affections accented by fits of vomiting and cramps, a description which fits cholera (Robertson, 1966).

Abu'ali Al-Husayn ibn 'abd Allah ibn Sina, the man whom the West called Avicenna (980-1037), highest ranking of Arabian philosophers and scientist, became known as the "leading wise man" in the eastern world and "prince of physicians" in the western world. His medical history, the Canon of Medicine, included earths such as the above-mentioned Armenian clay of Ani, Samian and Lemnian sigillated earths, and, curiously, one from the island of Lesbos, another of the northeastern Cyclades islands. I found no other reference to an earth from Lesbos.

The basis of Avicenna's erudition was Hippocrates. He, too, believed in the elements of water, fire, earth, and air, in the temperatures warm and cold, dry and moist (males are warm and dry, females cold and moist). He advocated yellow amber to stop bleeding and to reduce palpitations, to help humors of the lung and stomach, nausea, diarrhea and tenesmus (constipation?). Coral expands the chest, aids respiration and strengthens the heart. Armenian earth stops hemoptysis (coughing up blood), hemorrhages, bubonic plague (?) catarrhal dyspnea, asthma (really pneumonia?), and phthisis (tuberculosis?). It counteracts the pain of hemorrhoids (Wacker, 1935, p. 1279).

Between the 10th and 12th century AD, Salerno in the Campania region of southern Italy, had become the first organized medical school in Europe, predating many other schools by as much as a century such as: Montpellier (1289), Padua (1222), and Heidelberg (1395). Its knowledge was a bridge between Hippocrates, Dioscorides, and Constantin the African (1020-1087), who translated (or had translated) many volumes of Islam's extensive knowledge of Greek medicine into Latin.

The "Circa Instans" and other great herbals

About the middle of the 12th century, Mathaeus (or Iohannis) Platearius was a prominent teacher at Salerno. He either wrote or compiled the herbal of pharmaceutical plants entitled "de simplici medicine", commonly known as "Circa Instans" from its first two words. The oldest existing copy was written in the middle of the 14th century. The original volume, probably written at Salerno, has not survived. I saw the copy written in

Gothic miniscules at Erlangen University in Germany, where it is bound together with other collected texts of the time. An illustrated copy resides at the Pierpoint Morgan Library in New York. It is actually not just an herbal, but a pharmacopoeia of herbal, zoological and earth medicines such as *terra sigillata, terra lemnia, alumen, bol armenia, asphaltum, auripigmentum, coral, lapis magnetis, and sal gemma.* About 10% of all entries refer to mineral medications. Where a picture of the actual mineral would not be conclusive, the artist showed renderings of people mining the mineral, whereas in the Chinese Pen Ts'ao Kang Mu there are sketches of shapes of pieces of the mineral, which are just as inconclusive. The Circa Instans also has an illustration of *terra sigillata,* showing three clay coins with drawn rather than stamped six-pointed star that could indicate alumen, though not elsewhere known as sigillated troches, or it could indicate Samian "aster" earth, that, however, in other literature had an eight-pointed star. According to Anderson (1977) the Circa Instans is the prototype of the modern pharmacopoeia, the first attempt to establish nomenclature standards and the first attempt by medieval physicians to create a work that did not only copy the past. Actually, all great "herbals" of the middle ages recite not only medicinal plants, but also medicinal animal remedies and mineral medications.

Moses Maimonides of Egypt (1135-1204) systematized and categorized the medical material of 16 books by Galen that includes healing earths. He admired Galen's medical knowledge while disparaging his philosophy. Maimonides' modern attitude was "religion is too often confounded with theology - religion has not and cannot have any conflict with science" (Münz,1895, p. 27).

Another Arab physician (Jesu Hali, the oculist) used pumice stone to scrape eyelids and in a recipe for eyewash suggested cleaned hematite and Meerschaum clay, which is a hydrous magnesium silicate, sepiolite, also called pipe clay.

A *Book of Medicines* about Syrian anatomy, pathology, and therapeutics written after Galen (Budge, 1913) confirms the Syrian knowledge of *terra sigillata* (Tabh'êyamma), Cimolian earth (Kimâliâ), as well as gypsum, "Armenian nitre" (?), hematite and a "green" (fresh? moist?) earth (Khespê dhê Sapâ), which though appearing in literature in various places, has never been identified. As treatment for flow of blood from the nostrils one may have to smear the whole head with clay mixed with vinegar, if necessary.

The *Antidotarium of Nicolaus Salernitatus* (Van den Berg and Brill, 1917) of ~1100 AD mentions *bolus armenicus* as a sort of earth that, among other uses, was considered a stypticum, even though that would point to an alum rather than bolus. Additionally the *Antidotarium* lists *lapis armenicus* (copper carbonate?), alum(en), Terra Cimolia and *terra cretica.* 200 years later Gualteris Agilonis wrote in his *Summa Medicinalis* (Diepgen, 1911) of round, split, and feather alum and of frequently used Bolus armenicus. Roger Bacon (1220-1292) classified simple medicines as derived from plants and animals, while alchemy explains simple medicines found in things inanimate, such as *oleum benedictum* (oil of bricks) based on powdered, burnt, or roasted clay.

In the 12th and 13th centuries AD several other writers continued referring to healing earths in their voluminous manuscripts. In a "known world" society of at best a few million people at a time when "the common man" was rarely within reach of a trained physician, the mention of healing earths appears to indicate more a continuation of a known type of popular medication than a listing of oddities such as bezoar stone, unicorn horn, weapon's salve and beaver testicles which are also present in pharmacopoeias by the learned doctors.

Hildegard von Bingen (1098-1179) mentions the precious stone *ligurius* (yellow amber) and adjusts the story of the urine of the lynx by saying it is not of every urine, but only the one deposited when the sun is hot, when the air is light and mellow: the lynx digs a shallow hole in the sand and urinates into it, which then turns to ligurius. Hildegard also knew of the healing power of the pearl and suggests lime powder with vinegar when (and where) a worm gnaws on a human tooth (a good expression for a nasty cavity). Chalk with vinegar of wine is made into thin cement that is spread with a feather onto the hurting place.

Gilbert Anglicus (Gilbert the Englishman) wrote a *compendium medicinae*, one of the longest medical texts written in the first half of the 13th century. It covers medical theory and practice and is one of the first medical texts in the West to examine teachings of the Islamic physicians. It contains a huge collection of medical prescriptions sorted by their purpose: confortatives (strengtheners), repercussives (resistors), mitigatives (mild curatives), corrosives (strong curatives), strictories (hinderers), laxatives, subtilitives (gentle medications) diuretics and naturatives (natural medicines) (Getz, 1992).

Bech-I-Borràs (1987) in his commendable summary of medicinal earths, written in the Catalan language, cites Avenzoar (1094-1160) who mixed clays among bezoars and theriaks the ancient composite herbal medicine of 69 (read as: ∞ = infinite ingredients in Christianity) or of 40 ingredients (read in Arabic as understood to be indefinite). Averroïs (1126-1198), a disciple of Avenzoar, mentions medical earths and Armenian bole. Armond de Villanova (1245-1305?) mentions "argila", *bolus armenus* and a "bolus sigillated of the Holy Mary" known as "Mary's milk", that must refer to either. Geoffrey Chaucer (1342/3 - 1400) mentions *boole* and *sale armoniac* in his Canterbury Tales. Paracelsus (1493-1541) considered the virtues of coral, where red (male) coral is stronger than the white (female) coral. It stops fluxes of the uterus, eases delivery, stops nose wounds and hemorrhoidal bleeding. In his Archidox Paracelsus mentions Bol Armoniak to make weapon's salve, the weird ointment that could cure the injured at a distance when rubbed not on the wound, but on the injuring tool or weapon. Together with bezoar, beaver testicles (actually male and female beaver scent glands), this weapon's salve was the epitome of highly touted and virtually useless compound medicines, one more victory of hope over reason.

Hortus sanitatis - the garden of health

At the end of the 15th century another famous "herbal" contains most of the prominent healing earths. This is the Garden of Health (hortus sanitatis) written by the German physician Wonnecke (1483) in the character and style of Platearius' Circa Instans and of the Arab writer Ibn al-Baitar (Serapion). Wonnecke cites both and thus provides a bridge for the knowledge of healing earths into the late Middle Ages and early modern times: *Alum, Bolus Armenus, Bitumen judaeicum, lapis lazuli, lapis magnes, lapis margarita (pearl)* citing both

Albertus Magnus and Avicenna for the proposition that pearls cleanse and strengthen the heart.

Wonnecke's Hortus Sanitatis also contains a clay "from the island without a tree or weed", Lemnos, in the location where the clay was dug. Mixing as a drinkable potion defeats pestilence and poison. Mixed with rose oil it makes a good poultice for limbs.

Also at the end of the 15th century, Ricarrettio Florentino espoused sigillated earths, Armenian bole, a white clay from Elba and a red one of Alexandria. With the slow sunrise of the Renaissance and first attempts at original thought, the listing of earths changes from being mostly encyclopedic to being individualistic thought, even if the thinking process was still far away from reasoned deduction. In the history of medicine, at this point, we still look in vain for conjunctive thought such as "If he had this result doing that, then I should be able to duplicate it".They lauded each other's books and apparently never read or paid attention to them.

A typical example of the 200-year long incubation period of new medical thought is the mixing of clay with lemon juice as anti-scorbutic medication. We know it should have helped. We also know that nobody but the inventor tried and lauded it. The first president of the first German scientific society, the Academia Naturae Curiosorum, died of scurvy even though ironically it was he who first proposed that there is so much work in medicine that one man alone cannot solve all problems. It appears that this plea for division of labor and sharing of experience still stuck to ancient learning and teaching, closing its eyes and ears to modern evidence of better healing, such as ship captains' reports of controlling scurvy with citrus juice. At the end of the 17th century fascinating storytelling was still more popular among even prominent physicians rather than actual medical research.

The Badianus manuscript

In support of the thesis that has geophagy as a method of healing or medication in all populations of early time, the Aztec herbal of Badianus (Codex Barberini, Latin 241) is proof positive: "On two continents independently, the same type of medicine developed" states Henry E. Sigerist of the Johns Hopkins University Institute of the History of Medicine in the foreword to the Badianus Herbal translation by Emmett (1940). This herbal, including mineral medicines was written in Latin in Tlatelulco, Mexico, before any Western physician could contaminate the work with European thought. The little book, re-discovered after centuries in the Vatican library, lists sulfur baths, hematite, bezoars (especially of birds, but also of the llama), the cock-stone (*alectorus*) for stimulation of saliva, as enema to relieve stomach pain, for diarrhea and—quite unusual, but a good thought—as a lotion to combat fatigue in public officials.

Besides herbal and animal ingredients, the Badianus manuscript includes a wide range of stones, crystals, earth pigments, and soils of various kinds such as Yztaclalli (white earth, *terra alba*). In Mexico the white earth called Thicatlalli was considered good for drying and cleansing, for ulcers of the pudenda and for washing hands (Reinbacher 1998, p. 53 ff). Purple and reddish earths were used, so was alum (tlalxocotle) as astringent and to clean teeth, and dry up ulcers. Powdered shells from the ocean were used as antacid and stomach treatment. Stones and earth minerals in the Badianus manuscript are beryl, white clay, white earth, pale and purple earth, emerald, amber (or copal), and stones found in lakes and rivers. The ailments cured are virtually the same as were experienced all over the world, the earths also were spread all over the world and they found entrance into the treatment of maladies. Except, possibly, the curing of tired government officials, that is unique to Badianus.

Comments and Explanations

[1] Christian Gottlieb Ludwig (1748) called Galen by the first name Claudius, most writers don't, because it is not even sure that that was his first name and not the usual abbreviation C1. for the honorific "celeberrimus" – the most celebrated, who Galen certainly was.

[2] In the repeated battles between Venetians and Turks, the island of Lemnos was repeatedly razed, including all trees.

[3] There are confusing inconsistensies in the literature about Mosychlos having been a volcano. See Chapter 16.

[4] Robert R. H. S. Robertson did not believe that the Arabic lettering was meaningless; he believed that the spoken sound of the Turkish seal was an alliteration of the Greek words "Tini-ma-chton", meaning "from your mother earths". Ludwig (1748) in Table X divides clays into "BARR" (a friable, brittle earth) and "THIN" (a soft clay-like earth) and they have names like Mohabbab and Machtum or Maktum, thus "Thin-machtum" would be the clay earth Machtum. The real explanation may be lost in the haze of time. But, yes, a number of so-called Arabic seals sold in Europe were imaginative forgeries.

[5] Bech-I-Borràs (1987) puts Anazerbos erroneously into Sicily, it is located in Cilicia in Turkey. Classic literature gives Dioscorides the first name Pedanius, a German translator called him Pedacius, and one of my readers pencilled in Pedemius. I don't really care, but I lean towards the majority with Pedanius.

[6] I have not been able to locate either a German edition or the supposed Latin original of 1583 that was still cited in the middle of the last century. The entire English version is included as addendum.

[7] Roasting is done to be able to pulverize the clay better.

[8] Nowhere is a description of the mechanism of clay being an antidote for venom, unless it meant to reduce a swelling and thus minimizing the spreading of venom.

[9] I have consistently used the German 1992 Berendes translation (here chapter 173).

[10] While clays generally are combinations of silicone dioxide and aluminum oxide, there are no healing earths with a higher than 50% share of aluminum oxide. Ruby and sapphire and bauxite have 100% aluminum oxide, used for corundum or emery, but not for medical use.

[11] Not to be confused with Eritrea, once part of Abyssinia, now independent.

[12] Cavities result from long deep wounds unsutured, therefore always spreading.

[13] The word combination earth, cave, and replenishing suggests the material as calcium carbonate which is known for its "growing curtain-like folds on cave walls". I observed this in the moonmilk cave in the Swiss Alps.

Chapter Eleven: Medical Earths in Commercial Uses.

Most minerals, although occasionally used for medicinal purposes, reached their economic importance somewhere else in the course of history. This contributes to the prevailing ignorance of physicians as well as geologists about healing earths. The truly valued medical earths in antiquity were often worth their weight in gold. Most industrial or commercial earths are traded around the world now for pennies to the pound. This did not come about all at once.

Geologists rarely pay attention to the miniscule amounts of some earth products used in medicine, and doctors often shy away from very old medications. The present exception to this rule may be semi- or hemihydrated gypsum ($CaSO_4+ ½ H_2O$)) for fracture setting, more commonly known as Plaster of Paris, because it was found in large deposits in the Paris basin. Theophrastus coined the name gypsum for both hydrous calcium sulfate and plaster therefrom. In its mega-crystallized form gypsum is also known as selenite for its resemblance to the pale light of the moon; in its fine-grained condition it is known as alabaster, carved and polished into shapes such as grave crosses and decorative objects. In agriculture, gypsum is prominent as an enrichment for marls and clay soils. In all such uses it is valued by the ton, not by dram or gram.

We don't often think of "earth" or "clay" when we think of china dishes or porcelain toilet bowls. Millions of tons of kaolin are used annually for these uses as well as millions of tons for plain "stoneware" or pottery from red clay. Bentonite is found today in cat litter and also in cattle feed to guard against myotoxins. Diatomaceous earth is used in planting mix. These rail car quantity earths have become successful within less than 250 years.

There is alum, a volcanic or lava weathering decomposition product found often as slate or crystallization product in shale that contains sulfates. Then there is fullers' earth, a calcium montmorillonite originally from the island of Kimolos and its counterpart sodium montmorillonite, generally known as bentonite.

Alum and its history

Alum in history was primarily used as a mordant (from Latin: mordere = to bite, in the sense of holding fast), as a fixative for dyeing cotton, wool, and silk cloth. Since few natural dyestuffs have an affinity for fibers, particularly not for the cellulose of cotton, they could only be applied with the aid of an auxiliary chemical (or mordant), which precipitated the coloring matter in a less soluble form. Alum increases color fastness and enables a wider variety of hues than could otherwise be produced from the then ubiquitous vegetable dyes[1].

Alum's second commercial use was and is the preserving of leather, a method going back to 3,000 BC to all societies then developing: Chinese, Indian, Sumerian, Egyptian, Greek, and Roman, then finally Western Europe. Leather is the first of man's manufactured goods. Long before Christ was on earth, Chinese cured skins with mud and alum (as superior substitute for salt), practiced "tawing"[2]. The first mineral (alum) tanneries functioned in China, Assyria, Babylon, Phoenicia, and India.

There are three basic tanning processes: (1) using animal derived oil rubbed into dried and hard skin (Eskimo kayak sealskins, baseball gloves), (2) using vegetable tannins such as oak bark, roots, and galls, and (3) using alum.

Natural alum is mostly potassium aluminum sulfate (a hydrated double salt, $KAl(SO_4)_2 + 12\ H_2O$). It generally evaporates from solutions and is found in a variety of such crystal forms as sheet (split) alum, feathered, or round alum. It is astringent (styptic) as medicament, often ameliorated with white vinegar, honey, or sodium carbonate. From Egypt came roasted alum, from Yemen white alum. Syrian medicine used alum as well as borax and bloodstone. Almost all classical writers—Galen, Dioscorides, Pliny, and Celsus—suggested alum to cure "rotting teeth," probably endodontic problems. Georg Friedrich Most (Most et al., 1843) reported alum as used for the treatment of diarrhea, to gargle the throat, to wash frost boils, and to promote alum ointment for blisters of burns. Emil Isensee (1840) listed alum, but not any bolus or terra of old.

Alum is found almost everywhere from China to Turkey to northern Europe. Singer traced its importance (Singer, 1948) through history. The ancient hieroglyph BN or IBN is interpreted as alum. Its ancestry goes back 50 centuries before the present. Alum was not only used for general dyeing, but also for a color printing process similar to batik. Various papyri explain alum as prescription for eye infections and as a prescription against coughing. But much more prominent was the use as a mordant necessary for dyeing bright colors. The best mordant must be free of iron, which is a frequent contaminant in mordants other than alum.

The word alum is first mentioned in the encyclopedia of Varro (116-27 BC) (Singer, 1948, p.1) and is often associated with sulfur. He calls it "aluta" meaning alum leather, known later as cordovan or English Atlas leather. The Cairo museum has a piece 2,000 years old. Large quantities of alum were exported from Egypt, mostly for tanning, a little for medication, and some for polishing silvered copper to look like silver or yellow oxide of lead to look like gold. Alum was needed by Rome to dye cloth to the desired purple, because the mollusk dye by itself is not suitable for dyeing cotton.

An early classical source of alum was the Greek island of Melos (now Milos), which also provided a china-like clay, sulfur, Bentonite, gypsum, and pumice. Melos also exported much of it as grindstones (Singer, 1948, p. 17). Dioscorides of Anazerbos mentions that alum occurs in Melos, Macedonia, Lipari, Sardinia, Libya, and Armenia: "it has warming, astringent powers, purifies the pupil from darkening and melts superfluous flesh…[it] stops all kinds of mortification and hemorrhage and, if mixed with vinegar and honey, comforts flaccid gums and tightens loose teeth…with honey it relieves thrush and eczema… it is good against lepra (scurvy?) when cooked with cabbage juice…with water it is a fomentation for itch, psoriasis, ingrown nails and chilblains" (Singer, 1948, p. 19). During my visit to Melos in 2000 it seemed paradoxical to sit on a hill near a small deposit dug for medical use, and to watch huge quantities quarried from the surrounding mountains being loaded on freighter after freighter at the local mining company's pier.

From early on, the volume of alum required by the trades led to taxation, monopolistic surcharges, and customs duties. Great quantities of alum continued to be used in the early Middle Ages for dyeing cloth and preparing leather. These crafts spread to other countries even though those lacked the wool for cloth manufacture and the hides for the leather skins. Florence in the later 14th century is an example: It imported alum as well as wool and prospered with dyeing (Singer, p. 107). The trades, crafts and materials manufacture spread by sea to the Netherlands and England and by cart across the Alps via Chur, St. Gall and Constance to Basel and Cologne, which became a center of dyeing in Europe, exporting its wares along the rivers Rhine, Main and Danube to the North Sea and the Black Sea.

In the middle of the 15th century, when Turkish alum became too expensive and its alum trade went into decline, alum was found in quantity at Tolfa in central Italy, not far from the papal enclave. Indeed, the pope at once entered into the alum trade and tried to monopolize it. Not quite succeeding, the papacy still gained somewhere near 300,000 gold pieces a year from alum (Singer, p. 142). Pope Paul II (1464-71) decided to use all the alum revenue for war against the Turks.

For three centuries after 1450 a major medical application of alum continued to be in the sudatory baths at Pozzuoli. Today it is even rare to find a styptic pencil in a drug store, because you cut yourself rarely with a safety razor and not at all with an electric one (styptic pencils are sticks of alum used to stop bleeding from minor cuts quickly).

Cloth makers' earth

The name "fullers' earth" can be traced to the Latin word "fullo", meaning the person who made clothes white or at least prepared cloth for whitening and coloring. The earth substance used was called "creta" or "terra fullonica". In general, fulling was—and is—the trade to scour and felt[3] cloth. In historical importance using fullers' earth is comparable to the use of alum in the dyeing of leather and wool. Particularly wool had to be cleansed of its lanolin-like oils and of its dirt. For that a strong detergent was needed. The city state civilization of Sumeria was the oldest in Mesopotamia about 3,000 BC and it had the earliest fulling vocabulary. In Sumerian times the choice of detergent was either river mud or stale urine and persons walked or trampled the wool in the fulling medium (Robertson, 1986, p.8). Modern fulling still uses calcium or sodium montmorillonite (bentonite) and used stale urine until 1935 in England.

Generally, according to ethnologic studies, the walker or fuller received the woven material and trampled it thoroughly in a fulling pit so that the threads became felted together. He then beat it with a club or cudgel and raised the nap with teasels. This club is the chief tool with which the soiled cloth is remorselessly beaten after most of the dirt has been removed by washing the cloth with soap or a mixture of potash, lime, and alum (Robertson, 1986, p. 13).

In Egypt, the Nile mud was rich in montmorillonite and served not only as fullers' earth but also as detergent for washing hair. Montmorillonite is a clay and is an essential part of the mud from the White and the Blue Nile. Felted woolen garments have survived in Europe

(Switzerland and Scandinavia) from 1500 BC. Fulling was universal and where fullers' earth was not found, as in Israel, it was imported, in this case from Cyprus. In classical Greece a large deposit of fullers' earth was discovered on the Island of Kimolos (*Terra cimolia*) and became the source for the entire Mediterranean area. There was no other product that could whiten wool as efficiently as Cimolian earth. We trace the word "candidate" to aspiring Roman politicians who dressed in the whitest of white cloth (Latin: *candidus* - brilliant white, spotless) and who, like other politicians, were always candid with the people.

Some means of fulling were known in Europe since prehistory, but the occupation by the Romans transferred their technology of fulling cloth. Montmorillonite has been found in Gaul near Vaucluse (east of Avignon), in Montmorillon (not far from Limoges, type locality of this earth) and Ivre (near Paris). The clay near Vaucluse contained the clay mineral palygorskite of pharmaceutical fame (Kao-Pectate®). Fulling practices in England utilized local fullers' earth deposits. Fulling in the passing of time became mechanized between the 13th and 17th centuries[4]. In modern times fullers' earth was promoted for the original dry cleaning, cleaning without wetting, to take spots and stains from dresses (placing the clay over the spot and ironing with a very hot iron), cleaning straw hats (rubbing with earth on a piece of velveteen), removing dirt from kid gloves, (rubbing with India rubber, then with a mixture of pipe clay (sepiolite), with alum and fullers' earth). It was further used to dry clean ermine or fox fur, eiderdown and feather boas (Robertson, Ch. 8ii). Modern dry or French cleaning does not use water, it uses naphtha, benzene, carbon tetrachloride and similar liquids.

The island of Melos today mines and exports enormous quantities of Bentonite, but in this case the local mineral mined is calcium montmorillonite "activated" by about 3-6% by weight of Romanian dry soda to convert it to sodium montmorillonite. Its main uses are flower pot earth, cat litter, fertilizer, filler for paper and textiles and some plastics to combine the inertness and low shrinkage of the mineral with the properties of plastics such as polyolefins.

These two mineral materials are used by the hundreds of tons every day. In the olden days it was clay as such that has been used much more for building than for anything else, either as sun dried clay or as burned clay bricks. Unfortunately many poorer countries that try to make their own brick actually deforest their nation for wood to make charcoal to fire bricks.

Ruins of towns built of clay dot the landscape of Masar-I-Sharif in Afghanistan. In Mali (West Africa) the most awesome example of natural clay architecture is the huge mosque at Djénné and a beautiful smaller one in Timbuktu at the edge of the Sahara. In the towns' market places clay medications are still being sold by the gram or dram.

Comments and Explanations

[1] Such as the madder family of the order Gentianales.
[2] Tawing: To prepare or dress hides, making hides into leather in a solution of alum.
[3] Felting: thickening of fibers by trampling while fulling.

[4] In the fulling district of Rome, urinal pails were set out at street corners, inviting contributions (Robertson, 1986)

Chapter Twelve: Earths of Early Modern Times

My grouping of centuries by chapters is not accidental. It roughly parallels customary arrangements, but I will admit to purists that I have ignored the centuries of Cimbrian or Gothic invasions, the centuries of total confusion during the re-building of the Western world. But after having placed about two centuries of Renaissance into Chapter Ten I must somewhat belatedly include here most of the "copying encyclopedists".

To compensate for this liberty I start this chapter with the arrival of printing, the advent of individual thought (Georgius Agricola and René Descartes immediately come to mind). I will pass through the beginning of scientific enlightenment (Robert Boyle and Isaac Newton immediately come to mind), and I will go on through the 18th century when medical knowledge first showed repetitive success of curing. Not much was written about healing earths between 600 and 1,000 AD; what might have been written is deep in monastery archives and is, probably again, only repeated thought of earlier times.

Beginning the 16th century

The sudden outpouring of printed matter beginning in the 16th century gave access to thousands of books on alchemy and medicine. Everywhere the language of the learned was Latin. This allowed for substantial editions for printers because educated customers in every country could read the same books printed in Latin. Thus without loss of prominent proponents of healing earths because of (later) language difficulties, we can now enter the period from 1500 to 1900. This time reiterates the valued applications of classical earths in pharmacopoeias, libraries, collections in artificial and natural history (artificial being: man-made), and it brings forth the new healing earths found in Europe[1].

The newfound earths were not subject to transport costs, customs duties, price, and availability irregularities from the Mediterranean region of the "old" earths. They were no longer for the exclusive use of the noble and affluent. But the names *terra sigillata* and *bolus armenus* were kept, even when the clay came from a local pit and was judiciously sigillated or coined. "Doctors of Physick" started patenting their own medicines, some with tens to hundreds of ingredients, usually with one or two healing earths among them. The sad commentary to this money oriented medicine is that no two doctors' patent medicines for the same illness had even approximately the same ingredients, and that a doctor's prescription for an aqueous solution or a "water" against a specific illness, had entirely different ingredients than the oil dispersion ("oil"). Of course, many of these medications were for illnesses which were not curable in years past and many which are not even curable today, so it did not matter except for giving hope.

The great collectors

The 16th century became the age of a new breed of thinking encyclopedists, of a beginning of acceptance of the new heliocentric Copernican world order, and the rise of great collections of "things natural" and "things created by human arts". Scientists, literary dilettantes, noble personages, created their "rarity cabinets" (Kunstkammern). Usually they were called by imposing names such as *gazophylacia, thaumateca, pinacotheca,* words which differ from each other like "bacon and fat pork" (Major, 1967) The size of these collections varied from display tables and cabinets to rooms and even museum-like space in palaces. In those days a museum was a place dedicated to the muses, locations where knowledge was pursued, a library, a study, an academy. Then access was free, later the definition of museum required an entrance fee as a qualifier. Most kings and dukes proudly maintained collections, which always included samples of healing earths. A few even had a true and valuable unicorn horn.

Ferranto Imperato, an Italian museum fanatic (1550-1625) had a famous collection as basis for his *historia naturalis* which included the classic earths. The collection of Andrea Cesalpino (1524-1603) found later expression in his *De re metallicis* that mentions the white earth of the island of Elba. A third avid collector of renown was Ulyssis Aldrovandi (1552-1602) who created his *Museum metallicum,* in which he proposes a systematic scheme for grouping healing earths (see Chapter Seventeen). Other collectors of renown were Caspar Bauhinus of Basel (1560-1624) and Olau Wormius (1588-1654) whose book *Museum Museorum* serependitiously resides close to my home in the Rare Books and Special Collections Department of Stanford University in the Cecil H. Green Library for the Humanities.

A little known giant: Johann Daniel Major

A barely known trilogy about *Kunstkammern* or rarity cabinets (Major 1674, 1675a and b), is contained in three books by Johann Daniel Major (1634-1693), a professor of medicine in Kiel Germany (listed under three titles in my bibliography here, but really a trilogy). In one introductory volume Major describes the physical requirements of a museum (security, cleanliness, light, proper display), in another famous collections in America and Asia, in Africa and at the borders of Europe, and in Italy, especially Naples and Rome.

Major also expressed the need for a new philosophy of the world, the need that long existing problems deserved new scrutiny and new answers instead of the excuse of the "but, it is so difficult" attitude towards creative thinking. On the other hand the expression of new thoughts contrary to church edict could expose a writer to painful inquiry and death. Major hid his thoughts about a heliocentric world in a fable about the goddess Urania and Daedalus:

> "And isn't it easier in all reasonableness / that compared to the sun / the earth is small / and turns once in a day and a night / and that it, following Nicol. Copernico' rule / moves only a degree in its annual circle / to believe this than that a probably liquid body / everyday runs such a frightening Circle, without flying apart / or falling from the sky. "My good friend Daedalus [says Urania] think of this yourself / 860 German miles is considered half the diameter of the earth / and from

earth to the sun is generally thought to be 1150 *semidiametros* of the earth or 909000 miles / take this six times plus one seventh of the whole diameter (282817 miles) [the approximation of the circumference of a circle before π = 3.1416] gives us 62211977 miles / which the sun runs around the earth every day / that would be 259249 miles per hour / or 72 miles per second / about in a beat of the heart / and if you also speak of the fixed stars that are more than ten times as far / they have to travel 720 miles per second / well… let everyone believe what he wants.

The most heretical argument Major assigns to Urania is that the Earth is the same as every other star, and is a planet in her opinion (with "star", Major did not mean our sun, just the other planets and the fixed stars).

Of the scientifically inclined encyclopedists, or those "learned in all sciences", Conrad Gesner[2] (1516-1565), the "Swiss Pliny" only refers to the cave material "moonmilk" (calcium carbonate) that was dug in a cave on Mt. Pilate near Lucerne (Gessner, 1555). His 1565 book on minerals was bound together with a compendium by Johann Kentmann (1565), who also mentioned sealed earths. Kentmann lists 10 marls and 6 boles, including a *bol of Juliers* (Juelich, Nord-Rhein-Westphalia, Germany), a *bolus pannonicus* (from Pannonia, part of Hungary). He calls the Armenian bole the bole of the Levant. Quite prominent at the time, though he exclusively copied others verbatim, was Anselmus Boethius de Boot (à Boodt)[3] with his history of gems and stones. Many used him as a reprint generator for books as much as 100 years old.

Besides the classic healing earths (and a record of false ones) Johann Kentmann listed a rare dark gray clay from Giessen[4] (Gisela) in the region of Hesse in Germany, a red friable earth from Waldenburg. He loosely used the terms *terra* and *bol* and *argilla* interchangeably for clays and earths. All the other mineral knowledge from antiquity—hematite, cinnabar, gypsum, pumice, bitumen, atrament—is found in these writings.

Beginning with the 16th century also came the discovery of new local earths for medicinal application, spurred by the need for them and the difficulty of obtaining the classic earths. The terms "bolus armenus" and "terra sigillata" were rediscovered (Kegeler, 1529), even though particularly in the first half of the 16th century there was no agreement on the English spelling of *bolus armenus*: bolos in 1527, bolus armenicus or armeniacus in 1543, bonementum in 1564, according to Lehman (1985).

The Father of Geology, Georgius Agricola

A very prominent scientific, thought-out and enduring description of earths and their medical significance is the Textbook of Mineralogy (*De natura fossilium*, Agricola 1546) in 10 *libris* (book sections, not volumes). Agricola considered distinctive features and the origins of all mineral matter in the first book. The second deals with earths, the third with congealed juices generally, the fourth with the congealed juices amber and bitumen. The fifth book touches on stones, gems, marbles and rocks, metals and metallic substances, and finally on "combined" substances. This work brought the German Georg Bauer (latinized to Georgius Agricola) later recognition as the Father of Geology. His new thinking, his major achievement, was a systematic classification, a significant feat in the absence of chemical knowledge regarding geology.

In his classification by colors, none of the earths are included, probably because he covered that subject 15 years earlier (Agricola, 1530). Color has really little or no bearing on the physical properties of an earth. His first identifier after color is luster (for instance: *Creta argentaria*), his next is taste. Some minerals such as *galactites* and *melitites* have a sweet taste, Samian earth and marls taste oily, nitrum is bitter, halite is salty, lime is acrid, and red ochre astringent. Some earths are acidulous, moonmilk has no taste. In the property of touch Agricola distinguishes unctuousness and roughness, heaviness and lightness (then also two different properties discussed earlier together with hot and cold, dry and wet).

Agricola says that minerals that are taken in food or drink, may either be a remedy or a poison. Minerals that act as a remedy heal the body in part through an essence characteristic of all such minerals, and in part through some efficacious quality of purity. Some minerals are rich in this essence and counteract poisons or cure diseases.

Continuing, Agricola says that regarding medical properties, it appears that all earths are "drying out". Some warm the body (such as alum), some cool it (Eretrian earth). Jet and *galena* soften hard places on the body, nitrum opens pores, Samian Aster and other glutinous earths close them.

Agricola had studied medicine in Leipzig, Bologna, and Padua where he worked on an issue of Galen's books. Later he became a mining and geology expert. In hematite he saw both a drying out and astringency and considered it beneficial for treating external ulcers and to reduce "fleshy" growth. Mixed with water, hematite stops bleeding from an open vein. Mixed with egg and smeared on eyelids it reduces roughness there. Just as hematite and *schistos* (clay? shale?) form from red rocks, *morochthus* forms from white calcareous rocks. This earth is found in Egypt and is also mined in Saxony. Because it possesses property of dispersing swellings and reducing bleeding, physicians use it to reduce menstrual bleeding. Because it dries out and is not astringent and does not "draw a bite" when taken internally, it relieves pain in abdomen and bladder. It is used in eye medicines, it is used to fill hollow ulcers, and it stops the flow of humors.

Furthermore Agricola states that earth from the island of Milos (*terra Melia*) is of the alumen (alum) species, gray and harsh [Agricola confuses two different Melian earths here]. Egyptian mud that is used to treat tumors contains soda. An aluminous earth is mined near the town of Lüneburg in Germany.

Grouping by use

Earths are distinguished by the different uses they offer: One of the major uses is to fertilize [agricultural] earth; other clays such as Lemnian, Samian and Armenian are used by physicians. Sculptors and potters use red clay, fullers use Cimolian clay.

Of course, some groups overlap in uses. Agricola writes that Egyptian earth is used in agriculture and as medicament, red ochre is used by physicians, artisans, and painters, Cimolian earth is essential for physicians and fullers. Agricola classifies most earths by their place of origin, very much like today's type locality concept.

Poor soils are improved by marl (marga, derived from medulla, marrow, found in fractures or fissures and joints of rocks), but marl, when dissolved, can be drunk to stop bleeding, very much like Samian earth. An earth called Tripoli (tripela, German: Trippel) was used to polish brass. It is diatomaceous earth.

All dry earths have the property to dry moist things[5]. Most of them are so drying that they can pull skin off your tongue and they are cooling, but acrimonious earth has a taste characteristic of heat, it warms the skin. Dry earth will stop bleeding from any part of the body; wet earths are good for ulcerated wounds and burns. If these earths had been more abundant, the ancients would have put them to more uses, but they commanded a very high price. Earths similar to Armenian bole are found in Bohemia, Silesia, and Hesse. There was also Wildenburger Ton (clay) and the red stone marrow of Röcklitz. Where newly found earths were used, a doctor only had to taste the earth in order to determine its medical properties. Agricola's *De natura fossilium* is a lucid discussion of earths for medical uses (Agricola, 1565).

New drug manuals

The first pharmacopoeias or drug manuals appeared. 1535 saw the appearance of the Concordia pharmacopoeia Barcinonesis (Barcelona), 1546 brought the first Nürnberg and the first Augsburg pharmacopoeia, 1559 the one from Saragossa, 1565 Cologne. All of these contained many fanciful compound medicines. In 1574 the physician Andrea Mattioli became famous for his wonder-theriak with 123 ingredients, including three red earths: Armenian, Lemnian and Stalimene [Mattioli was confused, Stalimene was an old name for Lemnian]. Even the early theriak, which Andromachus made for Nero, included sealed earth with wine, lots of wine.

Valerius Cordus (1515-1544) wrote a dispensatory in 1540 wherein he lists alum, borax, asphaltum, bitumen judaeicum, lapis armenis, lapis terra sigillatae (4 pages), terra cimolia, bol armen (also called oriental or levantine), red and white coral. Prescriptions included pearls, hematite, bole from Blois in France, stag's horn powder (a good source of calcium). An error appears to be that he mentions "terra sigillata <u>vel</u> bolus armenius", vel meaning "or", not "and". The two names were never equated as pertaining to the same earth.

In 1574, Michele Mercati created and organized the Natural History Museum of the Vatican and wrote a *Metalloteca Vaticana*. Museologically he was the first to divide the subject into I. earths, II. salts and nitre, and III. alumina. In section I he carries Lemnian earth, Armenian bole, friable red earth (*rubrica*), Alana earth, Samian earth, Chia earth, Selunesian earth, St. Paul's earth from Malta, Cimolia earth from Kimolos, *cretica* (but he assigns the term to Crete*)*, *argilla* (clay)*, margis et medullae* (marl), *triple* (diatomaceous earth)*,* and *arena* (Bech-I-Borràs, 1987, p. 39).

Georg am Wald (1581) glowingly reported the "invention" of a new terra sigillata and universal medicine. His endless title, almost as long as his four pages, reiterates all the previously exaggerated "cures", invents some new ones (strengthening of the head and memory, all unrecognized illnesses). He touts his new invention as just as good as unicorn horn, Theriak, mithridate, and we all know by now how well they worked. He suggests his coined earth to be taken in warm soup or vermouth against pestilence of the eyes. Placing his earth on glowing fire to smoke out illnesses or drinking his earth with many juices (much juice?) will help against the English sweat[6] and will bring you help, so God will, unless the illness was sent to punish you.

This useless and seldom cited report of healing earth invention was soon followed by a serious report on earth coins from Silesia (now Poland) by Andreas Bertholdus (1587 in English). It was the start of the 200-year reign of the Silesian earth coins. Whether a newly found local earth became prominent depended very much on the promotion it received. Strigian clay from Striegau, a hydrous silicate of aluminum, one of about 60 earths from Silesia was reported in the 18th century by Ludwig and by Volkmann (discussed in detail in the Chapter of Illustrations). Two papers by Florian Heller reviewed them in 1961 and 1964.In 1984 Karl Dannenfeldt wrote a paper about Berthold. Again, these will be included in the discussion of the world of earth coins in Chapter Seventeen, where the subject and its chronology can be treated easier without interrupting the basic history of mineral medicines.

A modicum of progress

Upon entering the 17th century, we can continue to trace the healing earths, but the 17th was not yet the time for all good physicians to leave Galen and his humoral pathology behind. Those who did face the new world need to be segregated from those who still propounded weird and totally off-the-wall medications. In 1601 Wittich combined newly discovered "balsams, miracle plants, and roots" with the grease of the sun, *axungia solis,* (probably better called salve of the sun, a promoter), supposedly brought to Germany within the last quarter century from India. Actually axungia pertained to all the planets' respective planetary metals: Gold to the sun, silver to the moon, and the derivative, axungia, was generally applied to various healing earths. One healing clay coin named itself not only *axungia lunae* but also *mineral unicorn horn.* Advertising was not restricted in the 17th century.

The first London Pharmacopoeia was published 1618, still a list of 2,000 weird and useless medicines with only a few recognizable simples. In 1689 the second London Pharmacopoeia had not really improved. Athanasius Kircher (1665), in his chapter IV about the various uses of the earths, almost exclusively mentions only the classic Greek earths and St. Paul's earth. Gideon Harvey (1678) proposed in his "Family Physician and the House

Apothecares" a description of the river crayfish *Astacus astacus* and the powder made of his button of calcium carbonate. Harvey also suggested coral powder, white amber (?), harts horn, and oriental bezoar.

He does give an insight into prices: Bezoar cost 30-40 shillings per ounce, oculi cancri (5-6 shillings per lb), human skull (8£ 11s each), lapis judaeicus (1s 6p per lb), ambergris (18s per lb). These few prices are sufficient to show that these medications were not accessible to the poor, but England established dispensaries of free medicines for the poor from funds supplied by the more affluent.

It was still a period of ghastly imaginations by many of the medical profession. Prescriptions included snake meat, fox lung hachée, ant oil, butter made in May, ointment from live boiled frogs and smoked toads, earth worms cleaned in manure and mashed baby swallows. Human medicines were blood, fat, moss scraped from the head of those hanged[7] (especially male and red-haired), human gall, intestines, sweat, and the saliva of a fasting man (Reinbacher, 1998, p. 159-160). Not far from these medications were the offerings of the "Dreckapotheke", the filth dispensary, which advocated feces and urine for certain cures. Medical, especially physiological thinking was not one of the great accomplishments of this century.

The highly regarded Johann Daniel Horst, personal physician of the Duke of Hesse, published his Pharmacopoeia Galeno-Chimica in 1651. Regarding healing earths it is probably the most accurate and extensive at the time. His *terrae* include all known and several new earths such as *terra Brundisiaca* from Bohemia, but the most prominent were still the old stand-bys *terra lemnia* and *bolus armenus*. Typical for his time, his drug list is indexed twice, first by the form (oils, aqueous solutions called "waters", ointments, cataplasms are some) and second by the illness cured such as "water against the falling sickness" together with the name of the physician who patented that medicine.

A "standard" theriak[8] always included at least one earth. They always were very complicated compound medicines: Aqua bezoardica had 22 ingredients, aqua theriacalis 37, electuarium pectorala 50. Proprietary (patented) medicines included Mynsicht's *Marmelada stomachia* or his *Confectio opiata Mynsichtus* that was composed of ground coral, Armenian bole, "salt of the human skull" (?), bezoar stone, and unicorn horn (the "real" one, not the marine one). A standard grouping of precious stones are part of Horst's pharmacopoeia, as well as crushed eagle stone, alabaster, feather alum, Armenian stone and moonstone (*lapis specularis*)

Moonmilk

Surprisingly, what with the centuries old use of calcium medications, there is only one dissertation on the subject of the cave deposit calcium carbonate (Major, 1667), ignored by all but one biographer of Major (Reinbacher, 1998), because Major chose the less well known local name for his title *Dissertatio medica de lacte lunae* and other biographers assigned it to the realm of the magical. Actually, "moonmilk" is still the scientific name for soft, fine-grained calcium carbonates, and its type locality is the moonmilk cave

(Mondmilch-Loch) in the Pilatus mountain near Lucerne, Switzerland, named after Pontius Pilate. In his dissertation Major compares other white earths with moonmilk (*morochthus, galactite*) and mentions some of the other antique earths. He copied his knowledge of moonmilk from Boethius de Boodt who himself had copied it from Conradus Gesnerus. As wound treatment he recommends:

Moonmilk	7 drachma
Calamine stone	11 drachma
Armenian bole	5 scruples
Terra sigillata	5 scruples
Myrrh, mastic, olibanum	5 scruples each
Camphor	10 scruples

Make a fine powder; if desired, add a few drops of Camomile oil. Put in layers on the wound.

He used this prescription to cure a festering ulcer of the tibia (shinbone). In a case of nosebleeds, Major recommended blowing moonmilk into the nose through a silver or ivory tube. Moonmilk mixed with various herbal essences and seeds (such as anise) was a popular medication to increase lactation in women who had just given birth. In Major's time, during the Little Ice Age, food was scarce and peope often were severely undernourished. Barely edible foods may have been made more palatable by moonmilk, but at least moonmilk paste helped still hunger, herbs may have improved digestion, even lactation in famished women with a new baby.

Levy (1908, p.7) regrets that healing earth was also used for what we now know to be useless endeavors to cure and that therefore bolus acquired an unfair reputation as a quack remedy. When we today view medicines like stag's pizzle and whale penis (*priapus ceti*), skull moss and ambergris, we must conclude that many medical treatments were ineffective. Even bolus was unsuitable for many applications. This does not reduce the success of bolus in those applications which Hewson and Stumpf later pioneered and which are still effective, although not much prescribed today.

The London Dispensary of 1679 by Thomas Newcomb with annotations by Nicolas Culpepper lists *terra lemnia* and *terra samia* side by side with *terra silesica, bolus armenus,* and *bolus bohemica.* "The clays were in a class known as simples, and had, as we now know, some virtues, but the craze for elaborate formulations of umpteen mainly useless ingredients was accelerating towards a peak of stupidity" (Robertson, 1986, p.140). The pharmacopoeia of the Medical College of London added *bolus gallica* to *bolus armenia* besides the standard calcis, styrax and *lapis medicamentosus.* It also contained the elusive *terra japonica* that was later identified not as an earth but as an Indian plant juice; one source had claimed it was found in the Levant, another that it is green bark of a thorny tree in Japan. The latter may be the correct identification. *Terra adamis* dug near Babylon from great depth was the pure clay, untouched by human hands, from which the Lord made Adam.

The Jesuit scientist Athanasius Kircher describes in his *Mundus subterraneous* (1665) salts, "concretionized juices" (hardened juices such as amber), minerals, and other fossils and discusses sealed earths, our earth-coins, very much like Agricola.

The second London pharmacopoeia of 1689, or the "New London Dispensatory", translated into English by William Salmon, said:

> "There are several sorts of sealed earths, viz. that from Constantinople, which is ash in color (?) and indeed the best of all earths known to us, though the [earth of] Lemnos, which is red, is often used for the true. The best earth is known by (1) sticking to your tongue, (2) if cast in water it rises up in bubbles. Terra sigillata is drying, binding, sudorific and resisting plague, poison, putrefaction, and all kind of malignity, and venom. It is chiefly used against the plague, malignant fevers, diarrhea, dysentery and bites of venomous beasts."

It needs to be remembered here, even if anachronistically, that comments regarding the aid against the bubonic plague per se, as we know it today, cannot be considered accurate, but because many illnesses were considered "pest", there is no assurance that it always was bubonic plague, even if some texts refer, in translation, to "buboes". Rare detailed case histories made during a plague epidemic in Braunschweig, Germany (Giseler, 1657), including prescriptions of Armenian bole, showed that it had no more effect on plague deaths than did country air bottled and taken to the city by an enterprising physician.

Earths in the 18th century

Pomet (1712) had a very complete collection of classic and new European earths. In his Book IV he combines "earths", bituminous and sulfurous materials, such as the *terra ampelitis*, the so-called vine earth that drives vermin from the leaves of vines and also drives worms from the human intestinal tract. Pomet distinguishes *terra sigillata* from the earth of Lemnos connection in view of the availability of sigillated (coined) earths from Germany. Similarly, while he knows of Armenian bole, he advocates use of the fine bole from Blois, Saumur and Bourgogne (gray, red, and yellow), saying they are fine, too, as fine as butter melting in your mouth.

I am indebted to the late Robert R. H. Robertson (1986) who discovered *bole armoniack* in the "Family Household Companion" (London 1710): "To prepare Bole Armoniak for use you need not do more than moisten it with May-dew, or any other dew not too gross, and dry it in the shade. Rainwater will do well. You may give a scruple to half a dram against heart burnings and vehement pains in the stomach".

Quincy, Schröder, Ernstingius

John Quincy included *bole armoniak* in his *pharmacopoeia officinalis et extemporanea* or Compleat English dispensatory. Previously I have referred to the monumental (65 volume) Zedler's Universallexikon of the same period that contains about 1,000 columns on various healing earths, their provenance, and prescriptions for use against a multitude of illnesses. The dissertation entitled *terras medicinales* (Rivinus 1923) with Gottfried Miekisch as respondent, aside from being one of the few who cites from Johann Daniel Major about moonmilk, added some of the newer earths to the repertory of the old one: *terra basiliensis rubra* (red clay from Basle), a chalk from Cologne, earths from Hesse, Saxony and Silesia, as well as "foreign" earths from Spain and China.

From Ulm, Germany, came the pharmacopoeia of the renowned physician Johann Schröder (1744). His major earth categories were headed *I. terrae argillacea* (white earths from antiquity and Germany), *II. Bolus* (red earth imbued with mercurial spirits, from Armenia, from the orient and also from Germany), *III. Creta* (which dries out, hardens and can be made into a plaster, *IV. Marga, V. Ochra, VI. Rubrica* (red earth, possibly hematite) and *VII. Tripolis* (diatomaceous earth). For each category Schröder gives descriptions and suggests applications in medicine.

Also in Germany Arthurus Conradus Ernstingius (1770) published an extensive dispensatory of all medicines. Among 21 earths all but two have been previously mentioned: (1) *Terra bituminosa torfacea* (tar containing peat earth) which was in use in peat producing regions, and (2) *terra nitrosa* (dug in animal barns or shelters; it draws a parallel to the Chinese "earth from the defecation hole" and "earths from the urination hole".) Ernstingius mentions chalk from Crete (?) by various names such as *terra argentea* (polishing earth), *terra cretica, terra primogenea* and *terra candida* (all probably sedimentary calcium carbonate). He also resurrects bezoardica from cattle, monkeys, elephants (?), stags, mules.

The Middle Ages had not obscured knowledge of the earths or clays in medicine, rather Early Modern Times increased the awareness of newer local earths that were begun to be used frequently enough for their names to be entered and maintained in medical and pharmaceutical handbooks of the period. Clay throughout time remained the people's choice of home remedy when access to doctors was difficult. Since clay was also used successfully to cure farm animals, it was but a short step to use the same medication for the farmer and his family.

Comments and explanations

[1] There is a record of finding deposits of feather and rock alum in Virginia, and a report about healing earth similar to *terra sigillata* in use by Native Americans, who called it *waipek* according to Thomas Hariot, 1560-1621, reprinted privately in 1900. It is now contained in a National Park Service Heritage Education Program "Roanoke revisited", at Raleigh National Historic Site, Rt. 1, Box 675, Manteo NC 27954.

[2] Latin Conradus Gesnerus, Swiss-German Konrad Gessner. In many citations the first and last name spelling gets mixed up between languages.

[3] De Boot was archiater (personal physician) to Emperor Rudolf II. His book was published in 1609 in Hanau. I did not use it, preferring to go to the original writers.

[4] This dark gray clay is still used in 1950 for stoneware pitchers (usually with a dark blue decorative glaze) to purchase off-premise draft beer and apple wine from a tap room.

[5] With the previously mentioned difference between wet and dry, the question always was whether a dry earth had become wet or whether a wet earth had become dry.

[6] A curious fever, *sudor anglica*, the English sweat, occurred fairly frequently in England during the latter part of the 16/17th century. No cause was ever found, eventually the disease disappeared.

[7] *Usnea cranii*: Some Usnea lichens are considered today to have antibiotic properties.

[8] Probably no two theriaks were ever the same. A story goes that an apprentice had made a mistake mixing a certain medication and fearfully reported it to the apothecary, who calmed the boy and told him: "Don't throw this away, we can use it in the next theriak".

Chapter Thirteen: Progress with Medical Clay in the 19th Century

It was the 19th century when man made great strides in science, started developing revolutionary thoughts until then deemed heretic. He slowly eliminated many of the unsupported introspective beliefs of olden times. The picture of the universe was now routinely seen in the new concept of a heliocentric world. Medicine advanced onto a more scientific plane. Governments began to see the need for public health and sanitation. New discoveries boosted the knowledge of mineralogy, which enhanced the value of the healing earths. By 1807 Brogniart explained in his "Traité élémentaire de minéralogie" new chemical concepts such as borosilicates, fluorosilicates, aluminosilicates. The healing earths continued doing the healing of ailments for which they had been known for millennia. Some names changed; *argilla nativa* was now calcium carbonate, *argilla de porcellana* now described kaolin, some old earths were grouped under *argilles fines.*

Advances in Science

In 1825 Berzelius (1799-1848) devised modern chemical symbols[1] With those symbols one of the first analyses of clay gave the result 46% SiO_2, 19% Al_2O_3, 6% $MgCO_3$, 5% $CaCO_3$ and 5% Fe_2O_3, a very close approximation of the red[2] Lemnian earth. The Encyclopädie der Gesammten Volksmedizin (Most, 1843) included alum for unabating diarrhea, as gargling water and washing medium for frostbite, alum salve against blisters of burns. It mentioned Armenian and white bolus, chalk, borax, pitch and a curious green "Amazon" stone that is inserted into a surgical slit, totally different from the Amazon stone referred to by Alexander von Humboldt which required belief in a warrior tribe of women.[3]

The "Treasury of Drugs Unlocked" (Berlu, 1860) included alum from England and other parts of Europe. *Alum plumosum*, feather alum, came from Germany, alum roch (rock) arrived as *allum* from Italy. *Bolus verus* originated in Armenia or came from Wirtemberg in Germany (fattish, red, sticks to the tongue, therefore very adsorbent, dissolves in water like butter melting in your mouth). Red and white talc came from England. A green talc (probably a magnesium silicate) came from Venice. Erroneously Berlu said *terra Samia* came from Armenia near a city called Samos (not from the Aegean island of Samos).

Hager's basics of pharmacy

Hager's handbook on pharmaceutical practice (Hager, 1876) became the German bible of pharmaceutical knowledge through at least 8 editions from 1876 to 1919 as a manual for pharmacists. Its first and the subsequent editions read like a Rosetta stone of clays, because all headings are in English, French, and German and include all variations of local use. Each item has paragraphs on provenance, description, chemical nature and a paragraph of apparently authentic medical applications and industrial uses. After that follow numerous sample prescriptions showing the applicable use of the chemical and then a final listing of commercial products made from this material. In its listings it has synonyms and explanations of the meanings of ancient terms such as *medulla saxorum*, rock marrow, that mostly exists in veins as fine, soft magnesium silicate, also known as soapstone and steatite.

When Julius Stumpf started experimenting with clay for wounds in 1898, the British Pharmacopoeia had resurrected kaolin. Ten years later the American Pharmaceutical Association and National Formulary (Chicago Branch) contained *Cataplasma kaolini*, a clay poultice that was sold under various proprietary names. Hermann Schelenz (1909), aside from other historical citations, mentions that in 1909 the *Bole d'Armenie* (Armenian bol) was in the official Pharmacopoée Française as an ingredient in an emplâtre céroène, a wax and clay plaster.

The Episode of the Earth Toilets

Little has been discussed so far about clay's ability to deodorize organic smells. For that it helps to take a look at the phenomenon of the history of earth closets: toilets with a clay reservoir to eliminate odor. Indeed clay could adsorb totally the organic odors associated with human waste as well as the smells associated with putrid wounds. The invention of earth closets had a brief rise to fame. In contrast to its successor, the water closet (the toilet on each hotel floor was marked WC or Room 00). The earth closet could be put on wheels and accommodate people even at bedside and could be hidden inside a closet [French: *cabinet d'aisance*, abbreviated "le cabinet"].

Population growth by the middle of the 19th century seriously threatened public health. The deposit of increased quantities of waste products due to human metabolic processes had created not only an atmosphere rich in ammonia, carbon dioxide, and sulfated hydrocarbons, but made streets virtually impassable. "Night soil" was dumped onto the streets and even in the rare cases of street cleaning, the sludge disposal pits often were near city wells where the heavily contaminated liquid infected well water. Medical terms for "water" were still distinguished by degrees of pollution, the best being morning dew on the fields, next best being cleanly collected rainwater. In many towns the well water was evil smelling and polluted with putrefying animal carcasses (Reinbacher 1998, p. 194 f). Real water mains properly separated from sewers were still either nonexistent or in their earliest beginning, which made the first water closets ineffective for dispersal of effluent. In the first community water systems the pressure was low and the sewers could not cope with flushing. The problem of removal of human bodily waste loomed as a major problem.

The size of the problem

A survey[4] revealed that the volume of solid human discharge per person averaged 0.083 m^3 per year per person (~ 250 kg or 500 lbs), a rather generous estimate assuming an average of one bowel movement per day. Daily waste was estimated at 0.3 kg of solid waste per person per day[5.] Due to the known property of clay earth to deodorize organic matter effectively, the amount of clay needed per person per day was calculated as 0.5 kg, giving a total of about 1 kg of "deodorized matter". A small town with only 2500 people (~1,000 households) would need to acquire almost 500,000 kg/year of dry earth and would have to dispose of over 900,000 kg/year of dry deodorized clay-manure mixture per year. To achieve human excrement removal on such a scale, it was proposed that farmers would sell the neat clay earth to families and buy back the manure-enriched soil. It was envisioned that earth would be delivered similar to coal delivery to the basement and there were few proposals just in what manner to pick up the end product. The economic advantage for the "nation" would be that the collected manure soil would replace fertilizers imported to America from Germany at about 400 million marks per year, then about 50 million dollars. Even more important would be that all smells associated with the human manure would disappear in the earth closet and subsequently, since the clay also dried the matter, infectious diseases such a typhus would be minimized. Household servants (there were plenty available then) would carry the dry soil upstairs (same as coal) and night soil in clay (same as ashes) downstairs. Nowhere is mentioned what effect toilet paper (invented about 1860 by Scott) or its predecessor would have when it was suggested that the deodorized matter could be dried and thus could even be reused in the cabinets several times to reduce the quantity of clay needed. Even septic tanks do not always take kindly to toilet paper or other "foreign" substances.

The secret in the secret place

Invention of the "earth closet" is credited to the Rev. Henry Moule of Fordington Vicarage, Dorsetshire, England (Waring, 1868). The proposed toilet facility would consist of a wooden commode, the seating area backed by an upright container filled with dry earth, not really that different from having a water tank at your back. The dropping of the deodorizing and drying earth would be effected either by pulling a handle or by a mechanism that would release the required amount of earth into the bucket under the seat upon the user rising from the seat (the reservoir would be designed for about 25 use times). If properly designed and installed, no odor will be evident for 30 days or more. This mechanism can be placed in a closet or tiny room referred to as *Secretum* (the secret room out of sight). If built with wheels it would be usable wherever it was required (e.g. at sickbed side).The commode would be made of galvanized steel and have the shape of a coal scuttle and could be carried downstairs with no more offensiveness than a scuttle full of common earth (Waring, p.19).

It was recommended that the earth, dried as suggested above, could be used about 4 times over—thus the cost for earth is diminished and the manure value is raised. Just as water works must be adjusted to the population, so must the earth works:

> "Let one fall of earth be in the pail before using.
> The earth must be dry and sifted, sand must not be used.
> No slops must be thrown down.
> The handle must be pulled up with a jerk and let fall
> sharply*.
> Rise from the seat quickly** (Waring, 1868, p.22)
> (* in the pull-down model; ** in the self-acting model.)

George Waring's enthusiastic vision extended over the entire United States: On the basis of a population of 35 million, the USA would no longer need the annual amount of fertilizer of 200,000 tons of phosphoric acid and 900,000 tons of bone meal, worth over $50 million even then.

Waring designed systems for railway stations with several adjoining earth closets and also a chute system for use of earth closets in multiple-story buildings. Attached to the engineering drawings and suggestions are numerous testimonial letters which attest to the value of the earth closet system installed by companies such as the Novelty Iron Works, New York; the University of Pennsylvania Medical Department, the US Army Corps of Engineers, the Maryland Hospital in Baltimore and many others during the years 1869 and 1870 (Waring, 1868, p. 95-104). We do not need to go further in determining the deodorizing value of clay[6].

Resurgence of clay treatment in Europe

In Germany a priest became a proponent for hydrotherapy and for external treatments with clay. Born in 1821, Sebastian Kneipp overcame the rigors of a very poor youth and managed to study for and graduate from a catholic seminary. He was ordained a priest in 1852; by 1880 he was the parish priest and confessor to the nuns of the Wörishofen (Bavaria) convent. He became most famous the world over for his water cures and tight regimen of restricting food intake to simple meals, no stimulants. He suggested roast barley as coffee substitute[7] little meat, but an abundance of cereals[8].The books about his endeavors were "Mein Testament" and "Codicil zu meinem Testament"[9]. Foregoing Kneipp's comments on herbal medicines and his detailed water cures as outside the realm of this book, the interest is in Kneipp's thoughts about clay, his clay poultices and clay-water wraps. He was the first who resurrected systematic clay treatments for sprains and swellings (Kneipp, 1955).

Growing up in the country, the young Kneipp, then a weaver's apprentice, noticed that farmers would place clay poultices on their ailing animals, sometimes mixing the clay with vinegar instead of water (*essigsaure Tonerde*). Animals with sprains or crush-injured feet were easily treated with clay. When either bovines or horses had a "hot swelling", treatment with a clay poultice would soon remove the heat of the injury.

Both animals and humands respond

Kneipp considered that the same treatment should be effective with swellings from contusions or crush injuries of humans, that it would reduce the swelling and in general reduce the fever. Even after he had learned herbal medicinal treatments, he thought that no other method was faster than a clay poultice in healing external damage.

He tried thick clay bandages on swollen twisted, or sprained knees. The patient was told to replace, respectively wet down, the bandage whenever it had dried out. In a specific case history, the patient could work as before within three days. Kneipp was not a physician, but as village priest those around him would always have consulted him, especially the poor in the village and those living in forest and field outside the village proper.

"Anybody who has ever been stung by a hornet, knows how quickly the bite area will swell up, vomiting occurs and danger of blood poisoning exists." A colleague of Kneipp was badly stung, the whole head swelled up and the eyes swelled shut. "Clay mixed with vinegar was used as poultice, changed hourly. The heat decreased, so did the pain and complete recovery was observed" (Kneipp, p. 122). For milk fever of cows Kneipp had the backs of the cows rubbed with a clay paste until the hairs were barely visible and then he had the animal covered with a blanket. When the clay had dried, he had the cows wetted down with water or vinegar. In a few hours the sick animal was saved (Kneipp, p.123). For human patients, for fast heart beat or for strong "blood pressure in the head" he recommended applying cloths wetted with clay water over the heart and in the other case wrapping the lower legs with this cold bandage of clay water to draw the heat from the head.

Other applications of a similar kind were used for serpigo, herpes, lupus vulgaris and other dermatological complaints such as shingles. Wrapping clay cloth around the throat helped reduce the heat of sore throat. Kneipp mixed the clay to a pasty consistency and added herbal remedies such as horsetail *(Equisetum)*, tormentilla (*Potentilla tormentilla*), marigold (*Calendula officinalis*), ribwort or plantain (*Plantago lanceolata*), coltsfoot (*Tussilago farfara*) and other herbs. He also took dried clay and sprinkled it on old wet eczemas and on open ulcers. "Such powder absorbs the rotten, evil matter and acts astringent and healing." He insisted, though, that the clay be properly sifted and reduced to such fine particles until the eye cannot tell whether the substance is an ointment or pure clay. Heating the clay on a hot plate allows pulverizing to remove all particles larger than fine dust.

Sebastian Kneipp's final exhortation regarding clay was not to leave dry clay on the skin, too long, because that might increase the heat again and act adversely. While Kneipp even today is remembered by thousands of followers more for his water cures, his work with clay re-emphasizes the fact that clay has been forever a remedy of the "common people". Kneipp's uses of clay parallel those from 5,000 years ago and a quarter century in advance of Julius Stumpf, he advocated 1-2 spoonfuls of "healing earth powder" daily for cleansing of the intestines and to stimulate appetite. It is not different today in West African nations.

The "healthy soil" theory of Max von Pettenkofer

The 19th century became the time of what truly can be considered bacteriology. The antecedents had been the theories of Varro, who thought about unseen "animalcules" in 100 AD. Fracastero mentioned similar little things in 1546, and the renowned Jesuit Athanasius Kircher saw what he thought were microbes about 1650.

The first one to actually observe miniscule living things in his tiny microscope lenses made of amber and to report this to the London Royal Society was Antoni de Leeuwenhoek. He made representative drawings of the little things he would call "bacteria" in 1683 (Meyer, K., 1998).

Major credit for sterilization effects on bacteria was earned by Louis Pasteur (1822-1895) in his recognition that living organisms (bacteria = little sticks) cause putrefaction in tissue. Bacteriology, as branch of microbiology, was furthered with a classification of bacteria by Ferdinand Cohn (1828-1898). The prominent German professor of hygiene, Max von Pettenkofer, published his work on the interdependence of earth and human health in 1882. This was the year that Robert Koch (1843-1910) had discovered the bacterium causing tuberculosis and a year later had discovered the comma bacterium causing cholera. Together with his 1876 discovery of the bacterium causing anthrax, he would receive the 1910 Nobel Prize for medicine. Pettenkofer was not convinced: The bacteria had to come from somewhere.

Pettenkofer reached back to Hippokrates' thoughts on air, water, and earth. Humanity mostly believed that the ill-making propensity was in the air (mal aria, bad air) and in the water rather than in the soil of the location of the illness. According to Pettenkofer the influence of the air had to be discounted once it became known that the average speed of the atmosphere at ground level is 3 meters per second, and even when it feels totally calm, the air still travels at 0.5 m/s. "Stagnation" of air at a specific location is error. Illnesses (epidemics) are tied to the locality where they occur. It is the same with water, which starts out as rain and does not absorb peculiarities that have their origin in the localities through which water courses. (Pettenkofer, 1882, p. 6).

As one example Pettenkofer cites the river Trent in England which was polluted by sewage of two million people of Nottingham upriver, yet the river below Nottingham is clear, tastes good and is chemically free of all dirt that had been deposited in it. As second example, in Paris below the bridge of Asnières, water from Clichy flowed into the Seine so polluted that neither fish nor plants could live in it, yet a few miles below Paris, at Meulan, the Seine has lost every trace of pollution.

The cause of epidemics must be in the soil. It takes the longest and it is hardest to remove pollution from the soil:

> "It has been known forever that malaria comes from the soil[10], but now it is certain that illnesses that were thought to be independent of the soil actually in some way are dependent upon it…The frequently sharp localization of cholera and typhoid was believed to come from the influences of air and water that cause these illnesses in humans, but it appears now [1882] that the causes of epidemics must be investigated in the soil."

Pettenkofer particularly wondered why certain areas were cholera-prone and others, not that far away, never had an epidemic. While Paris and Marseilles suffered cholera epidemics, Lyon, between the two, never did. Even more so: Versailles, but an hour from Paris, never had a cholera epidemic, either. He believed in "sickness bearing" and "sickness void" soils, just as the draining and drying of the earth and subsequent fertilization and cultivation of the Pontine marshes led to a reduction of malaria. "Fireplaces and chimneys suck contaminated air from the soil into houses. It is well remembered that the most dangerous thing in the Pontine marshes was to spend a night there and to sleep in this fever promoting region."

Sickness bearing soil

To understand the reason for the appearance of sickness-bearing soil, Pettenkofer studied the level of groundwater in cities. Often typhus occurred in Berlin and in Munich when the water tables were low, but that doesn't happen in both places at the same time of the year. Was there a coincidence with increased illness[11]? Pettenkofer attributed the illnesses such as cholera to bacteria from the soil but did not regard the probability of massive infection from human to human. It was not known until six years after his treatise on the soil and human health that Italian researchers found that mosquitoes carry malaria. It was not until 1928 that the Pontine marshes were finally completely drained and malaria there ceased.

Other researchers, among them Addinell Hewson (before Pettenkofer) and Julius Stumpf (after Pettenkofer) found that illness-causing bacteria are rarely found in the depth of soil from which aluminum silicates should be unearthed for medical use. Even hookworm is on the surface of the tilled depth of soil permeated by feces and urine. Bacteria infections due to clay treatments with earth were rare, and if the earth was sterilized, there were none at all[12].

Clay treatment of wounds by Addinell Hewson in America

The whole matter of earth closets and the deodorizing power of clay would only be an anecdote in sanitation history had not an American surgeon recalled reading about it in 1869 (Hewson, 1872, p. xi). The surgeon, Addinell Hewson, had been "zealously engaged" in search for a disinfecting dressing for offensive wounds and ulcers during his tour of duty at the Philadelphia Hospital in 1869. Having read Waring's book on earth closets, he wondered whether the earth might have an advantage in surgery.

A case that Hewson encountered brought back to his mind the deodorization power of clay: A young man had been run over by a cart loaded with a ton of coal. The injury had required a resection of the tibia. With the wound enlarged, the leg swollen, there was "a free escape of pus and broken down blood" (Hewson p. xii). Additional incisions to free accumulations were made and discharge of pus into the "fracture box" of bran necessitated removal of the dressing twice a day. The stench from the wound became intolerable in the ward, the case was offensive in the extreme (Hewson xiii):

> "I felt it was one [case in which] to test, in the severest
> manner possible, the power of the earth as a disinfectant. I had
> had some earth taken from a heap in the hospital lot, left there
> from the excavation for a new lecture room, and had it well
> dried and sifted. This earth was rich in yellow clay."

With a bandage of waxed tissue paper sufficient to envelop the limb from ankle to knee, Hewson first placed the back of the leg on a layer of clay and then made a correspondingly thick layer around the whole leg. The clay bandage was held in place by a rolled bandage, and the knee was elevated and suspended. The patient was pleased with the success of the earth bandage and everyone in the ward cheered the almost instant deodorization.

During the night some pus had seeped through and after midnight the evil smell returned, but not as offensive as before. Covering the pool of pus next morning with earth immediately stopped the odor once more. Hewson found the clay wet throughout, but saw less evidence of pus than he had expected (Hewson, p. xiv): "The earth looked like it had been wet with water, except where it was directly in contact with the suppurating surfaces, where it had a thick film of pus."

Hewson was not only satisfied with the clay as deodorizer but was impressed with its power to effect a beneficial healing of inflamed ulcerated surfaces. By the 12th day of treatment, the shin opening that had been made to allow escape of pus and clotted blood, showed that the 2 in. ulcer had completely cicatrized.

The second opportunity to try this yellow clay earth came with a patient with painful varicose vein ulcers. Upon receiving a clay bandage, the first thing the patient noticed was that he was greatly relieved of pain each time the ulcers were dressed. It happened so clearly after each dressing change that the conclusion was quite plausible that it was due to the earth. This induced Hewson to try the clay as a primary dressing after an operation, this time it involved the removal of a mammary gland leaving over 40 square inches of open surface. The wound was dressed with an earth bandage. Within seven days the patient was up and about. The wound had closed except for a minor discharge of icorish pus, but that was due to a shred of oakum (fibers) left from the cleaning of the wound of coagula (Hewson, p. xvi).

At the end of his introduction Hewson cites a ten year old letter that the steward W. G. Malin had found in the files, which refers to fullers' earth and to the Eastern custom of using scented clay instead of soap at their toilet as well as to the custom of using earth for ill-conditioned sores. "Perhaps the profession might fear being dubbed mud doctors, but they are unfit for their profession who object to the simplest means which nature offers for restoratives" (Hewson, pp. xvi-xvii).

Hewson was aware that some of his colleagues came not to see what he was doing and how successful he was, but to express their criticism and hostility, sometimes injudiciously in the presence of patients being treated. Hewson responded to this with the following case history:

> "One of the most significant of these cases was that of a
> woman with an epithelial ulcer on the side of her nose. She
> had heard about Hewson's clay work and solicited admission
> and was treated. At first she improved quite rapidly and then a
> lachrymal abscess formed and she became frustrated and
> asked to be discharged. At home the original ulcer began to
> spread again. Not being able to find relief with a variety of
> ointments and being quite despondent, she dug into the subsoil
> of her garden, extracted some, and dried it and applied it to the

sore as had been done in the hospital. At the end of three
weeks she was healed and presented herself to the hospital
(ten miles distance for her) to show her cure by the dry earth."

Before going further into Hewson's case history comments and the modus operandi of the clay treatment, Hewson clarified that at all times when he used "earth", "clay", or such description, he always referred to deeply dug, well-dried but not roasted clay, sifted through a fine flour sieve. "The yellow subsoil is common everywhere in our city and its vicinity, rich in ferruginous clay entirely free of all sand, grit and foreign matter" (Hewson, p. xx).

His case histories total 74, but only a few need to be listed here. The number of the case history in Roman numerals precedes the page number in his book where the case history begins:

II/30: Compound fracture of metacarpal bones with extensive laceration and contusion of soft parts—sulfite of soda without effect on fetor—fetor disappeared under dry earth and complete cicatrisation occurred without bone loss in 22 days.

IV/34: Extensive and deep burns from coal oil—189 days of dry earth dressing with positive relief of pain when earth was dry—decided improvement in ulcers—patient died from exhaustive diarrhea [which might also have been cured by ingestion of the same clay had he but known].

LIX/132: Cauliflower growth on Os uteri with offensive discharge— fetor destroyed by dry clay applied to vagina and renewed at end of four days—ulcer looking less angry but patient declined further treatment "because of something said about her in the ward."

LX/133: Axillary abscess opened and poulticed for two weeks— reopened and filled with white clay—some pain—subsequently dressed with yellow clay—no pain—healed in ten days. [Lacking an analysis and definition of either clay, the color of the clay alone should have had no effect on the case].

Expected and unexpected

In his comments on cases, Hewson addressed first the effect of contact with the earth. He compared other medically approved dressing materials such as bran, carron oil[13] and molasses against the decidedly favorable impressions of patients with the earth dressing (Hewson, p.189). The effect of earth dressing on pain was also salutary with all kinds of wounds whether great or small. The relief continued even when there was an abundant discharge of pus (Hewson, p. 191).

Hewson lauded the deodorizing, distinguishing it from disinfecting. Hewson addresses only the power of earth to destroy "morbid emanations" floating in the air. No measures were taken to arrest the gaseous emanations, but what flowed into a basin was instantly deprived of all odors by the earth. This was demonstrated repeatedly. Hewson also received a comment from a colleague that trials of "earth" as deodorizer in the washing of hands after dissecting and demonstrating upon a cadaver "showed it a complete success"[14] (Hewson, p. 195). As historical aside, Hewson mentioned the habit of certain native inhabitants of America to bury opossum meat for a few days to remove its horribly offensive odor and offers the conjecture that wild animals bury prey and bones to avoid leading scavengers to the meat by its smell. (Hewson, p. 195/196).

Regarding inflammations, Hewson stated firmly that there was no instance when there was any evidence of the earth either provoking or aggravating inflammatory action (Hewson, p. 196). Case history LXXIX was an operation for cancer of the breast. The wound healed without the faintest trace of irritation:

> "...even at the one minute point, where the union did not take place, the hemorrhage which prevented it, may be said to have failed to excite such action, for although there was discoloration, bogginess, and tenderness from the coagulum, there was never any heat or other sign of inflammation (Hewson, p. 197)".

After investigating numerous tests on various soils as to their deodorizing character, there is no doubt that soil has an action upon coloring matters and substances producing the smell of putrid urine. That the power of the soil is in all cases due to the clay contained in it, there is not the slightest doubt (Hewson, p. 233). Trials with sand produced not the same results as white clay. Hewson recalls that alum earths possess ability to combine with coloring matters as is proven in dye-works where it is used as mordant. Since compounds of silica with alumina exist in the clay, Hewson attributes the deodorizing effect of clay to them (Hewson here confuses alum with aluminosilicates, but he recognizes an absorption mechanism.)

Clay under glass

Hewson deduced that what the clay absorbs is the "pathological milk" of pus and then the pus corpuscles become shriveled and disappear. He asked Dr. Tyson to do experiments with pus and clay, without telling him what he, Hewson, had observed. Tyson put a little earth mixed with water on glass slides and added "healthy" or normal fresh pus. Within a few minutes, or seconds even, the pus corpuscles started shriveling and became altered so they would not have been recognized as the remains of corpuscles had they not remained constantly under view. A little later they disappeared altogether. All this happened so fast that the result could not be attributed to desiccation by the minute air spaces, but must be the effect of the clay. (Stumpf or Megele never made this investigation).

Hewson's successful earth treatments were mostly ridiculed by colleagues, even those who had come to observe; thus Hewson's research did not enter the mainstream of curative knowledge. There is no readily discoverable evidence of similar work in the English-speaking world. In Germany, Julius Stumpf had not discovered the record of Hewsons work, it was not reported under foreign news in the prestigious Münchener Medizinische Wochenschrift. Today this title is hard to find on computers because the word "earth" in the search phrase connotes our planetary home instead of a geological substance.

Stumpf was aware of the work by the two German non-medical "healing practitioners" about the last quarter of the 19th century. One was the above-mentioned Sebastian Kneipp, and the other proponent of natural healing was Emanuel Felke (1856-1926), who advocated clay for his regimen of health by the virtues of air, water and earth. His patients or adherents sat naked in shallow pits dug into a meadow and filled with clay, and spread the clay all over their bodies. In the first quarter of the 20th century this method was ameliorated to include treatment indoors.

The 19th century ended thus with Kneipp and Felke, Pettenkofer, Koch and Hewson, but its last years brought also the beginning of the clay treatments of Dr. Julius Stumpf of Würzburg who early in the next century would defeat cholera.

Comments and explanations

[1] Berzelius also discovered the elements cerium (1803, selenium (1817), thorium (1828). He isolated silicon in 1823, discovered zirconium (1824), titanium (1825) as well as aluminum, a constituent of clay as aluminum oxide.

[2] Different striations in the Lemnos clay pit account for occasional reports of Lemnian earth other than red. At the time of my visit the hill was thickly in grass and weeds and even a sample digging was not possible. On most bare surface the clay had a pink-brownish tinge, probably from weathering.

[3] Elsewhere (Reinbacher 1998) the Amazon warrior tribe of women is described as located in Africa in the mysterious kingdom of Monomotape, still shown on maps of Africa in the late 17th century. It extended southward into the Kalahari desert and northward towards the snow mountains of East Africa, where their male children were educated and trained. The female warriors were said to cut off one breast for better shooting of arrows, but I could not get a comment from modern bow-and-arrow societies.

[4] Meyer's Konversations-Lexikon, 4th ed. Leipzig & Vienna, Vol. 5, 1890, under "Exkremente".

[5] Recently I discovered a citation of a report by the city medical office of Montreal (Canada) of 1885 that said that the daily total amount of human solid waste in the city was 170 tons of 374,000 lbs. The population of Montreal in 1900 is reported by the1977 Encyclopedia Britannica as 270,000. This averages about 1.4 lbs per person per day or 0.6. kg/day. Thus the estimate of 0.3 kg/pp/day is not excessive.

[6] No one mentions that toilet paper was not invented until 1857 and not really commercially available until years later. No question is raised by Waring about the addition of toilet paper or equivalent to the value of the "returnable" earth mixture. In many places in this world today, where sewers are not available and septic receptacles not encased, the WC has a waste paper basket for deposition of toilet paper after use so as not to clog the septic tank.

[7] Use of roasted barley as a coffee substitute was quite common among less affluent folk in Germany. During WWI and II the roast barley was replacement for shortages of imported coffee; roasted fig powder was added to make the barley "coffee" look black and richer.

[8] Catholic Encyclopedia: Sebastian Kneipp, available on several search engines.

[9] I have used the 1955 edition of "Mein Testament und Codizill von Sebastian Kneipp", a new commentary by Dr. med Christian Fey, physician in Bad Wörishofen, Ehrenwirt Verlag, Munich.

[10] In 1898 three Italians, Amico Bignami, Giovanni Batista, and Guiseppe Bastaniele first proved that human malaria was transmitted by mosquitoes—actually 200 years after quinine was found to cure it.

[11] This was at different times of the year. Berlin is drier in the summer, Munich often lacked water after completion of the annual snowmelt in late summer and fall.

[12] In the case of cholera, infection with tetanus was not really a concern, since without treatment with clay the prognosis was fatal. For treatment of wound infections, yes, the clay should be sterilized.

[13] 50% linseed oil with 50% lime water, first used in the ironworks of Carron, Scotland.

[14] T.H. Andrews, letter to Hewson, March 7, 1871. A similar hand washing application was described by Burmeister 1912—bolus as slip agent in surgical gloves.

Chapter Fourteen: Earths of the Early 20th Century

We have previously entered the early part of the 20th century with Dr. Julius Stumpf's success with the curing of cholera and the widening acceptance of this therapy by his peers. The clay treatments described by Sebastian Kneipp in 1894 continued effective well into the new century: "In case of varicose veins, bind lower legs with cloth drenched in clay water from ankle to knee, twice a week overnight, to alleviate hardening of the calf due to venous congestion of blood" (Kneipp, 1955, p. 227).

For peat's sake

19th century methods of bandaging wounds before Stumpf's clay application were anointed again when Benade (Benade, 1937) advocated loose dry peat as a bandage material, even though it had been found wanting 50 years earlier. None of Benade's literature references were less than 24 years old at the time, that is: 1913. Early drying tests (see Chapter Four) with peat moss (sphagnum) and with wood shavings (excelsior) had been shown to be inferior to clay as bandage medium (Megele, 1899).

Benade and Teichmann's peat bandaging system (1944) involved finely sifted peat (<0.1 mm particles) mixed with urea, glycerin and distilled water. The cited case histories at best show a cleansing and wound stabilization, but not a healing of wounds, not after 14 or even 120 days. Then they admitted that their peat bandage method cleansed wounds in the short run, but in the long run irritated and "provoked" tissue.

Bandages of moss (Kronacher, 1890) and of peat moss or moss-peat (Miele and Leisrink, 1882) showed that sphagnum dressings would reduce wound infections, but sphagnum was no longer a factor in the 20th century. By 1944, sulfonamides and antibiotics had begun their career as fighters against infections.

Mudpacks and baths did not lose the place in natural healing. Still today "fango" from natural lakeshores or from finely pulverized volcanic rock, sometimes mixed with paraffin to affect a cleaner release from the skin, is the staple for hot treatment of arthritic complaints and general physiotherapy, if only to give temporary relief from chronic pain.

Unsupported research statements

In the aftermath of World War I., political stability was regained and medical research flourished. Clay treatment receded from mainline medical journals to natural healing advocates. Such ill-defined publications as the clay book (*Lehmbuch*, Meyer-Schlatterer, no publication date given) took up the promotion of clay treatments. The book's preface cites Hippocrates "Do not shy away from asking the common man whether a thing is useful as medication", but in its second argument states a non-sequitur: "It would be highly unusual if peoples who built houses from clay, made bricks from clay and wrote on clay tablets should not have known the healing power of clay". This ignores that clays or earths evolved as medicines together with plants and animal products in many areas of the populated world where there were no great rivers, where people did not built houses of mud and where they did not write on clay tablets.

The problem with early 20th century natural healing publications is that diseases considered treatable are expanded ("nervous" digestion, bladder and kidney "problems") to include all categories of complaints: gall bladder and liver infections, lung and bone tuberculosis, inner inflammations and exterior eczemas of all sorts, diabetes and arthrosis. Even after failure of cure and resultant death, it was suggested to hide some wet clay under the shroud to reduce the smell of the decaying body.

Drinking a mixture of clay and water was promoted for cure of stomach and intestinal catarrhs as Stumpf had successfully done, but now clay was also suggested for constipation, excessive flatulence, and to remove "slag remnants" from the body (*Schlackenausscheidung*). There was even a suggestion in the *Lehmbuch* to drink clay water with buttermilk against appendicitis.

Abbreviated research

All these claims were supported by statements of "abbreviated" patients, i.e. ABC from Bonn or DEF from Hamburg. Reference was made to unreachable experts such as "I believe it was said by a health councilor in Berlin", and even the treating doctors were hidden behind initials. There is no way to check the validity of a claim, particularly not when it is shrouded in the oxymoronic statement "I have had someone tell me that..." implying an incognito source of unproven knowledge, never revealed. Similar to many present-day natural herb medicines, one can neither reliably pinpoint maximum dosages nor a specific claim for cure, just opinions by ephemeral people.

In cases of chronic kidney inflammations, the Lehmbuch suggests flannel bandages (shades of another century) and cooling clay packs, but only after (!) all causes of the inflammation have been eradicated which is the job of the physician (!). The 6th edition of the Lehmbuch mentions a testimonial on page 71 dated to 1927. In part II, the sales pitch for a new AION A "earth"[1] in a newspaper article from 1948 is cited. Thus the Lehmbuch contentions fall into the revival period for clay between 1927 and 1948.

A publication about healing earth by a geologist and a pharmacologist (Röpke and Peyer 1927), after acknowledging that the term "healing earth" was coined by a company called Luvos in Blankenburg (Germany), discusses new offerings of curative earths, all either of the bolus group or the loess group. Three earths, identified as "Jusch" yellow, gray, and brown, are weathering products of sandstone relatively rich in aluminum oxide. "Dr. Hähle's healing earth" is fairly pure silicon dioxide such as from the island of Milos. Two earths, *Hannosol* and *Medizinalerde* are loess products, the latter one with a higher calcium content is dug from loess washed down from the mountains into lake deposits. "Terra nova" earth has an iron oxide coating rather than quartz. The healing earth "Luvos" has no taste, a minimal smell, consists of 70% (crystalline) silicon dioxide and 9% aluminum oxide.

Röpke added two earth preparations made by a manufacturing company in Stuttgart. They were basically loess with herbs added, called "earth power", and typed as #1 for eye maladies, #2 for blood cleansing (!), #3 for lung illnesses, #12 for dropsy, #21 for goiter problems. Röpke found sugar, linseed, and senna leaves in #2. These mixtures fell under an imperial ordinance and could only be sold by licensed pharmacies, but did not need a prescription. An "earth power skin cream" was exempt from any dispensing restriction because it made no healing claims.

In 1928 Röpke distinguished between bolus and loess by classifying bolus in the Al_2O_3 or SiO_2 (or both) containing group, and loess, with its fine covering of quartz dust blown off ground moraines after the ice sheet retreated, in a separate group. Röpke states that loess would not cause coproliths (intestinal blockages). Over a decade later Jung (1939 and 1948) is the only one raising the specter of coproliths that were not observed in clinical practice with bolus or loess[2].

Kunze and Vogel (1936) stated that loess neutralizes less stomach acid than clay and thus leaves some stomach acid to aid digestion, another marketing oxymoron: If diarrhea indicates use of clay, it is not concerned with digestion in the first place, but with elimination of pathogens. Adolf Just promoted it mainly in his treatment spa *Jungborn*. In his theory, even though he did not know "under which specific conditions the body works", it appears possible that earths can physiologically add minerals in solution (see also Volkheimer, 1933). The then favored "radioactivity" property actually was weak in evidence and well below any biological effect and was not mentioned again in medicine other than as a general scourge of mankind.

Kunze and Vogel correctly claim that bolus is a weak acid, essentially neutral and totally useless for stomach acid neutralization, but that calcium carbonate excels very much in this property. Excrement analysis showed possible adsorption of intestinal poisons such as phenol, creosol, indol, skatol, kadaverin and putrescin. It didn't help the promotion of Jung's loess product Luvos *Pro-Terra*.

The promotion of clay and loess products in medicine was eclipsed by other medical innovations, which made the former a lesser choice of treatment. However, during the first quarter of the 20th century, clay was firmly ensconced in the pharmaceutical environment. The American Pharmaceutical Association and National Formulary (Chicago Branch, 1908), after first denouncing private proprietary specialties with superior claims and little tangible evidence for them, listed *Cataplasma kaolini* as an antiseptic clay paste similar to like products marketed under the names Antiphlogistine, Anydrosine, Thermofuge, Thermaline, Unguentum terralis, all secret nostrums which had to be taken on trust. Few patients were aware of their mineral nature.

In Germany the 1919 edition of Hager's Handbook of Pharmaceutical Praxis (Hager, 1919) still listed Lemnian earth, miraculous earth (from Saxony), Armenian earth, *Bolus alba* and *rubra, terra argillacea pura, terra infusoria,* and *terra ponderosa* and gave their names in four languages: Latin, German, English and French. The pharmacopoeia of Japan of 1927 listed the minerals or earths called potassium alum, copper alum, borax, burnt gypsum (exsiccated calcium sulfate), prepared chalk, magnesium oxide, liquid tar ointment, talc and *Bolus alba.*

The only "new" earth beyond these is an amorphous (precipitated) silicon dioxide anhydride, which will be discussed in Chapter Sixteen on new research.

Comments and explanations

[1] *Lehmbuch*, p. 87 translated:…besides the proven clay earths known to us today, such as "Meyer-Schlatter" clay and "Anliker" clay, Just's "Luvos" and "Hähle's medicinal earths" another product, a powdered species of stone—prepared in Switzerland—caused talk by its "amazing successes". This new substance that has not only the known effects of clay, but in addition the efficaciousness of the Baden healing spring waters, is called AION A. Since this stone powder is found near a "healing water" spring, it was believed that the stone embodies the healing power of the water in concentrated form and has the ability to premeate the skin. [An analogy to astrological pronouncements is fairly evident and of equal believability.]

[2] Most likely one would choke to death trying to swallow a mouthful of dry clay before any coproliths even mattered. In his self-tests Stumpf once almost choked to death because he ate fine dry clay that not only invaded his lungs as dust but started clotting to a hard mass in his oesophagus.

Chapter Fifteen: Healing Water, Healing Mud

Since prehistory, humans and animals have searched for mineral waters as a curative for agues and pains. The mineral waters from both warm and cold springs contain combinations of one or more minerals. Some springs have mostly sodium chloride (86%), others are high in carbon dioxide (60%), most of them have combinations of several ingredients. In Germany, as many as 11% of the waters contain iron, 15% fluor, 11% iodine, and 28% of them sulfur. All contain calcium or sodium in various combinations[1].

Humans and animals have long used mud baths (mud wallows) to achieve amelioration of specific health problems, usually eczemas and escape from insects. Both humans and animals searched for hot mud to relieve arthritic pains, sore muscles, and pains of injuries.

Zedler knows everything

A monumental work of historical detail, written and assembled, during almost the entire first half of the 18th century, is the "great complete universal lexicon" of Johann Zedler, 65 folio-size volumes of indeed anything worth knowing then: history of people and peoples, locations and happenings, current sciences summarized, and the knowledge explained. Each volume has about 1,500 pages of two columns of about 750 words, all volumes together over fifty million words. Among its subjects is the devil, the making of soap, healing baths and their medical effectiveness since long before 1750.

Bathing in health-giving waters of natural springs was equally important as taking mineral medication from solid earths, mainly because spring waters pass through mineral layers and pick up mineral particles that are endowed by the local people with a belief in a variety of cures or treatments. Springs or wells that come forth after passing through or near veins of antimony or gold were said to be efficacious in curing eczemas and sprained limbs (Zedler, Bäder, Vol. B., cols. 1305 ff). Those having been enriched with silver (mercury?), called *Mercuriales* (ibid, col. 1307) help heal open wounds and ulcers. Spring waters containing salts address gout, cramps, cold and wet limbs, infertility and like complaints. The relationship between the mineral content of a spring and the illnesses it cures has always been—and still is today—mostly conjecture based on perceived benefits for the economy of the town where the bath is located.

Sulfurous waters attack stomach ailments, liver complaints, pains in the loin and uterus. They "correct" illness of the spleen, stomach, eyes and ears. Alum waters help blood circulation and the "golden artery" (hemorrhoids), minimize belching, relieve constipation of the liver and spleen, dissolve bladder stones, reduce spitting blood, and treat all "cold fluxes."

Chemists, Zedler says, are trying to determine what affects the cures. They boil the waters to see what sediments they create. They distill the waters and add oils and spirits. They use scales to determine heaviness or lightness (as the reader recalls, they were then two different properties).

Zedler divides health-promoting bathing into dry (*sicca*) and wet (*humida)* baths. Dry baths are immersions in ashes, common salt, or sand. Wet baths are divided into steam baths (*vaporoso*) and into tub baths (*aquosa*). The water in either may be improved with boiled herbs, roots, flowers or seeds from which the vapor is desired. There may be 20-50 ingredients in medicated steam. Tub baths were divided into those with natural waters (*naturales*) and, again, those with added secret herbs and spices for specific curative effects (*artificiales*).

The "balneum" is a sitting bath in a tub, usually up to the navel. Doctors of physick were given to patenting bath prescriptions for specific ailments (though no two of them ever agreed on even the key ingredients), but the natural springs were the ones marketed to the people. Then patients might be offered Mynsicht's sleep-promoting bath, Rolfinck's sweat box, Rondeletti's nerve-steeling bath, or Gockel's bath to remove kidney and bladder stones: "It will help if the patient has taken "stone-breaking" medication before the bath and continues to take it during the often lengthy immersion". Even five hours of bathing per session were not considered excessively long.

By 1750 (and a good while thereafter) baths were mostly segregated by sex and rank: There were baths for nobility, baths for gentle persons and baths for the burgher. Further, the same classifications of baths existed for noble ladies, gentlewives and common women. Some facilities were set aside for the poor people as sort of a social contribution. There were baths for noble men's horses and probably baths for the noble ladies' pets, too. Some baths were accessible only by steep climbs down ladders glued to steep rocks; others were readily visited on river embankments or higher meadows bordered by the forests' shadow.

Bath towns come and go

Every community hired experts and hoped for the assets of a "verified", "certified", or even a "licensed" health spring and could then advertise. It would add to the towns' coffers, provide employment and income for the citizens who could provide room and board for the bathers. Popular physicians were engaged to judge the medical value of the waters. The trade also firmly maintained that health waters could not be bottled, since they lose their potency shortly after opening the bottle due to the shaking of the bottle in transit, which perturbs its medical value[2]. This helped to establish famous "baths" and the contention that such a bath cure there (including drinking the water) needed to be repeated at least twice a year. The arrival of famous people "to take the cure" enhanced the reputation of the bathing town. They expanded curing visits to a healthy local climate if they had no mineral springs or local peat or mud. This community involvement was essentially the same as for newly found earths since the importance of provenance made the location site more popular and hopefully attracted more affluent clients. Typical examples are the health spa of Pyrmont in lower Saxony, the Seltzer wells and the source of Schwalbach water. Often these waters were mixed with wine to make the water more palatable for ingestion. Doctors recommended "promenades" in between, gentle walking that most likely also helped the local businesses. It is generally known even today that those seeking loss of weight eat special (expensive) diets in the morning, and during the afternoon perambulations gorge on fancy baked goods and whipped cream in the ubiquitous cafés. The luxuries and amenities varied and were priced accordingly. Towns that had prominent spas and later also rail service (for instance, Baden-Baden, Wiesbaden, Aix-les-Bains) had great advantages to attract affluent visitors.

In this sense of pride in the community health wells, it was also widely disseminated that chemists cannot artificially reproduce natural waters with the same quality, strength, and virtues (Zedler, Bäder, col. 1308) because the "particles" in the water are too small and too effervescent to be analyzed and because the unknown factor of earth's internal heat on the mineral waters is indeterminable (ibid, col. 1309).

Health wells

The health wells usually were accompanied by a story on how they were created: In the hamlet of Hornhausen, during a strong rainstorm, a rivulet or creek in town washed away a wooden pier. When the local shepherd tried to fix it, he found a deep cavity filled with greenish water. The usual community leaders, priest, and teacher, and mayor, inspected it and had the water in the hole bailed out until they found a clear and thus obviously healthy water spring. This was followed by a report of a woman who had been suffering from terrible abdominal difficulties and could only walk on crutches. She heard about the new health well, went there with a large pitcher. She prayed and then confidently drank a pitcher full of the water at the well and took another pitcher full home with her. She was comfortable at night, felt better in the morning. Daily she returned to the well, prayed and drank of the water. She passed bloody urine and calcified material, and soon she was able to walk without crutches. A counter argument arose saying that nitrous salts had been found all around Hornhausen and the "terrae nitrositate" contained alum, a laxative salt, saltpeter, and liquid bitumen. Thereupon the curative powers increased in the advertisements, now included help for arthritis, convulsions, fevers and cleansing of "bad harm".

The health well of Hornhausen enjoyed public acclaim in 1647, was forgotten until 1687, and was discovered a third time in 1718. People wondered why the flow of the well ceased at times for years on end[3]. Beggars found more alms from local people when they claimed they had come for the waters to cure them, and therefore had to quit their work back home. One complaint was that one of what by now were 14 different wells in town was at the side and below the wall of a cow barn and that the healing water smelled and tasted heavily of ammonia.

In spa villages[4] many citizen made room and board available to visitors for drinking cures or bathing. A whole medical specialty "bath or bathing doctor, balneologue" developed among whose members competition was fierce (and still is today). Testimony by competing physicians about the healing earth waters of a well could be diametrically opposed. Statements of relief alternated with those of no help.

Within the mass of approximately 1,000 bath towns in Germany alone by the end of the 19th century, all vetted by the imperial bath authorities, it is not difficult to find baths that had similar minerals as people had found in earths. The German word *Kur* can be translated as "cure" but in a modern sense, that is, since the demise of the Middle Ages, it means to go to a bath town to be cleansed by the waters (internally or externally) generally once or twice a year. This health period, the "Kur", was recognized as acceptable claim by the majority of government health insurances and was not charged against vacation time by the employer. Health spas generally had the town name prefix or suffix "Bad", like: Bad Orb or Schinznach-Bad. The Latin original of "Kur" is cura, which expresses the need to pay attention to well being, to care for, called wellness today.

In the 17th century, the Swiss town named Schinznach-Bad in the canton of Bern, situated on the river Aar, not far from the city of Brug, was known for its mineral springs. It boasted of delightful warm health-giving waters. Jacob Ziegler (1663) of Zurich first described the minerals involved. Ziegler, a physician, himself tested the waters and found that they extracted minerals during its course underground such as gold, iron, lead, vitriol, salt, sulfur, alum, terra sigillata and asphalt, a veritable liquid geopharmacy.

"Gold is the strongest and most perfect mineral, helps internally and externally and thus strengthens the nature, takes away vertigo and absurdity, cures melancholy and sadness, epilepsy, pluralgia, heart ache and unconsciousness. Gold aids lame limbs, fills the queasy stomach, cleans the blood and resists fevers. It cures intertrigo, scabies, eczemas and it battles dropsy and jaundice" (Ziegler, 1663).

Iron was said to dry out open wounds and ulcers and to stop fluxes of the stomach, liver and spleen. Lead was favored since Galen to heal putrid "old harm", fistulas, and to reduce fever, to improve the face, to take away heat of infections and swellings. Lead cures injury from high fever, hot oil, hot water, gunpowder and the like.

Vitriols warm or dry out or still or pull together. They strengthen the stomach, eject worms. They dissolve and remove sand and gravel from kidney stones. Sulfur in the waters cures everything else plus bites from rabid dogs, and it is a good way to open the pores of podagra.

Bathing cures (almost) everything

The most prominent ingredients of this water are the bath salts that renew the entire person, make everything taste better, reduce three-day-fevers and gallic (venereal) diseases. Alum cures old wounds, closes open wounds, and heals ulcers, cleans the mouth cavity and thus cures rotting teeth and improves stinking breath. These ailments are frequently transcribed from antiquity to modern times.

Terra sigillata, internally, strengthens heart, brain and liver. It promotes perspiration, heals "congelated" blood, bee stings and poisonous scorpion bites. Asphaltum opens fluxes and strengthens, warms, softens and improves ulcers and "open damages." With his claims, Ziegler was very persuasive.

One concern of the Jesuit scientist Athanasius Kircher was that obviously the mineral waters flow down to the ocean that already has become very salty since the creation. It is further polluted by fish excrement, black amber, bitumen and agstein (confused with amber, succinum). He then propounded a theory of the recirculation of water that required the return of ocean waters to the mountains. In his *Mundus subterraneous* of 1665 he drew a map of Africa where all ocean waters returned to a huge under-the-mountain lake called *hydrophylacium* from where the springs of all the African rivers were fed with new water. A similar mechanism must exist in all other parts of the world, wrote Kircher.

The Swiss physician, author, and naturalist Johann Jakob Scheuchzer (1717), wrote about Schinznach-Bad in the second part of his Natural History of Switzerland. His somewhat more modern analysis still confirms the previously mentioned minerals in the water. A curious matter, other than the expanded descriptions of what the waters are good for, are purported case histories to support the apparent qualities of "the waters": They are inexplicably few:

1695: One gentleman from Zurich cured of "weak limbs".

1697: Two gentlemen from Basel, one cured of sciatica, the other cure unknown.

1698: A lady cured of arthritis

1700: A gentleman from Basel (?),

1706: A pastor cured of gas in the stomach, a nobleman cured of heartburn, a case of kidney cleansing, a burgher from Niedau (?), a gentleman from Büren (?), a gentleman from Bern cured of sciatica.

1707: A case of cleansing kidneys.

It is doubtful that Schinznach-Bad survived on only twelve clients in twelve years. There are no reports in libraries between 1763 (a doctoral dissertation was written then) and 1852 (Amsler, 1865). But then, keep in mind, Schinznach Bad was almost 11 hours distant by coach from Basel, from Bern 16 ½ hours, from Lausanne 33 hours. The water of the spring contained a high value of sodium chloride. The sulfur component could cause annoying sulfur smells during inclement weather. Water temperature was recorded as 36° Celsius, 28.4° Réaumur., or 96° Fahrenheit. Amsler's booklet gives successful case histories of chronic skin diseases, gout, scrofula and rachitis (rickets), joint pains. An unusual side of this spa report is that it does specify when the waters could be deleterious: internal infections, various "old" or chronic conditions, pregnancy from the fourth month on, and great care and supervision for those very young and very old. The report also points out that some bathers could develop an allergy or other reaction to the sulfurous salty water, eye irritations from steam bath vapors, and, though rarely, development of furunculous skin conditions.

But we are getting ahead of our general chronology here. In the Middle Ages bathing in town or village pool was often a virtual coeducational community affair with music, food (as much as a dozen eggs eaten in 6 hours are mentioned) and occasional erotic activities (Pictorius, 1650). Cold spring waters were used only for brief dipping in a natural pool; in naturally and artificially warm waters the bath might take hours or days. Frequently used for bathing were tubs or pools where the water was mixed with aromatic herbs.

Pools of mineral waters frequently invited tempted bathers to use this opportunity to cuckold their spouses. Some public baths lost their licenses when they permitted gambling, rough behavior, drunken screaming and excessive sex. After too many complaints, sometimes the sexes were again segregated by dividing the pool into gender specific halves to regain the bath license. Part of the bathing ritual was rubbing the body with wood ash lye (soap was unknown then) by bath maidens and bath lads. Frequently bloodletting was practiced by the cupping method, sort of a mechanical leech, in a hut by the pool side: Bathing in warm water dilated the blood vessels and supposedly made the bloodletting easier. Medical advantages of bathing were published frequently in medieval times[5].

In modern times, though, the "cure" or "Kur" was taken as an annual toning up or "system refreshment" rather than as a specific course of treatment. That is why all spas advertised the cultural amenities and the beauty of their surroundings. One could promenade along the esplanade and at the beautiful drinking well take several glasses of the mineral water while passing it in one or the other direction. Old woodcuts only hint at other entertainment. The waters remained a popular vacation at insurance expense.

By 1933 a journal "Der Balneologe" appeared in Germany, and about the same time the International Society of Medical Hydrology was founded. From it we can try to glean some of the then scientifically examined bath benefits. Looking at the journal (Balneologe, 1937, # 2, p. 39f) we encounter the society. Its most pressing problem was to judge the efficaciousness and dangers of bathing in radioactive waters (radon). One knew that there probably was a problem with dosage of radium emanation, and one tried to understand how much was beneficial, at least which doses were stimulating to the body and which were deleterious, but the society swept it under the rug, because most bath towns had no way of measuring that.

An Eastern European physician compared radon exposure to light ray exposure and supposed that these rays, too, changed physiologically ineffective forms of inorganic and organic bodies to an active form (?). Then it was considered that naturally radioactive sources of water might also contain still unknown materials with biological effects, and that different individuals could be affected differently. Therefore, it is not enough to know the exact composition of the springs, but the sensitivity of patients to allergies must also be explored.

Attempts to put science into bathing

Almost every representative of a bath town at the hydrology meeting would maintain that his town's water was a different type and could not fall under any attempted classifications. The Prussian government physician Benade appointed himself the watchdog of nomenclature. Bathing as a cure became big business and called numerous societies into life, such as the Association of German Spa towns (Deutscher Bäder Verband), a society of bath- and climate-healing, and in due course, by the mid-1930s, the International Society of Medical Hydrologists. It appears that by 1937/8 this society had operated a Peloid Committee. Whatever the committee decided, it continuously ran afoul of Benade, who knew everything better. Eventually he succeeded so well that the Peloid Committee was disbanded by the society shortly after the definition "a dry material obtained by drying a natural peloid may be described as a "dried peloid" was proposed for consideration. (Lewis, 1938, p.76).

Lewis decided to determine what a peloid actually was besides a refuge in Latin. Intended as a generic name for all kinds of mud and peat, the Council of Medical Hydrology decided that "a peloid is any naturally produced medium consisting of uniform mixture of finely divided organic and/or inorganic solid matter and water, such as is applicable in medical practice as a cataplasm for external treatment". This immediately raised the question whether a peloid was still a peloid if the water was added later, such as for a mud or peat bath. The answer was: no. Then was added the requirement that the peloid must be of geological origin, but the multinational committee (representing Sarasota Springs, Berlin, Bath, Talinn, London, Dax, Wiesbaden, Vienna, Prague, Lisbon, Florence, Buxton, Pistany, Bloemfontein, Odessa, Belgrade, Héviz-Fürdö, Sofia, Breslau, now Wroclaw, among others), decided that "all information shall either (!) be scientifically sound or be firmly established and acceptable in all countries". The same international committee decided at the same time that it is apparent that a strict classification (as propounded by Benade) was neither possible nor desirable.

The Champion of Mud

First Benade (1937) created the distinction between "healing sediments" and "healing earths." Then he split each into those with preponderantly mineral content and those with preponderantly organic substances. The organic substances he collected under the heading of "concretum vegetabile", the inorganic ones as "lutum", which in turn was divided into lutum naturale thermale (an inorganic healing substance created by a thermal spring), lutum naturale thermalisatum (not a thermal mud, but minerals mixed with thermal water), lutum naturale simplex (the sediment not within a thermal spring) and lutum artefactum commune (it does not occur in nature, supposing this to be, for instance, a mixture of volcanic ash, peat, and thermal water as is available in Calistoga, California). Benade seems to have got lost in the finer points of meaninglessness.

His suggestions caused an outcry that not all therapeutic sediments or earths exist in the form of a mud, but Benade insisted that if it is not a mud, don't call it mud (Schlamm). The difference between healing sediments and healing earths is that the former is an underwater deposit and the latter a weathering product. Sediments he divided into bioliths and abioliths[6], and those again into kaustabioliths (of plant origin, can be burned when dry; they contain mineral substances besides organic carbon) and akaustabioliths. Kaustabioliths are either peat (humolith, such as from a flat moor, forest moor, high moor, but always mostly moor earth and weathered mineral rich peat), or organic mud (Saprolith). Akaustabioliths are low-tide muds, riverine muds, and calcium products such as chalk. Among the abioliths are clay, sand, and gravel.

In 1938 Benade faced considerable criticism, because he proposed a further change of the peloid definition to divide peloids into natural and artificial peloids, but kept under natural those to which water had been added, as long as there had not been any additional preparation of the mud. But Benade added the subdivision of "healing mud" which is not only any material in mud form naturally wet, but also those, which are no longer wet in nature. Benade was into precisity.

From a medical hydrology point of view the not so surprising major conclusion of the Peloid Committee was that there is no way to classify muds as to their therapeutic value. Almost everywhere in the world mud baths and fango packs still exist, and probably from the benefit perceived by the patient, are therapeutically of value even if it is primarily the feeling of soft warmth after physiotherapy.

Steel waters run deep

One of the more curious preparations of bath water was the "steel water." One immersed a red hot rod of iron into a bucket of water to make this steel water. One much broader version is the creation of mine slag water (*Schlackenwasser*) near active iron and copper mines. In the literature it surfaced in 1855 in the journal "Balneologische Zeitung" published by the German Society for Hydrology as internal house organ. Erlenmeyer (1855) appears first as researcher into application of slag water to baths. First of all, the "slag baths" had to be near mines or smelters and that was usually not close to towns, so special bathing facilities had to be built and access to them had to be provided. From the smelter came the hot slag of which cake-like pieces were immediately thrown into a bucket of cold water: Steam rises up, water bubbles, the slag becomes porous like pumice. The water turns grayish. It was either carried to the bath cabinets immediately or reheated later. "A prominent chemist whose name I shall leave out for the time being (!) was kind enough to analyze the slag water and found siliceous iron, siliceous manganese, and much sulfur iron. Illnesses for which the slag bath is beneficial are (1) conditions arising from anemia and (2) conditions arising by profuse shedding of outer skin and mucous membranes, such as heavy perspiring, especially night sweats, eliminations from the vaginal mucous membranes, fluor albus (white flux), mucous hemorrhoids and other chronic catarrhs."

Slag bath case histories

As case histories Erlenmeyer presents a female patient of 53 years of age with advanced hysteria based on anemia. "She refused to take food (the throat felt restricted), her stomach had a lining (?), affectations of the vagus annoyed her and led to mental instability." To improve the mixture of her blood she was given iron preparations that did not help. Daily bathing in slag water cured her. "A young sensitive girl who suffered constantly from neuralgia of all kinds had a soft, richly shedding skin that caused her to perspire day and night. Bathing in slag water cured her".

Erlenmeyer continues to list possible applications for slag baths, such as digestive illnesses, discharges from all branches of the mucous membrane system, slow blood circulation in the veins of lower extremities and lower abdomen, illnesses of gallbladder, imbalance of intestinal juices, urinary gravel, anemia resulting from previous bouts with typhus, cholera, difficult birthing, loss of blood, muscle weaknesses, abnormal menstruation, stomach ailments, migraines, hypochondria, hysteria, and others. This leaves the dry comment that "contra-indications against the use of this bath are obviously none".

A year later Rupprecht (1856) reported on a slag water bath near Hettstedt. It was near a copper mine. Since the mined material contained a lot of bitumen, the raw ore was roasted over wood to melt and remove the bitumen. This produced a residue of 3-3½ % copper and some silver. The average amounts of other minerals were about 50% silicic acid, 12% clay, 20% calcium earth, 13% ferric suboxides and traces of vanadium and molybdenum. Results varied little between six different mines or shafts.

The slag, after burning out the bitumen, was at a temperature of 350-600° C. It was cooled off in a tank or pond. The mineral content was similar to the above percentage. The suggested indications for the slag baths were the same as are mentioned above, but early mental weakness, memory and "abating of male prowess" were added.

In addition to the benefits of the slag baths, it was recommended that patients seek out the smoke of the smelters to achieve easier expectoration and healing of their "grief". Equally favored were pleasant accommodations, hearty but inexpensive meals, sources of sumptuous coffee and cake combinations (probably including the *Konditorei*), and the availability of steam wagons to all destinations.

Moor and Mud Bathing

A second kind of medicinal bathing was promoted by availability of ancient bog material, in general peat. Peat-moss and moss-peat were distinguished from each other, peat-moss being the ancient, black, dry peat, and the moss-peat being primarily that created from the decomposition of sphagnum. In the early 1880s it was sewn into muslin bags and pressed against wounds to absorb wound secretions (Mielek and Leisrink, 1882). These gentle moss pillows replaced cotton pads when held in place by muslin bandages. The authors pointed out that it reduced wound odor, and in their experiments, they did not encounter a septic reaction. Two years later, Kronacher (1890) experimented with sphagnum, cotton, and wood wool to find that sphagnum with cotton adsorbed 22 times the original weight in five hours, continued adsorbing for 20 hours more than moss, cotton, or wood-wool by itself. The use of moss-peat as basic medium for medicinal bathing benefited from the moisture retention, the reliability of asepsis and also the slower loss of heat than with a mineral water bath.

The final type of spa bathing is the schlick type. *Schlick* in German is "gently flowing river mud", the very fine particle black-bluish clay layer exposed when ocean tides recede in low water depth areas such as the continental North Sea coastal shelves and river estuaries or the Russian Black Sea coast. The nature of the medium suggests that schlick baths are can be combined with the normal toning up cure of a sea shore environment.

Generally the water content of schlick is between 50 and 60%. Its heat retention is several times as long as that of water. Additionally it appears (Souci, 1937) that with schlick, too, the human organism can tolerate much higher bathing temperatures than in water. Depending upon the source of the aluminum silicate, the clay may contain additional minerals such as iron or calcium, which might actually enhance one schlick bath over the other (at least promoters say so in their brochure.)

Almost everywhere, the bath industry is in decline. Especially in Germany the health insurance companies, except in rare circumstance, do not pay for bath cures any more and the towns and hamlets having built their prosperity on medical purpose bathing are facing severe recession. Furthermore, even if bath-cure aficionados are financially healthy, they elect other forms of vacation locations than spending all or part of their accrued vacation time in a sleepy little village, when for an equal amount they can undertake charter flight vacations in salubrious exotic climates. Modern man and his automobile allow a wider range of bath town choices. An operator of a hotel in a well-known spa town in Germany reflects that for what people would spend for a week in his hotel, they can fly by charter to a Turkish resort and stay there longer[7]. Repeat customers, often the elderly, who chose one town and then come there each year, now even have a wider non-regional choice of a cure or bath town (Kurstadt) by traveling on the very high speed trains and by sending ahead luggage by the official courier companies. But there are fewer elderly customers every year who still have the Kur habit.

Not much has changed on the way to the 21st century. Using Germany as an example, the bathing or "curing" ritual, though no longer financed by the insurance companies, continues to exist in about 350 communities divided into sea water spas, mineral water spas, mud baths and "moor" baths and Kneipp water baths. The majority of these locations is found in and about middle mountain ranges and along the alpine slopes, except, of course, the sea water spas along Germany's coast on the Northern and the Baltic Seas. With the fierce competition for the aching aging population attracted to spas, sea water cures are renamed "thalasso cures" (thalasso is Greek for sea water, nothing else). Moor spas brag about their local kind of moor, when actually (a) moor is only a location and not the product found there, which is peat, and (b) due to natural environment concerns cutting peat has been prohibited in many moors. Peat is now shipped in from as much as 500 km away. As mud for baths and packs the term of endearment is "fango" (Italian for mud, fare i fanghi: to take the mud bath cure). "Fango" can be mud from the shores of mountain lakes drying out (*Eifelfango*), mud from riverbanks and sea shores (schlick), with or without added chemicals from sulfurous or other mineral springs. One patented version is volcanic fango ground finely from specific sites (*Vulkanit*) or fango ground from slate (*Jura fango*). Other countries, notably Japan, England, have similar histories of the bathing ritual.

Packaged brand-name clay mud mixed with paraffin is sold to physiotherapists to warm afflicted body sections with mud at the end of a treatment, but for physiotherapy few clients spend hotel time in a far distant location. In my youth, I was sent every June to an ocean spa to minimize my annual hay fever. It might have helped better if I had known I was accommodated to a thalasso cure.

Comments and explanations

[1] Deutscher Bäderkalender 1999, Deutscher Bäderverband, Bonn

[2] In Germany, still today, different health regulations govern waters available at spas, and bottled waters.

[3] During the "little ice age" (1450-1700) unusually heavy precipitation could have changed run-off and spring patterns more than the drier time through 2000.

[4] The word spa derives from the Belgian town Spa renowned for its baths.

[5] Pictorius cites almost every famous classic and medieval doctor: Avicenna, Aristotle, Averroës, Constantin the African, Dioscorides, Galen, Isidor of Seville, etc.

[6] If the sediment contained remnants of fossilized plants and animals.

[7] Personal communication from Dieter Adt, Hotel Orbtal, Bad Orb (Germany)

Chapter Sixteen: Research into the 21st Century

In the 20th century research into the history of *terrae medicinalis* and into the mechanics of clay healing continued. Though Stumpf's involvement took the reader past the first quarter of the 20th century, and the description of new earths and the story of earth in balneology is still ongoing, the following review on healing earths begins at the XIIIth Congress of Medicine in London.

Thompson in 1914

At this congress C. J. S. Thompson (1914) gave an independent paper in the section on the history of medicine under the title of "Terra sigillata, a famous medicament of ancient times." In 1912 Stumpf's success with wound healing and curing cholera was well known in Germany. The clouds of WW I had not yet gathered on the European horizon. Unfamiliar with Stumpf's work, Thompson opined "we must conclude that its [terra sigillata] virtues, like those of many ancient remedies, were chiefly due to the mystery surrounding its origin and the superstitions connected with its source." In the 20th century, both Thompson and later Priesner are surrounded by passive ignorance in many published histories of medicine.

Thompson correctly cites both Dioscorides and Galen about Lemnian earth, but leaves it to the reader to realize where Dioscorides was in error: The Lemnian earth is not mixed with goats' blood, and the site where the earth was dug by the priestesses of Artemis is not the side which is marshy in summer, but red and bare. Since Thompson apparently was learned in classical Greek or had an excellent translation of Galen's Virtues of Simples at hand, I thus cite Galen with all due credit:

"I was given a book written by one of that country, in which all the virtues and uses of Lemnian earth are given. I was pleased to experiment with them and took away with me 20,000 of these seals. The person who gave me the book, and who was one of the most important men on the island, used the medicament for many purposes, such as ulcers that were slow in healing, and against bites of snakes and other animals. He advised me to administer the earth after and not before poisons. He stated that he had experimented with Terra sigillata mixed with juniper as an emetic. I have used this in cases where people have been suspected of having eaten cantharides [Spanish Fly] and sea hare [Aplysia depilans, a mollusk] and as soon as they had taken a potion composed of Lemnian earth they vomited everything so they escaped the consequences of these poisons although they had eaten of both. I do not know whether the potion made of juniper and

terra sigillata has the same effects against deadly poisons, but
Hephaistos affirmed it for a certainty".

A question appears in a related text of Galen when he talks about Armenian bole. The person giving it to him called it Armenian stone, yet Galen's description is not that of the vitriol stone but of Armenian bole, i.e. clay. Possibly it is a mistranslation, the two substances could not be confused by their appearance.

Thompson, who has neither bibliography nor footnotes in his paper, cites Bartholomaeus Anglicus from a 13th century manuscript, but it appears to be a 1532 version of "Batman upon Bartholome, his booke, De Proprietatibus rerum, newly corrected, enlarged and ammended." It contains the lauding description of an earth "somedeal white, well smellynge and clere which Dioscorides calleth it *Terra Saracenica* and *argentea"*. The descriptive adjective *Saracenica,* however, does not appear in two translations of Dioscorides and is rather a name applied during the Middle Ages when Arabs and Turks, then called Saracenes[1], occupied Lemnos and took over marketing of the sealed earth.

For the proposal that the Lemnian earth was dug near Kotchinas (today's Kotsinas), Thompson cites Pierre Belon (1517?-1564) who describes a deep cave entrance which apparently did not exist in Galen's time, but Belon's location description appears the same as I found it in 2000 with the exception that in August the hill was red, dry and bare, whereas in May (the time of my visit) it was covered with high grasses and weeds about to dry out, and the right Agiochoma spring was still running. Of the two springs, Belon said, the left one dries out, the right one continues to sicker into the earth making a marshy trail downhill.

Tozer (1890 p. 261) confirms Belon's description regarding the hillside called Agiochoma (sacred earth) that is but the faintest remnant of the prehistoric volcano Mosychlos, where Fredrick (1906) erred. "On the hillside were two fountains, of which the one on the right hand ascent was perennial [it fills a bovine drinking trough now] and the left dries up in summer time [it had already dried up in May and the bath/wash house Kokola had only stagnant water]. No trees grew upon it, except a carob, an elder and a willow which overhung the perennial spring" [the willow was gone in May of 2000, two scrub-like trees grew in the hollow below the indent in the hill where on the left side the earth digging was done].

August 6th in liturgy

Though only a minor matter relating to the date of the digging of the earth, it should be clarified that the Eastern (Byzantine) rite of the Christian church since about 300 AD has celebrated August 6 annually as the Transfiguration (Metamorphosis) of Christ, when he appeared on a hill (Mt. Tabor?) white and heavenly, shining like a light to show his disciples that he really was one of the Holy Trinity[2]. Right by the hill Angiochoma are remnants of a temple or church called Metamorphosis. This liturgical celebration is a fixed date and appears to have been the same date under the Julian as well as the Gregorian calendar and accounts for mass being said (Tozer, 261). This date should not be related to the earth digging festival of the Goddess Artemis, though it is not improbable that the ceremony then also took place when the hill Agiochoma was dry and bare.

Historical research into healing earths and related subjects continued sporadically. While many papers, for instance Jung (1948), Spanudis (1945) and Black (1956) show some photographs or drawings of sigillated pieces of clay, they are reproductions from old documents and thus not readily discernible in all detail. The collections of medical sigillated earths of the German National-Museum in Nürnberg have been detailed meticulously by Florian Heller (1964)[3.] A major collection in Dresden was destroyed by a fire during the 1849 revolution, but the Ludwig 1748/49 text survived. Illustrations of almost 350 seals dating back at least to 1555 are added below in Chapter Seventeen.

Heller in 1964

Heller (1964) saw a revival of interest in the proven and good healing properties of earths, especially the aluminosilicates such as sodium and calcium montmorillonite which exhibit the special ability to absorb large amounts of water, similar to the calcium carbonate, but more than the "classic" sigillated earth kaolin. In his search for sigillated pieces of healing earth Heller found (a) that there is nothing in the literature as to how, when, and where the actual stamps or forms were made, and (b) there are variations of depictions which cannot be related to actual sealed or minted coins, and there is also a presumption that a number of the seals were counterfeit.

Heller classifies the German sigillated earths into those originating in Germany, grouped by regions, and earths that do not. His first grouping is about earths from lower Silesia (Niederschlesien): 1) The *terra sigillata strigoniensis* (Striegauer Siegelerde) dates to the 16th century and was lauded by Johann Schulz[4]. Montanus or Trimontanus: the appellation trimontanus refers to the seal of this earth, which shows the three mountains of the Striegau area, namely the Breitenberg, the Georgenberg and the Kreuzberg. The clay found there was a yellowish bolus. Its impressions, besides the three mountains, variously showed city seals of crossed sword and key, two crossed keys, or even two swords. Sometimes the seal has an added double eagle. While the crossed keys refer to the city of Liegnitz, a simple eagle over three mountain peaks is the seal of Goldberg. The actual provenance of these Silesian earths was not precisely represented. Thus the Liegnitz earth (*terra lignicensis*) is of three different colors of bolus sealed with three mountains with trees even without the seal of the city. Heller suspects that earths from completely different regions were hidden under this seal to grab a share of the Liegnitz marketing success.

The third earth from this region, *Terra sigillata goldbergensis* (Goldberg) always has an eagle above the mountaintops or crags. It is mostly white, but also yellow and red clay from the township of Grödizberg. Finally, an earth close by, *terra seichavensis* named after the town of Seichau was sigillated with the escutcheon of the nobles of Falkenhayn.

Earths not identified but believed to be from the Silesian region generally have a seal of a landscape under a sun and a half moon. Usually the alchemical symbol of a circle with a dot inside means sun or gold or axungia solis, and a half moon denoting axungia lunae or silver. In old beliefs the rays of sun and moon penetrated into the earth and created the gold and silver deep in the earth (Reinbacher, 1998, p.55). A blue clay of sedimentary origin with a sharply detailed single-headed eagle of Prussian connotation was called Saarauer Blauton (blue clay from Saarau). This clay was found not too distant from Striegau.

Not far from Silesia, in the region of Saxony, the *terra sigillata beyerfeldensis* was marketed from the city of Graul, sealed with an anchor, symbol of hope, and a half moon, symbol of silver. Other regions with sigillated earths were Hessen and Franken, today states of the Federal Republic of Germany.

Of dubious origin are sigillated earths with Arabic (Turkish) lettering. Same as Lemnian earth when Lemnos was under Turkish rule, the characters make little sense in Arabic. Many "arabicised" earths from Germany are blatant forgeries.

The Maltese connection

Outside of Germany or "foreign to Germany" healing earths were known from Bohemia (*Terra jablonensis*) and some earths sealed with just the words *Terra sigillata* and the year when they were sealed. Of the earths of the island of Malta there exist two dozen of a variety of counterfeit pieces which, though not marked "vera terra della Grotta di S. Paolo", have seals of saints or the thorn-crowned head of Jesus. These Maltese earths may actually date much later, about the 16th or 17th century. Seals with the prominent letters IHS (Jesus and Christ abbreviated in Greek, Salvator in Latin - saviour) and often with another cross arising out of the H crossbar and having three nails at the bottom were adopted as the sign of the Society of Jesus about 1555. No doubt the Jesuits were marketing some clay coins with elaborate seals.

Of the "classic earth" Heller lists *terra armenica* as a sigillated earth. This appears to be the only reference to a seal on the Armenian bole. He indicates it was a large seal (indeed troches of 10cm square were reported, the marketing of earths was highly competitive) - but does not describe it, apparently because few if any survived with legible impression.

The value of Heller's paper is not only in the detailed description of the earths, but also in showing the implied value and use of these earths in late medieval and early modern times. The quantities made for continued medical use are not known, but there are a number of different dates on basically the same earth coin which indicate repeated making, sealing, and marketing. Some coins were sold in specific Silesian pharmacies, we do not know how many were marketed in a wider area.

Bech-I-Borràs from Catalonia, Robert Robertson from Scotland

Two major works on the history of medicinal earths in this century were (1) the very thorough "Fullers' Earth, a history of calcium montmorillonite" (Robertson, 1968) which includes an enormous amount of detail on all classic and most European medical earths as well as on the history of fullers' earth as the origin of the dry cleaning industry, and (2) the very detailed history "Les Terres Medicinals" by Jaume Bech-I-Borràs (1987). Written in the Catalan language this book has not enjoyed widespread attention in most of Europe, but its bibliography includes Catalan, Spanish and Italian sources not normally found in books and journals in northern Europe. This enhances greatly the value of a his history of medical earths. I have had no luck contacting Bech-I-Borràs, having been apprised of the book by Robert H. S. Robertson, who as brilliant multi-linguist in living and classical languages had great confidence that I would work my way through a French-Spanish-Latin related language, but the idiosyncrasies of scientific Catalan were not always readily found even in dictionaries at Stanford University and translatable only because of great familiarity with the subject of medicinal earths in history.

Aside from history of medicine, research on properties of clays and earths continued especially with respect to Stumpf's cures and to determine the defenses clay offers against bacteriophages and poisons. In Stumpf's time the only defenses against illnesses arising from canned goods gone bad and from poisonous mushrooms were his *Bolus alba* and a treatment with animal charcoal, activated charcoal, proposed by Starkenstein (1915) and Wiechowski as cited by the former. Stumpf had been much more cautious with broad statements about poisoning and about efficacy in case of typhus than Starkenstein.

Black in 1956

D. A. K. Black (1956) analyzed *terra sigillata* in line with the reported human experiment by the Earl of Hohenlohe in 1581, where possibly terra sigillata protected against a dose of mercury chloride of 6 gr (2 gr, are normally fatal). Black considered that possibly the terra sigillata described by Thompson (1912) could have an ion-exchange action, taking up mercuric ions and replacing them with innocuous calcium or magnesium. Since in 1956 it was not possible to repeat the experiment from 1581, Black used sulphonated polystyrene resin charged with H, NH_4, K, or Na which effectively removed mercuric ions from aqueous solution.

After experiments with iron as a relatively non-toxic substance, the amount of iron recovered from the feces was half of the quantity given. The second experiment showed only a 10% uptake of the administered iron. Black stated that these results do not suggest a very bright future for exchange resins in the treatment of heavy metal poisoning. But since there was a significant difference between these test results and the recovery of Herr Thumblardt in 1581, Black argued that the need to recover from the feces required the use of coarse mesh resins. Coarse mesh resins are less efficient in taking up cations than fine mesh resin. (As mentioned before, the original story of the human experiment of 1581 was published by Andreas Berthold, translated into English in 1587 (See Chapter Eighteen).

Black's second explanation was that the resin recovered from the stools may be very different from its composition in the absorptive part of the alimentary tract. Black could not make strong claim for exchange resins as antidotes for heavy metals, but at least they are ten times more efficient than milk and active charcoal (wherein Black is also substantially more cautious than Starkenstein cited above).

Other than the belief that ingesting a slurry of fine clay particles to envelop the bacteria of cholera and lift them from their nutrient and flush them out with intestinal activity, there had been no knowledge of a mechanism how this can happen. In early 1980 a paper by Said and others (1980) confirmed that the causing of diarrhea by the enterotoxin of *Pseudomas aeruginosa* is due to a heat-labile protein. Adsorbents such as kaolin are used for treatment of diarrhea, alone or in combination with antibiotics, antispasmodics and analgesics. The authors reported that it was known that charcoal eliminated the effect of cholera enterotoxin but that the clay material attapulgite (the active ingredient in Kao-Pectate® in 2000) reduced the toxic effect of both cholera and *Escherichia coli* enterotoxins.

What, now, is the curative factor of clay?

The one question which had never been answered by Stumpf or anyone else was the one about the role of each of the two major clay components in healing - the aluminum oxide portion, the silicon dioxide portion, or both. We do know from the classical Greek times that several "earths" used for medication (and still being baked into bread on the island of Milos as stomach pacifier) were almost pure precipitated (amorphous) silicon dioxide with hardly a trace of aluminum oxide.

Whereas the earth sample I brought brought from Kotsinas on Lemnos showed about 52% SiO_2 and 14 % Al_2O_3, the earth sample from the 1581 human test purported to be from Galen's place on Lemnos had 37% SiO_2 and 13.5% of Al_2O_3. But the renowned white earth from the island of Milos, of which I brought a sample, tested fully 96.27% silicon dioxide and only 0.7% Al_2O_3.

The modern day "Mustachoma" earth had 43% SiO_2 and 13.5% Al_2O_3.

Can silicon dioxide (not as crystalline quartz), in the absence of aluminum oxide, effect a cure from cholera or *E.coli* or other infections? This subject was addressed in a German doctoral dissertation in quite some detail (Kugelmeier, 1980).

First she determined that normal stool has a water content of 60-80% (at 3 bowel movements per day to three per week the average evacuation was ~200 gr/24 hrs. In cases of diarrhea evacuations increase to 3 or more per day at more than 200 g/day and with up to 95% water. Pathogens and their toxins disturb the liquid balance and lead to diarrhea and so do protozoa, virus, fungi, yeasts and some medications. Typical bacteria are vibrio cholera and E. coli. Diarrhea is caused exclusively by a secretion. Travel diarrhea bacteria remain in the intestines for 24-26 hours, cholera bacteria 4-8 days.

A second diarrhea mechanism is the salmonella diarrhea. Its bacteria penetrate the mucous membranes (but do not damage them). Systematic salmonella infection is typhus which inreases water and electrolyte secretion in the ileum. This mechanism applies to Salmonella enteritides, Salmonella typhi and paratyphi. The third mechanism is the infection with Shigella creating actotoxins; Shigella dysenteriae penetrates the mucosa and damages them (surface ulceration).

Food poisoning (*Staphylococcus gastro-enteritis*) causes vomiting and watery stools. Parasites like amoebae can also be causes of diarrhea.

Non-invasive pathogens (cholera vibria, e.coli) lead to non-bloody watery diarrheas. Invasive pathogens such as shigella and amoeba dysentery (Ruhr) cause pus formation, mucous and bloody admixtures to the stool. But in any case the effect of any acute diarrhea is loss of water and electrolytes with life threatening dehydration.

It is amorphous silicone dioxide

Kugelmeier's research confirmed that amorphous silicone dioxide adsorbs 100% of the bacteria used for the tests in a few minutes. She points out, that to achieve the basic absorption of macromolecules onto amorphous silicon dioxide surfaces, the binding occurs only when the molecules reach the SiO_2 surface and can react with it. The absorbing surfaces have been shown to be boundary areas of a hollow space structure. The mechanics of the hollow structures allow adsorption of solutions in correlation between the hollow spaces (major and minor capillaries) for small and large molecules, allowing the removal of the toxins with the feces. The absorption of bacteria appears to obey a different mechanism much less dependent upon the structure, which leaves us with Stumpf's thoughts that the extremely fine particles of clay (i.e. including silicone dioxide), being smaller than bacteria like vibrio and E.coli, surround the bacteria and eliminate them harmlessly.

Following Kugelmeier's analysis, a study by Gardiner et al. (1983) found that terra fullonica (calcium montmorillonite) and kaolin, but not charcoal, significantly reduce systemic endotoxemia; clay protects the intestinal mucosa from many intraluminal pathogenic bacteria and endotoxins, including toxins which attack the mucosal barrier. The method of how this happens is the research result of Kugelmeier. Paul Nadeau (1987) suggests that fine films of clay would be useful to treat burns and that clay immobilizes bacteria. Brouillard and Rateau (1989) determined that the use of clays in the treatment of enterocolitis is justified by their ability to absorb viruses, biliary acids and bacterial toxins secreted into the intestinal lumen.

The 1993 British Pharmacopoeia lists a combination of kaolin and morphine, but a century earlier Stumpf had argued that the effect of clay is better if intestinal activity is not artificially interrupted and if the efficacy of clay treatment is not delayed or defeated by food intake. Said et al. (1980) had shown that certain foods including milk products and fats reduce the absorption capacity of kaolin by one-half to two-thirds (Sorbitan monostearate representing fats in the test gave 70%, skimmed milk 44.6 % and gelatin 37%). The absorption capacity is also reduced by various drugs by as much as 45%.

In 1995 S. M. Sondhi and N. Agarwal showed that among medicinal plants used to control or cure diarrhea, certain ones actually absorb clay particles, especially *alocosia indica* (almost 5%), *Heliotropium strigosum* (4%), and *imusops elengi* and *Tylophora indicaI* (both over 5%).

At the end of the 20th century we can conclude that *homo sapiens medicinalis* (the doctor) has essentially forgotten the practical use of earths for healing. *Homo sapiens patiens* (the sufferer) still successfully takes patent medicines as described in the introduction to this study. But the animals have not forgotten to practice intelligent pharmacognosy.

Animal geophagy

Amazon parrots have been shown to reduce toxins (alkaloid quinidine) by 60% by ingesting clay. The buffalo living on the slopes of Mt. Kenya in Eastern Africa have been studied for their habits of geophagy (Balkema, 1989). Mahaney and others (1990) and several other papers concluded that the major elements aluminum and iron "most likely" are chemical stimuli for geophagic behaviour (?), that clay was ingested for stomach upsets (even though aluminum oxide is stressed in these papers rather than the silicon dioxide in the clay). Soil was eaten by chimpanzees, elephants, and buffalo (Mahaney, several papers between 1990 and 2001).

The unresearched question is whether the animals, from small birds to large mammals, eat earth after they have an intestinal problem (ungulates and the fresh greens of spring) or before, since often their feeding routine cannot prevent or avoid all toxic and bacterial and parasitic effects of their selected and necessary foods. Aufreiter et al (2001) published data from Tanzania, where soils ingested by animals and tested for composition showed that in all of the tests silicon dioxide had the largest component percentage of the earth.

Recent unrelated, but very much to-the-point, research (Polette, L.A. et al, 2000) into adsorption of large molecules and bacteria in the interstices of amorphous silicon is a further indicator besides the German amorphous silicon patent medicine that it is the silicon portion of clay which effects the healing of intestinal distress.

And lest we forget: While we often disdain people we haughtily consider living in a third world environment because of our faith in modern drugs, we overlook that they have retained their faith in natural medicines including healing earths. You will find such earths in many markets today, far from the big cities enriched with modern medicine. It is how the people have survived not by relying on the flying doctors for 10,000 years, but by being familiar with the three legs of medicine. In Madagascar clay eases stomach problems, whereas even simple medicines like electrolyte powders (at US$0.30 per dose) are unaffordable. On a Greek island mothers still cook an earthy medication, because what the local pharmacy offers in modern drugs, costs as much as a day's wages. In Indonesia geophagy among humans continues (Mahaney et al, 2000), in Mali, clay rolls are used to ease insect bites and Niger clay powder to cure stomach ailments. I know, I bought samples in 2001. And yes, they, too, are high in amorphous silicon dioxide.

Comments and explanations

[1] Saracens were Muslim enemies, Turkish and Arab, invading Europe about the 15th century, until defeated by Christian forces in 1456.

[2] The Western Church (Pope Calistos III) took the Transfiguration of Christ into the annual liturgy for August 6 in 1457 to celebrate thanks for the victory over the Saracenes near Belgrade in 1456. Another fixed (not Easter dependent) liturgical date is the Ascension of Mary on August 14.

[3] There are some minor errors: 1) Using an unreliable source, Heller places the locus of the Lemnian earth to the hill Mosychlos, a barely visible rim of an extinct volcano. The error dates to 1906, whereas the correct

location as I saw it in May 2000, was correctly described in the 16th century. Heller places the Samian earths not in the Island of Samos but relates them to the St. Paul's earth from Malta.

[4] Scultet, scultetus, is a latinized version of the German Schulz or Schultheiss, an appointed community clerk or mayor (Killy Literatur-Lexikon, Vol. 10).

Chapter Seventeen: Minting the Coins of Clay
The Chapter of Illustrations

Through the whole book we have followed the searching for and administering of earth for medicinal purposes: The most prominently known was the *Terra sigillata,* clay dug up and minted into "health" coins. Regarding the digging of the clay we spent a few pages on the island of Lemnos and the location of the ancient site of one of this highly regarded healing clay. Alfons Lutz (Lutz, 1958) even went so far as to find a regular mine with deep shafts that seem to have been overlooked by writers for 2,000 years. To me, 42 years after Lutz, the hills didn't appear to offer much opportunity for deep shafts, because the hill Agiochoma is not that high and vertical shafts would come out the other side fairly soon.

Everybody also wrote that the dug clay was made into pastilles or trochisks or tablets or compressed little balls. They were either stamped or minted at the site or at a facility of Hephaistos nearby, stamped with Artemis' goat (not her portrait, a mistake by Dannenfeldt (1984) or the Turkish ruler's Arabic seal. Galen was supposed to have carried away either 5,000 or 20,000 clay coins to his ship in the harbor nearby (the second time he was there). All this is said to have happened on one single day of the year.

Accepting the modern value of about 2.2 as specific gravity for clay for the moment, and accepting the report that sometimes, but at least on one August 6th, either the priestesses of Artemis or the subsequent priests of the Eastern Christian Rites loaded a cart full of clay and transported it about 2-3 km to the temple site of Hephaistos. I would imagine that a two-ox cart probably carried no more than 6' by 4' by 3' or 75 cubic feet of clay, 2,600 lbs. Let us assume that each trochisk was 0.5 in. thick and 1 per square inch, per cubic foot that would be about 3,500 tablets or disk. The whole load of clay then represented potentially 75 x 3,500 = 262,500 disks. At half inch thickness the total rolled sheet would amount to 24 x 75 = 1,800 square feet of clay sheet rolled flat, then stamped out with a cookie cutter or knife and then carefully stamped with the seal. (We totally disregard here any washing and re-drying of the clay). If rolling and cutting just one square foot of 1 sq. in. "cookies", stamping them individually and packing them safely, is estimated to be only 15 minutes, processing the 1,800 square feet of clay sheet would take 450 hours. We have no report on how many people were engaged in the making of the trochisks. Possibly Galen could have got 5,000 per day, but it appears highly unlikely.

Having decided to make some cookies, we ran into the problem of where and how to keep the disks while awaiting being sigillated, and after they were stamped, how to store them without compressing the now cut and sealed disks. This type of parlor game calculation suffices to show that it is unlikely that Galen—even if he had time to wait—had any chance to carry 20,000 sealed disks, especially not if the disks had not been lightly fired first so they could be packaged. Even 5,000 seems improbable, and that surely is part of the reason why we don't read about the troops Galen cured, but only the gastro-intestinally challenged troop commander.

We must come to the conclusion that there was a reason, why the earth coins were so expensive and why it was difficult to transport them across the sea. Throughout the book we pointed out how well clay absorbs moisture. The whole matter of the *terra sigillata* can only have been much more relaxed and low volume.

The unusual thing about earth coins is that this concept of minting a medication and using an international term *"terra sigillata"* makes it the only medication in history with a generic "trademark" which is really a contradiction. But it has existed in writing for at least 2,000 years and the association of the words terra sigillata with being a trademark on the coins has been reinforced by governmental agency seals (city names, city coats of arms, noble names and coats of arms) and by secondary means of recognition (the provenance on the coin of a name, recognizable landmark or escutcheon of prominent feudal lord).

This historical implication is that any discussion without illustration such as the otherwise well-researched paper by Dannenfeldt (1984) becomes inaccurate or rather incomplete (he did have the illustrations of books between 1700 and 1750 available, he cited the volumes). Heller twenty years earlier (Heller 1964) at least had included representative graphic samples. With illustrations of coins Dannenfeldt could have reinforced his opinion of Johann Scultetus Trimontanus as introductor of Silesian earths and would have noticed the questionable statements by the promoter Andreas Berthold from Oschatz.

What made double sided minting of the coins even more impractical (there are only isolated records of such) is that unless the graphic is *recessed* in the coin, there is no way of stamping the soft clay on the other side without ruining the reverse side image unless one is very, very careful. Of all the seals Heller investigated, only one had recessed relief, because for that you need a difficult engraving job on the tool. If you engrave the image, the coin will be in raised relief, but then creating an image on the reverse side is very tough and the clay has to be of just the right dryness to accept the stamping and not to shatter. The minted coin would then have to be lightly fired to make it durable in transport.

In the chapters above I have traced the beginning of the passing on the knowledge of healing earths, herbs, and animal substances to tribal associates and their successors. Before writing of any kind, there is no record of this. Even cave paintings, petro- and geoglyphs do not contain recognizable depictions that could be interpreted as healing substances. At best they can be assigned to the fourth level of healing that required the intervention of the supernatural realm, gods or magic.

Early Chinese drawings

After advent of writing healing earths were described in words only if deemed worthy of memorialization, usually set down on wood, clay tablets, papyrus or other writing substrates. In time methods were developed of addressing the appearance of healing substances, not only by verbal descriptions. Pictorial presentations would not require the knowledge of reading, just the memorizing of appearance. The earliest drawings of medical substances came from ancient history of China. They included the most common minerals in healing or comforting use. Drawings of minerals are difficult at any time and a system needed to be developed which allowed these hundreds of "expanded ideographs" to be recognized and memorized and understood. I first saw them in a library in Munich (Germany) in a beautiful book printed on silk paper.

These approximately five thousand year old picture dispensaries or pharmacopoeias (the ancestors of the Pen Ts'ao Kang Mu) offered three basic kinds of drawings. The first kind were pictures that could quite readily be recognized, such as coral pieces, as stalactites and -mites in a dripping cave, or coal in a coal mine, or petroleum (naphtha) flowing from a rock crevice. The second kind of illustration are pictures of rocks assembled in different designs of carrying baskets such as for saltpeter, nitre, and green vitriol to facilitate recognition by repetition. Third are drawings that show several sizes of a rock-like or crystal-like mineral such as black crystal, sand stone, talcum, 5-color-stone (?), or "stone from a well. The fourth version would a drawing a single crystal, clump or rock of a specific mineral such as calcite, stone sulfur and the five kinds of clay.

From the early Middle Ages

The first Western drawings or depictions of earths and earth coins that I could find are illustrations from a 12th century manuscript attributed to Matthaeus Platearius and called the "Circa instans" from the first two words of this incunabulum. One drawing shows three round trochisks or coins with the identifying graphic of a 6- or 7- pointed star inscribed into the surface and identified as "terra sigillata". Two drawings, in concept similar to the Chinese "collection basket", are sketches of a human being using either pickaxe to dig in hillsides for the medical earth "alum" or other digging tools for the clay "Armenia bol". The fourth illustration shows the melting or recovery of pitch or asphalt in an oven structure.

From the later Middle Ages

With the beginning of the 16th century and the advances of printing, wood cuts became the means to depict minerals in several ways. One way would be to show pieces of pitch or tar floating on a lake, another would be a natural scene of rain (dew) dripping from the moon and clouds (moonmilk or dew-of-the-moon). A third way would be to show a human and a table with product spread over it, either as salesman for the shown minerals or as a helper for the uses the product (hematite) was intended for, such as to still a customer's nose bleed. Another method was to depict a mineral by the use to which it was destined, such as the eagle stone being brought in the beak of an eagle to the female in the nest. This stone as amulet assisted women in pregnancy or facilitated birth.

From early Modern Times

Between the latter part of the 16th century and the middle of the 18th the art of printing engravings had progressed to where accurate drawings (or imagined ones) of earth coins could be published in books or most likely in broadsheets as advertising. There were too many different and competing ones not to have required advertising. For 250 years earth coins were sold in Europe, many in Germany, in Italy. Religious ones from St. Paul in Malta and from the Company of Jesus included pictures of saints and religious occurrences such as

Christ rising from his sepulcher in resurrection. It is not inconceivable that such "health coins" were sold by the church in the same manner as indulgences. Quite a few more illustrations are drawings from a major collection of earth coins described by Christian Gottlieb Ludwig in 1748. Ludwig unfortunately must have disliked that job, not only because his descriptions are 90% referrals to other authors, but because the most frequently cited author is seriously in error, 5% are just descriptions of the color of the earth and only 5% actually useful source descriptions. One chapter exists 1½ times with different text. Still, his 12 tables of drawn illustrations (not all 350 are reproduced here) show an immense variety and the earth coin activity especially in eastern Germany and within the realms of the church or affiliated earth coin marketers. Malta and St. Paul are prominent sales points, but the ultimate advertising is the "earth from the sepulcher of Christ".

Later modern times

Because it was known in educated medical/pharmaceutical circles that the healing earths were "trademarked" as "terra sigillata", that the original once came from the Aegean island of Lemnos until the Turks occupied it, thus coins of clay were sigillated with Arabic lettering of which many writers assure us that most of them were faked.

After about 1850, when science allowed more modern chemical identification and analysis, healing earths were sold in powder form (or pressed as pills or trochisks) in pharmacies, still associated with the trademark "terra sigillata" plus a local name of provenance. In the 20th century the modern tribal members (citizens) could resolve their need for earth (bolus alba), their need for herbal medicines (belladonna), and their need of zoological medications (beef extract). Modern medicines ultimately still derive from minerals, herbs and animal (even human) products.

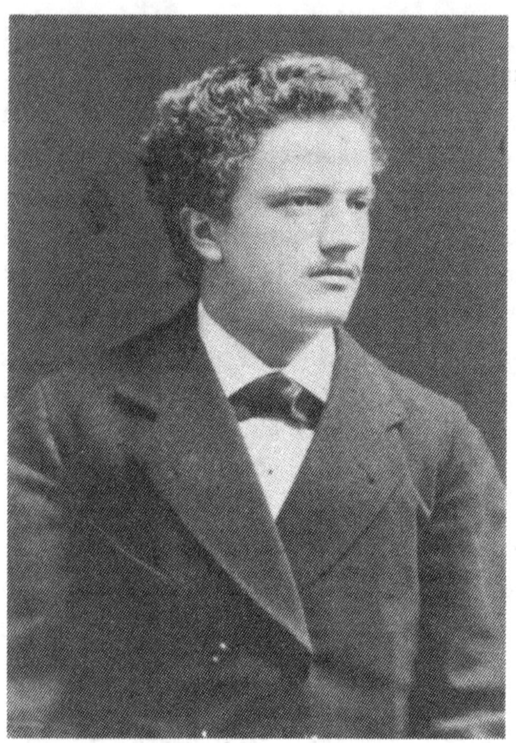

Illustration 201
Dr. Stumpf and Family

This studio portrait at left of Julius Stumpf probably dates to 1879, the year of his graduation as physician, of his license to practice medicine and of the award of a doctorate of medicine.
The family portrait below is of an older Julius Stumpf together with his wife Anna (née Schmitt) and their two sons Gottfried (seated) and Paul (standing) and the one surviving daughter Ella. (Daughter Madlon had died of diphtheria at age 4).
Anna died in 1902, so this family photograph probably dates from the period 1891-1902, the time when Julius Stumpf was appointed Assistant Professor of Medicine at the Julius Maximilian University of Würzburg am Main (Germany).

Incident to my work on Julius Stumpf in Würzburg, the local paper carried a story about an American author reseaching Dr. Julius Stumpf at the university and the city archives. A family friend mailed a copy of the article to Frau Irmgard in Munich who contacted me with an offer of records, photos and memories of her grandfather collected from her living relatives. She also had a duplicate made of Julius Stumpf's doctoral diploma (next illustration).

There had been doubt that Julius had obtained an M.D., it was not in records I found, but the family had a copy and entrusted it to me.

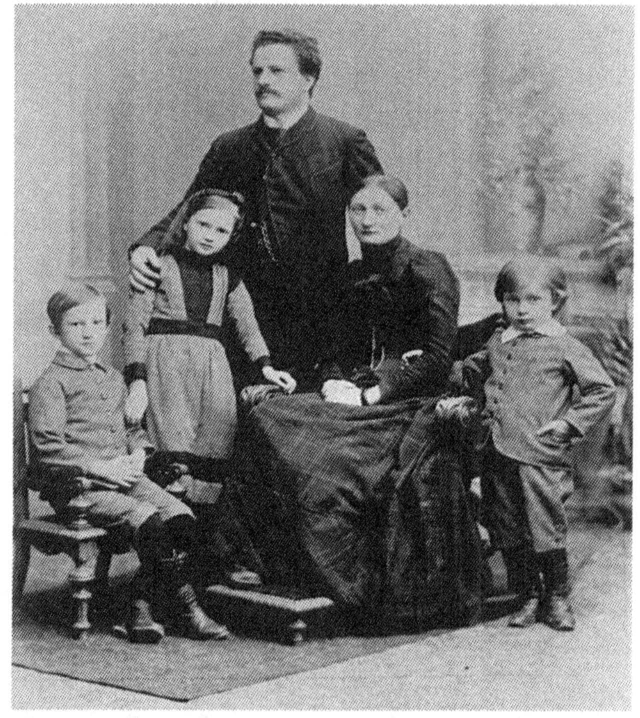

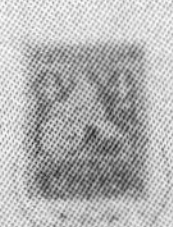

A. D. O. M.

AUCTORITATE SUMMISQUE AUSPICIIS

AUGUSTISSIMI AC POTENTISSIMI PRINCIPIS

AC

DOMINI DOMINI

LUDOVICI II.

BAVARIAE REGIS

COMITIS PALATINI AD RHENUM BAVARIAE FRANCONIAE ET IN SUEVIA DUCIS ETC.

ACADEMIAE IULIO-MAXIMILIANAE

RECTORE MAGNIFICO

ILLUSTRISSIMO CLARISSIMO ET CONSULTISSIMO VIRO AC DOMINO

ADOLPHO FICK

MEDICINAE CHIRURGIAE ET ARTIS OBSTETRICIAE DOCTORE PHYSIOLOGIAE PROFESSORE PUBLICO ORDINARIO

ORDINIS SANCTI MICHAELIS IN BAVARIA PRIMAE CLASSIS EQUITE

PROMOTOR

ILLUSTRISSIMUS CLARISSIMUS ET SPECTATISSIMUS VIR AC DOMINUS

ALOISIUS GEIGEL

MEDICINAE CHIRURGIAE ET ARTIS OBSTETRICIAE DOCTOR POLIKLINICES ET KLINICES PAEDIATREAE AMBULATORIAE

PRIMO HYGIENES PROFESSOR PUBLICUS ORDINARIUS

OGATIONE MEDICORUM ORDINIS D. T. DECANUS

PRAENOBILI AC DOCTISSIMO DOMINO

JULIO STUMPF

NATO IN „EBRACHSHOF" FRANCONIAE INFERIORIS

EXAMINIBUS RIGOROSIS SINGULARI AC PERINSIGNI STRENUITATE EXANTLATIS ET EXHIBITA

DISSERTATIONE INAUGURALI

„ZUR DIAGNOSE DER HERNIA DIAFRAGMATICA NEBST EINEM NEUEN FALLE"

DOCTORIS IN MEDICINA CHIRURGIA ET ARTE OBSTETRICIA GRADUM

EX UNANIMI ORDINIS MEDICORUM DECRETO RITE CONTULIT

WIRCEBURGI DIE XVIII. MENSIS IULII MDCCCLXXIX

QUOD QUI FACTUM SIT HOC SOLEMNE DIPLOMA SIGILLIS MAIORIBUS ET REGIAE LITERARUM UNIVERSITATIS ET FACULTATIS MEDICAE

NEC NON EIUSDEM FACULTATIS DECANI PORRO RECTORIS MAGNIFICI ET UNIVERSITATIS SECRETARII AUTOGRAPHIS MUNITUM TESTATUR.

Dr. Stumpf's Doctoral Diploma

Illustration 203
Drawing of Ancient Chinese Mineral Medications #1
From various sources within the Pen Ts'ao Kang Mu.

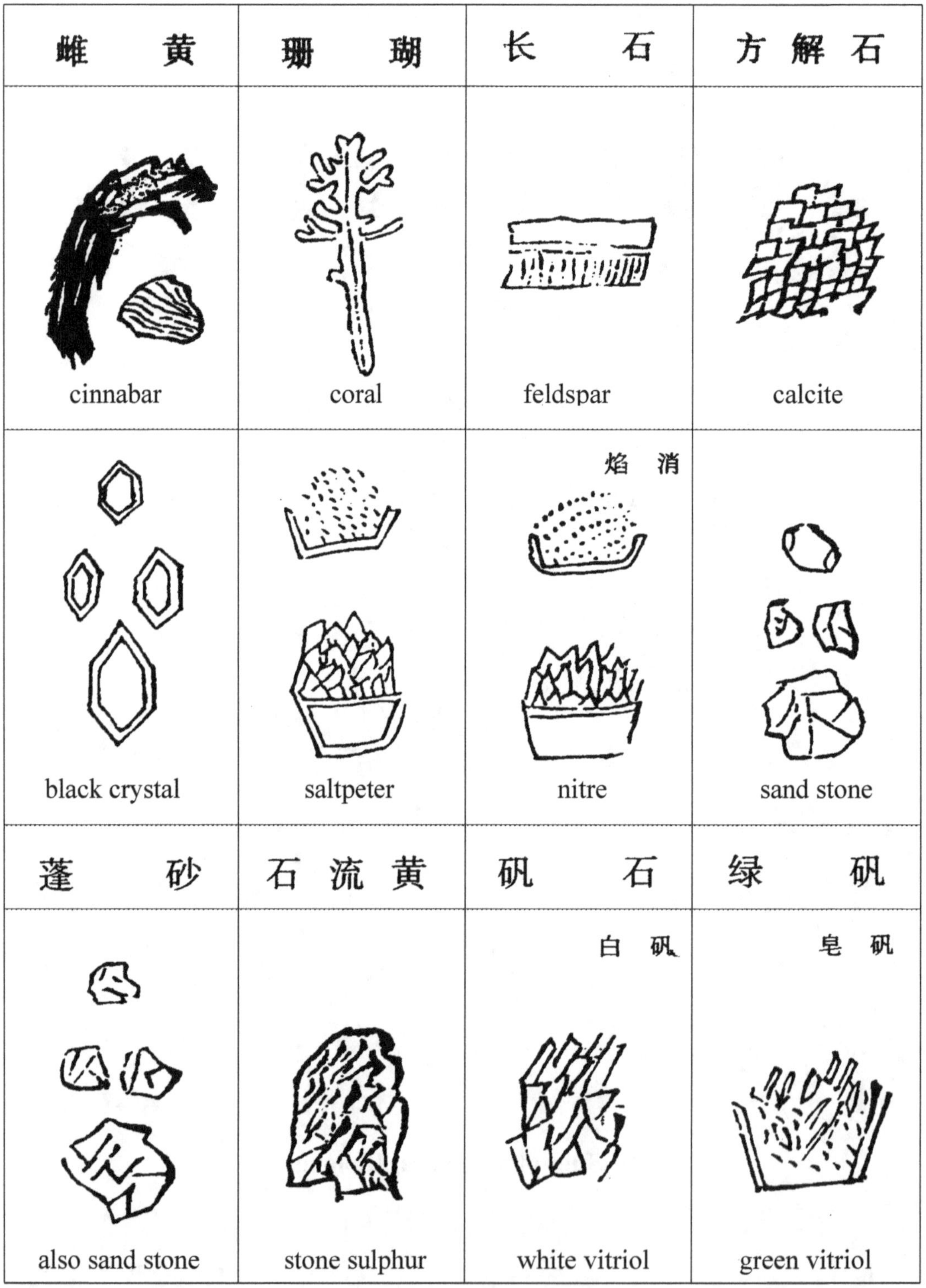

雌　黄	珊　瑚	长　石	方　解　石
cinnabar	coral	feldspar	calcite
black crystal	saltpeter	焰　消 nitre	sand stone
蓬　砂	石　流　黄	矾　石 白　矾	绿　矾 皂　矾
also sand stone	stone sulphur	white vitriol	green vitriol

Illustration 204
Drawings of Ancient Chinese Mineral Medications # 2
From various sources within the Pen Ts'ao Kang Mu.

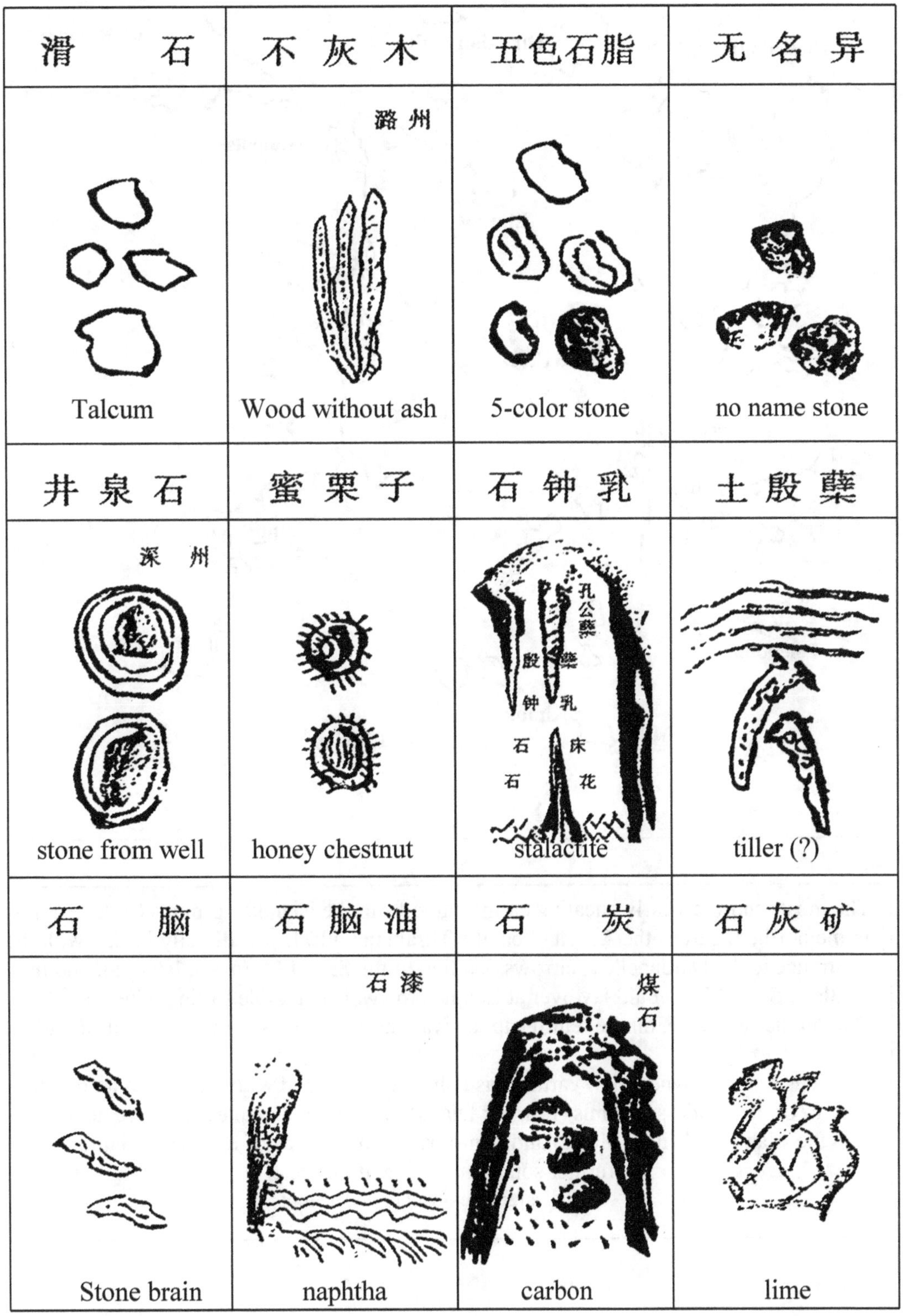

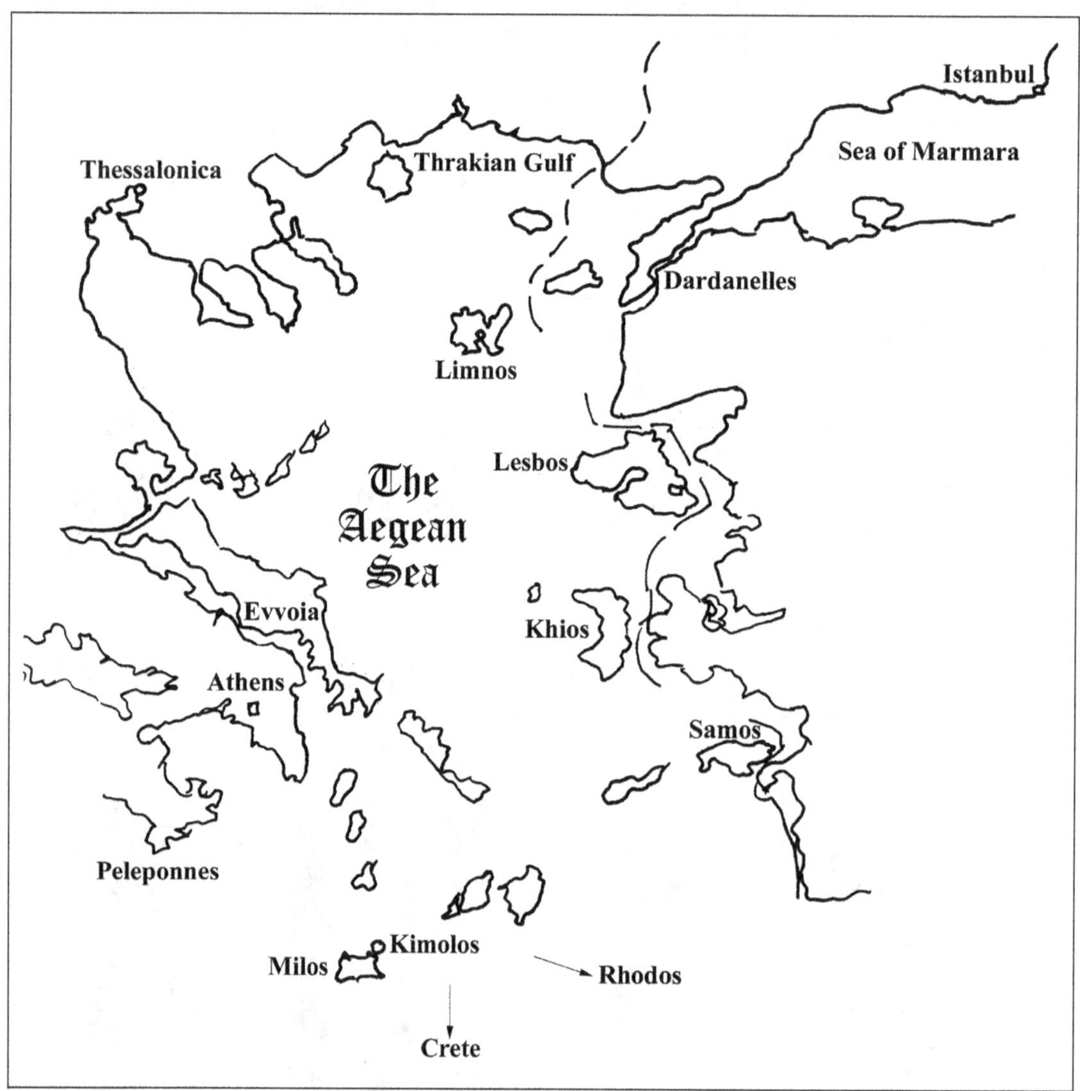

The most renowned early "healing earth" came from the island of Limnos (old: Lemnos) in the northern part of the Aegean Sea, the Thrakian Gulf. It was directly in line with the entrance to the Dardanelles Narrows, leading to the Sea of Marmara, Istanbul, and the Black Sea. Ships would lay over at Lemnos to await a suitable sailing wind into the Dardanelles entrance, on the return trip to await suitable winds for their next destination.

Besides Lemnos, where the "earth" was coined or sigillated with the seal of a goat, the mascot of the goddess Artemis (Roman: Diana), medically useful earths were also found on the islands of Milos (Melos) and Kimolos, on the islands of Khios and Samos, and further south on the island of Crete.
Map design: Reinbacher and Talbot

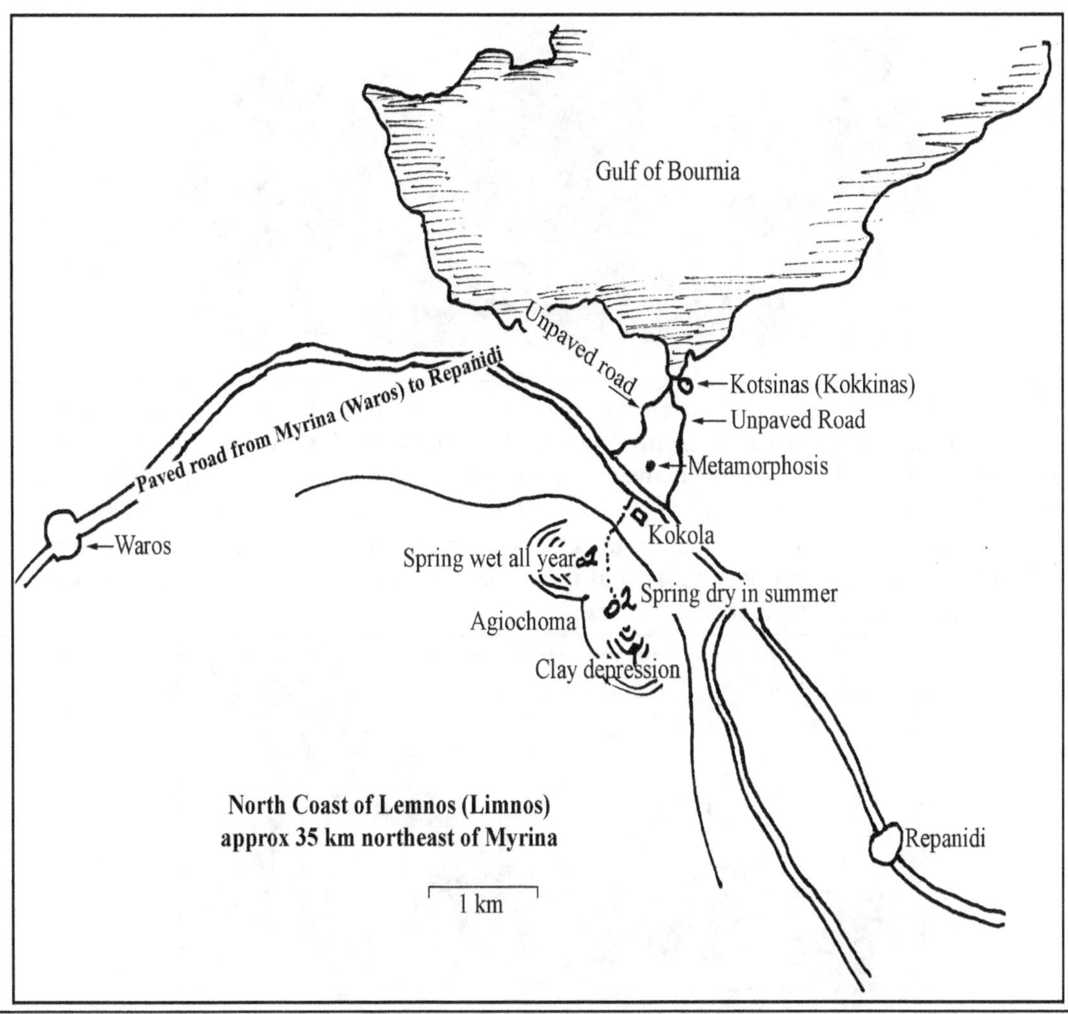

The famous physician Galen of Pergamum, practicing in Rome, visited the island of Lemnos (Limnos today) on the way to Turkey. He had hoped to see the annual digging of the clay of Lemnos, its conversion into coined disks with the logo of the goat of the goddess Artemis (Diana). But as his ship anchored in the western harbor of the island, today Myrina, his ship's captain would not let Galen leave the ship, respectively would sail when the wind was right, regardless of whether Galen was back on board or not. The second time Galen visited Lemnos, most likely on a return voyage, his ship anchored in the harbor of the Gulf of Bournia near Kotsinas (Kokkinas). From there it is only 2 km to the hill Agiochoma and the clay depression where the (#2) spring is dry in the summer. Reportedly Galen asked the priestesses about goats' blood being mixed with the clay and the answer was negative. Galen took either 5,000 or 20,000 earth coins with him, but the latter figure appears unlikely.

Map design: Reinbacher and Talbot

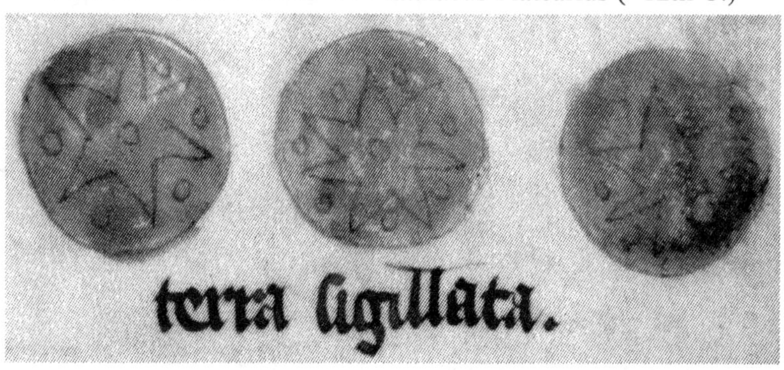

The upper drawing (*terra sigillata*) represents round troches or flat pills of sigillated healing earth. At least one surface of each has been inscribed with a hand-drawn 6-pointed and two 7-pointed stars with small circles in the recess between the points or teeth of the star shape. It appears that these "stars" may be a semblance to "aster" (star), the clay earth from the Greek Aegean island of Samos. Some sources say that the name stems from pieces of glitter in the clay, others believe that the sigillation of a star shape was the origin of the name. These are the only instances I have found of a hand-drawn sigillation on clay disks or coins.

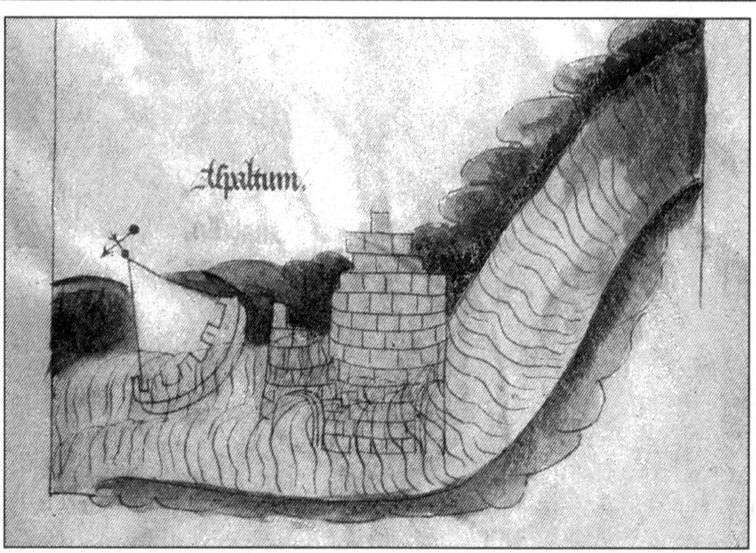

Tar, bitumen, pitch was a frequently used as wound treatment and occlusive protection against infection. "Aspaltum" (asphalt) is a heavy liquid to solid petroleum material. Natural asphalt (brea as in La Brea tar pits) includes other minerals. This drawing appears to represent an underground flow of "rock oil" (petra+oleum) and an oven where asphalt was heated to achieve a uniform density and formable pieces for wound treatment by battle medics. Asphalt was also used as water barrier between brick walls and to join bricks. (Its use in road building was not prominent until about the 1800.)

(The name "Circa instans" has been used because of the first two illuminated letters in the book. While this incunabulum is called an "herbal". its inclusion of animal and mineral with plant medicines technically makes it an "Alexipharmacon" or book of antidotes and healing substances, thus covering all three legs of medicine).

From the "Circa Instans" of Matthaeus Platearius (~12th C.)
The harvesting (mining) of Alumen)

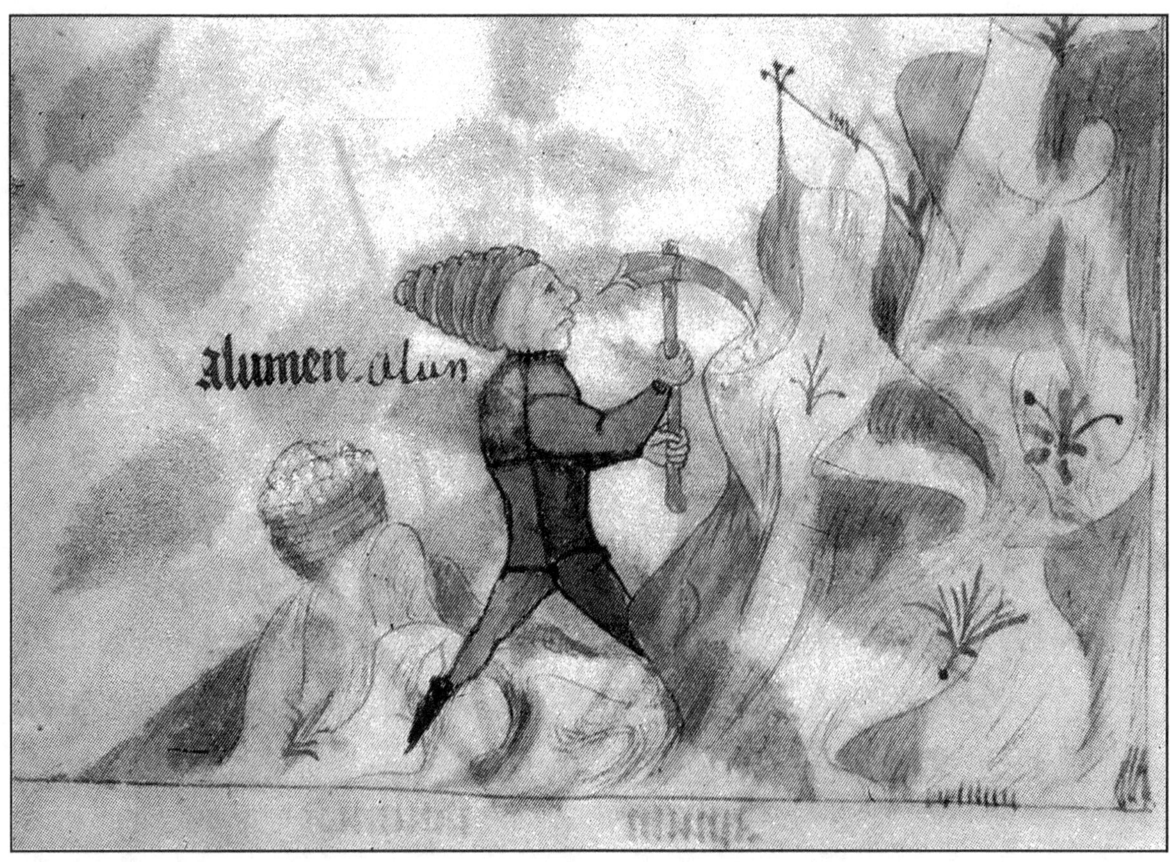

The faintly colored original of this drawing displays a rocky hill almost bare of vegetation from which a man with a pickaxe on a wooden handle mines alum. Most of mined alum was used in ancient processes of dying cloth with better color fastness (mordant) and the curing treatment of leather. As medicament it was used as an astringent (styptic) to control bleeding. Apparently the mined alum pieces were collected in a basket to be carried away. The quarryman wears a beehive type cap (turban?).The pants were divided into in red and green legs and a jacket and waistcoat of blue and yellow quarters alternates on each front and back. The harlequinesque dress might be indicative of the person's trade.

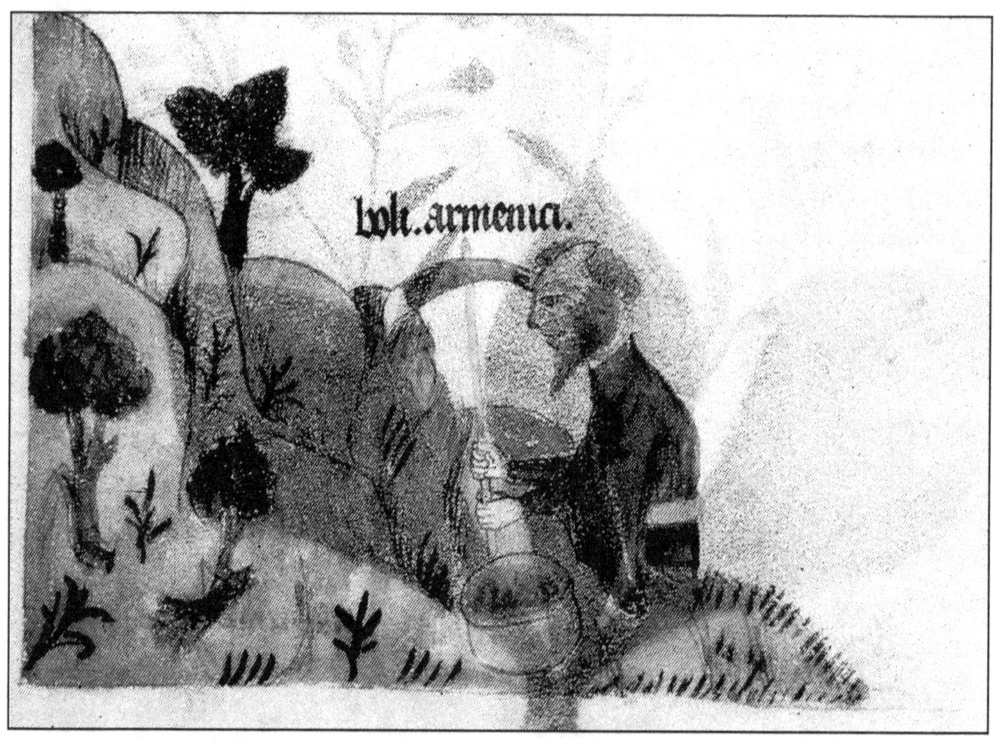

This drawing illustrates the mining of the famous antique "Armenian Clay" (*bolus armenia*). A bearded worker is using a pickaxe to loosen clay from a hill or pit side, well covered with stylized trees and bushes. He has a bowl or basket at his side to collect the loosened clay. It is red in color, the usually reported color of the Cappadocian clay which contains 3-5% of iron oxide. This medicinal clay was valuable enough to be a princely gift.

It appears the workman is wearing a red-orange jacket with a yellow sleeve stripe and a green sash across the breast. This colorful dress may signify a trade or occupation. He has two fists on the axe handle; dry clay can be very hard to dig.

Illustration 300
Alchemical Symbols for Minerals in Medicine

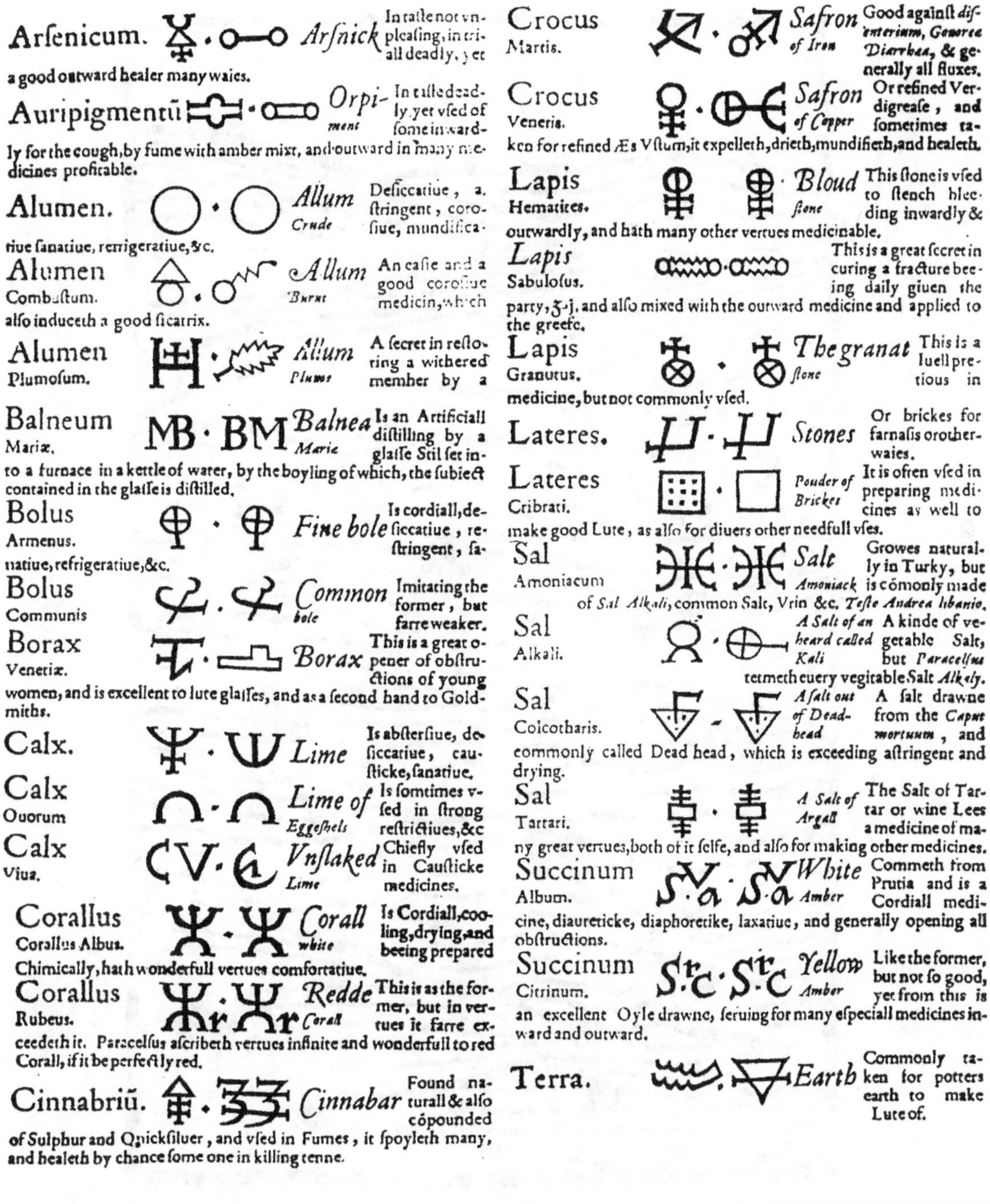

Arſenicum. — *Arſnick* — In taſte not vn-pleaſing, in tri-all deadly, yet a good outward healer many waies.

Auripigmentũ — *Orpi-ment* — In taſte dead-ly, yet vſed of ſome inward-ly for the cough, by fume with amber mixt, and outward in many me-dicines profitable.

Alumen. — *Allum Crude* — Deſiccatiue, aſtringent, coro-ſiue, mundifica-tiue ſanatiue, rerrigeratiue, &c.

Alumen Combuſtum. — *Allum Burnt* — An eaſie and a good coroſiue medicin, which alſo induceth a good ſicatrix.

Alumen Plumoſum. — *Allum Plumo* — A ſecret in reſto-ring a withered member by a

Balneum Mariæ. — MB · BM — *Balnea Marie* — Is an Artificiall diſtilling by a glaſſe Stil ſet in-to a furnace in a kettle of water, by the boyling of which, the ſubieɗ contained in the glaſſe is diſtilled.

Bolus Armenus. — *Fine bole* — Is cordiall, de-ſiccatiue, re-ſtringent, ſa-natiue, refrigeratiue, &c.

Bolus Communis — *Common bole* — Imitating the former, but farre weaker.

Borax Venetiæ. — *Borax* — This is a great o-pener of obſtru-ɗions of young women, and is excellent to lute glaſſes, and as a ſecond hand to Gold-miths.

Calx. — *Lime* — Is abſterſiue, de-ſiccatiue, cau-ſticke, ſanatiue.

Calx Ouorum — *Lime of Eggeſhels* — Is ſomtimes v-ſed in ſtrong reſtriɗiues, &c

Calx Viua. — *Vnſlaked Lime* — Chiefly vſed in Cauſticke medicines.

Corallus Corallus Albus. — *Corall white* — Is Cordiall, coo-ling, drying, and beeing prepared Chimically, hath wonderfull vertues comfortatiue.

Corallus Rubeus. — *Redde Corall* — This is as the for-mer, but in ver-tues it farre ex-ceedeth it. Paracelſus aſcribeth vertues infinite and wonderfull to red Corall, if it be perfeɗly red.

Cinnabriũ. — *Cinnabar* — Found na-turall & alſo cõpounded of Sulphur and Qnickſiluer, and vſed in Fumes, it ſpoyleth many, and healeth by chance ſome one in killing tenne.

Crocus Martis. — *Safron of Iron* — Good againſt diſ-enterium, Gonorea Diarrhea, & ge-nerally all fluxes.

Crocus Veneris. — *Safron of Copper* — Or refined Ver-digreaſe, and ſometimes ta-ken for refined Æs Vſtum, it expelleth, drieth, mundifieth, and healeth.

Lapis Hematites. — *Bloud ſtone* — This ſtone is vſed to ſtench blee-ding inwardly & outwardly, and hath many other vertues medicinable.

Lapis Sabuloſus. — This is a great ſecret in curing a fraɗure bee-ing daily giuen the party, ℥ j. and alſo mixed with the outward medicine and applied to the greefe.

Lapis Granutus. — *The granat ſtone* — This is a Iuell pre-tious in medicine, but not commonly vſed.

Lateres. — *Stones* — Or brickes for farnaſis or other-waies.

Lateres Cribrati. — *Pouder of Brickes* — It is often vſed in preparing medi-cines as well to make good Lute, as alſo for diuers other needfull vſes.

Sal Amoniacum — *Salt Amoniack* — Growes natural-ly in Turky, but is cõmonly made of Sal Alkali, common Salt, Vrin &c. Teſte Andrea libanio.

Sal Alkali. — *A Salt of an heard called Kali* — A kinde of ve-getable Salt, but Paracelſus termeth euery vegitable Salt Alkaly.

Sal Colcotharis. — *A ſalt out of Dead-head* — A ſalt drawne from the Caput mortuum, and commonly called Dead head, which is exceeding aſtringent and drying.

Sal Tartari. — *A Salt of Argall* — The Salt of Tar-tar or wine Lees a medicine of ma-ny great vertues, both of it ſelfe, and alſo for making other medicines.

Succinum Album. — *White Amber* — Commeth from Prutia and is a Cordiall medi-cine, diaureticke, diaphoretike, laxatiue, and generally opening all obſtructions.

Succinum Citrinum. — *Yellow Amber* — Like the former, but not ſo good, yet from this is an excellent Oyle drawne, ſeruing for many eſpeciall medicines in-ward and outward.

Terra. — *Earth* — Commonly ta-ken for potters earth to make Lute of.

Alchemical medicine developed symbols for many "earth" medicines. In alphabetical order they are: Alumen, bolus, borax, calx, coral (white and red), *lapis hematites*, *lateres* (brick and brick dust), salts, succinum (amber) and, of course, *terra*.

Medieval Woodcut - Bitumen Judaeicum - Asphalt floating on the Dead Sea

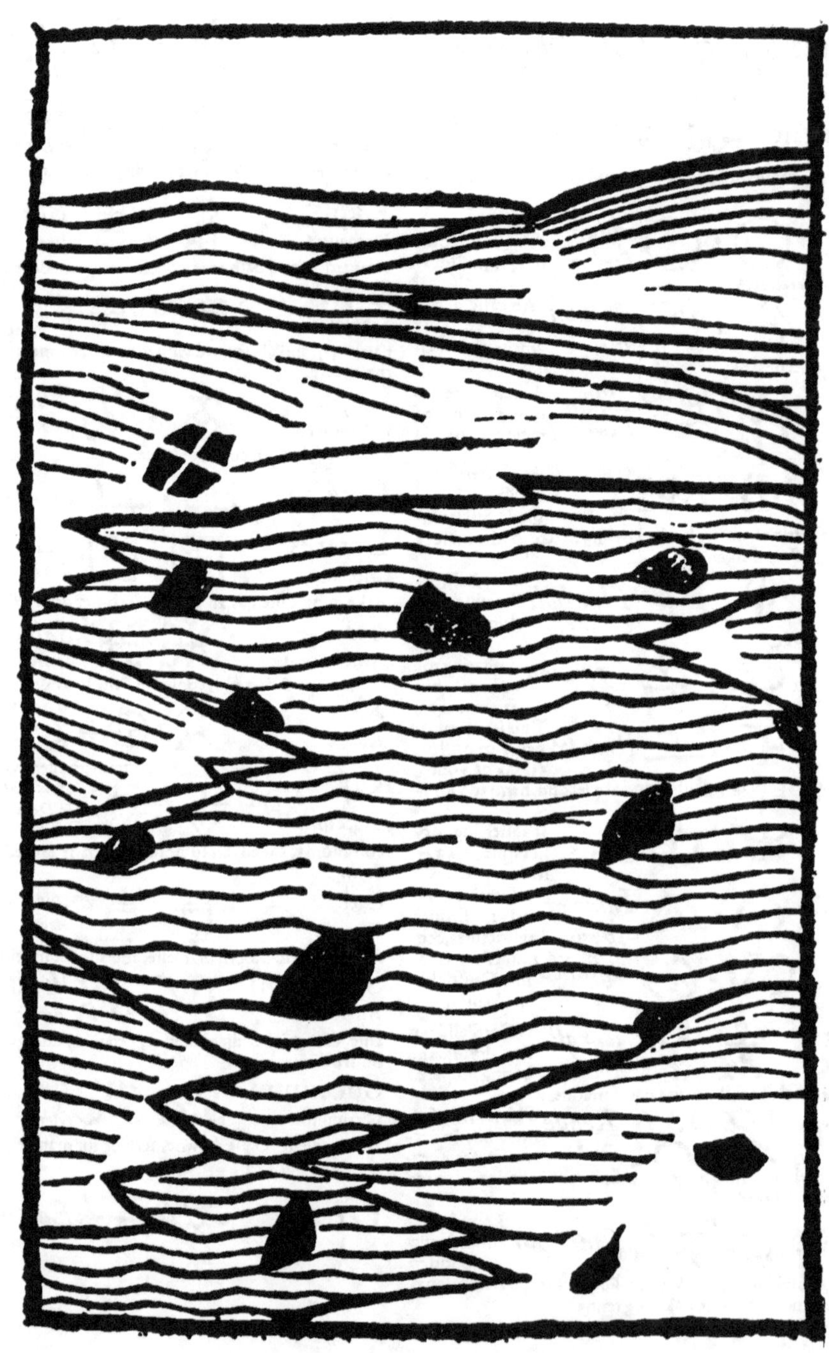

It was used as mortar for clay bricks, as medicament and wound treatment, and
as preservative for mummies.
Hortus Sanitatis (Garden of Health) 1507, from Lüschen 1969, p.181.

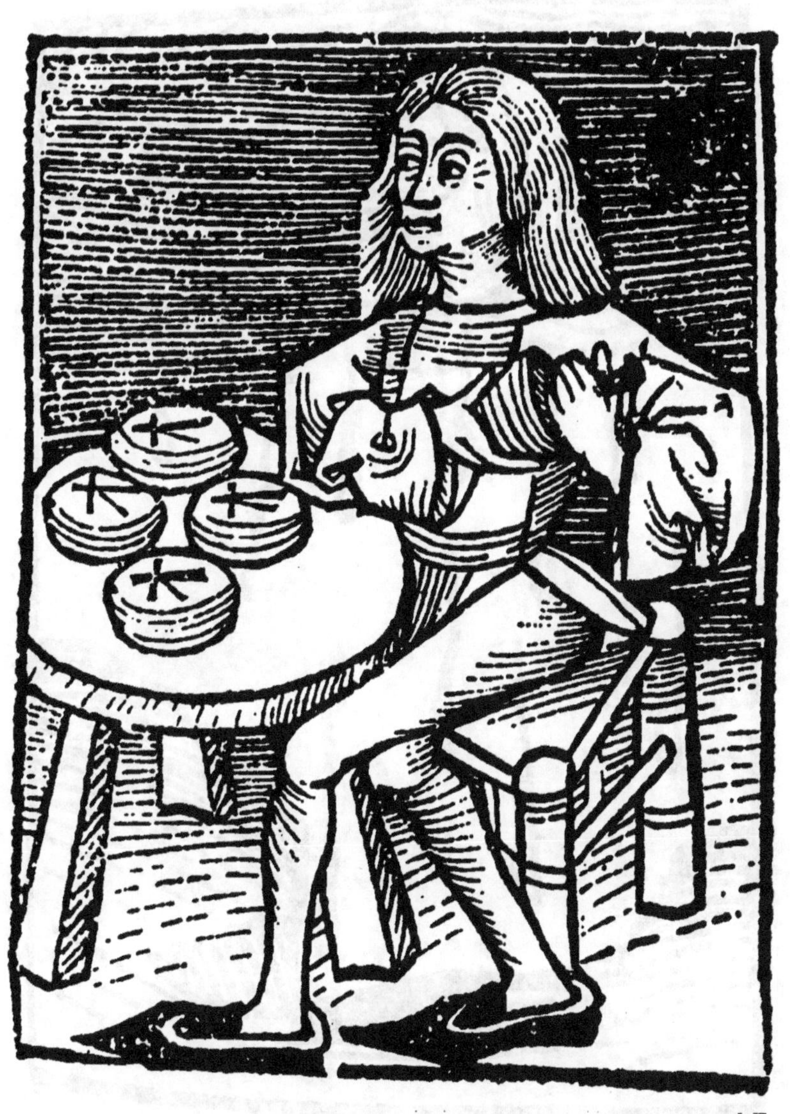

He is holding a bottle of wine with which to take the the
stamped coin of medicinal clay.
Hortus Sanitatis (Garden of Health) 1509
from Lüschen, 1969, p. 318

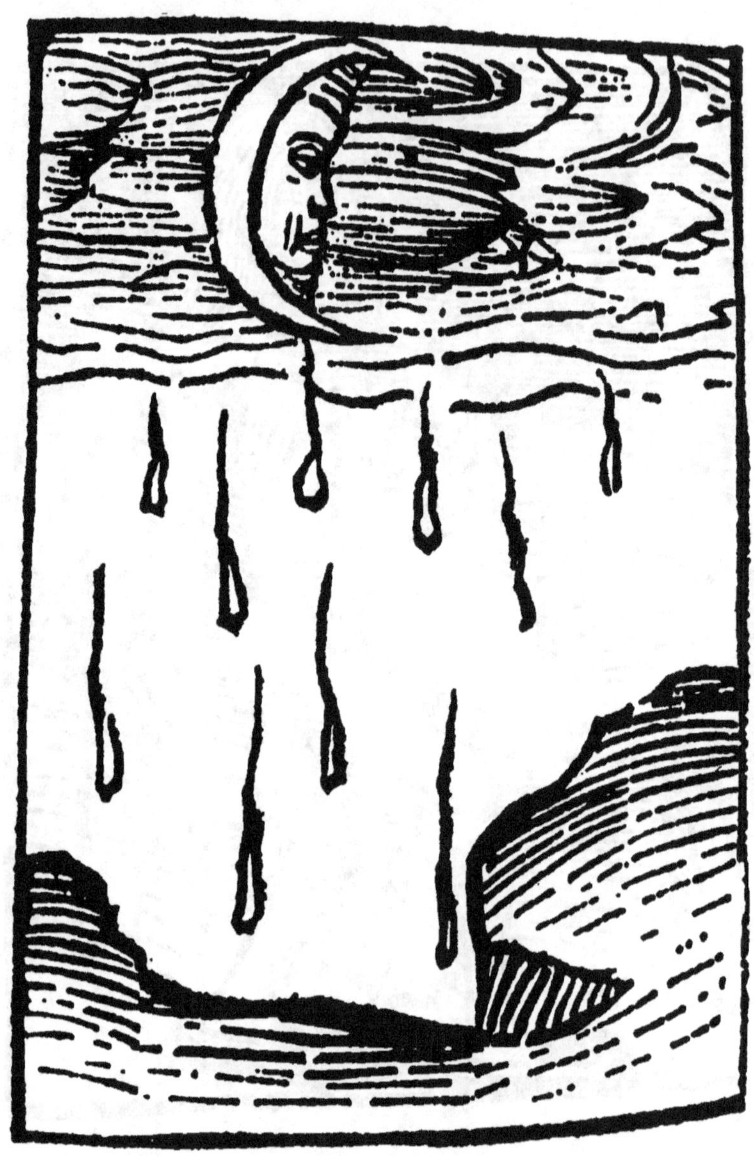

Dew from the moon penetrates the earth and becomes
moonmilk, calcium carbonate in cave, also referred to as
"Aphrosolinus".
From: Johann Daniel Major, Dissertatio medica de lacte
lunae. The illustration is from Hortus sanitatis (Garden of
Health) 1509, from Lüschen 1969 p. 279

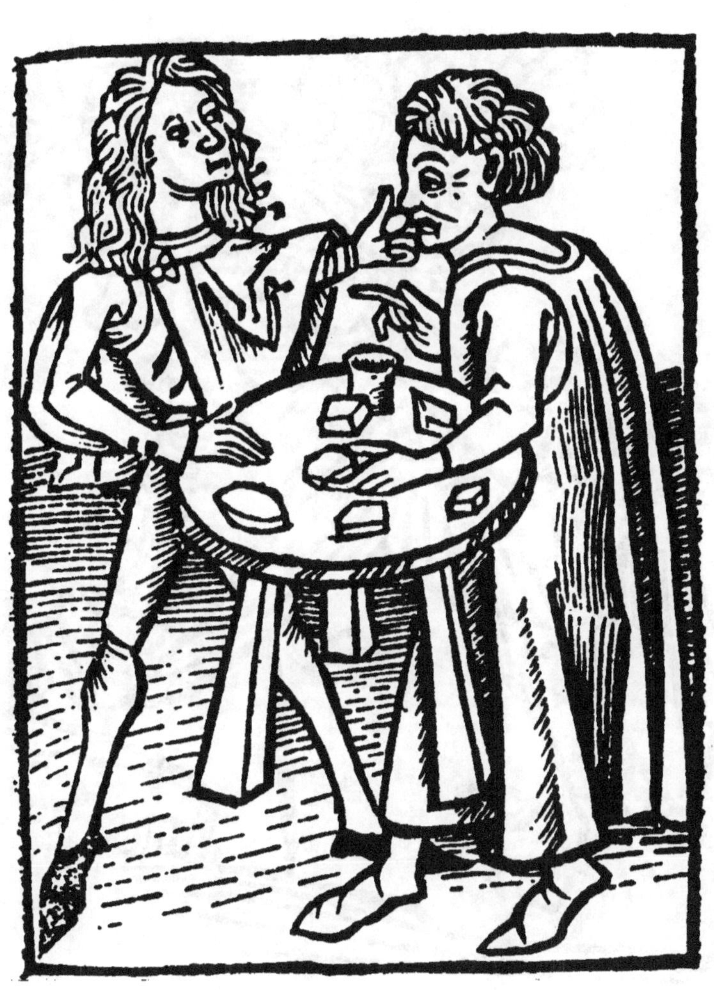

Blood stone (hematite, haematite)
being given by a doctor to still bleeding of all kinds,
external and internal. Here a nose bleed is treated. Use
of blood stone was known on all inhabited continents
since ancient times.
Hortus Sanitatis (Garden of Health) 1509,
from Lüschen, 1969, p. 235

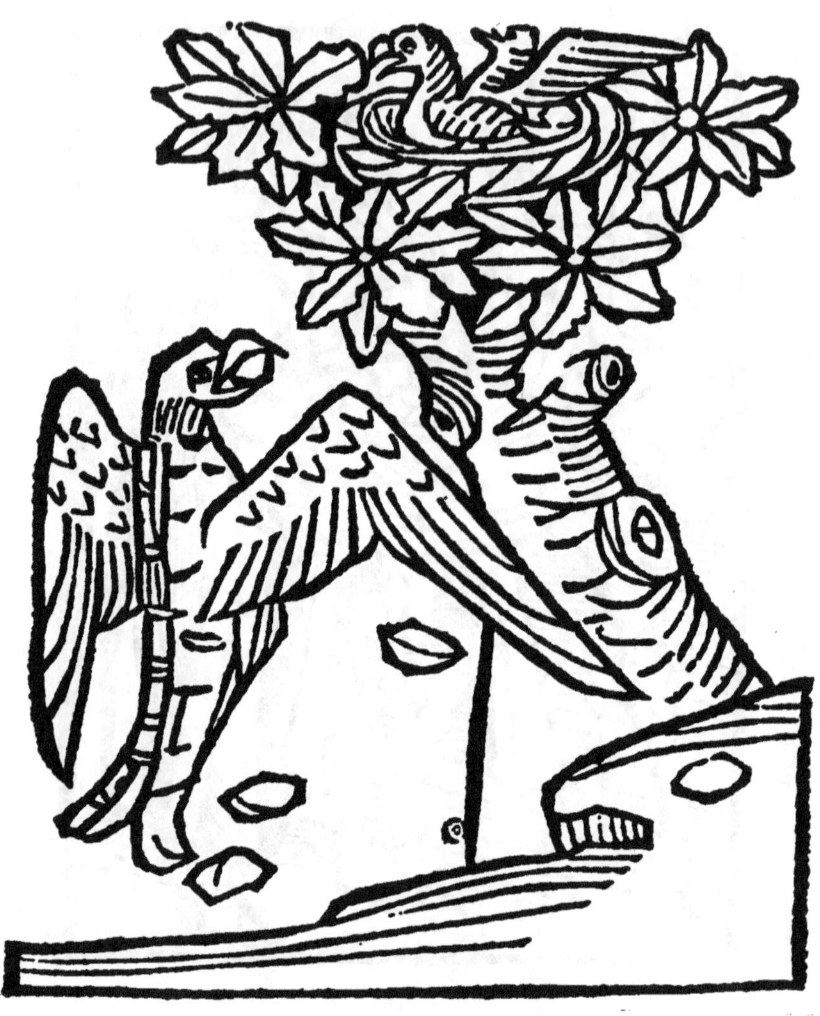

Eagle stone being carried into the eagle's nest.
The eagle stone is hollow and contains a pebble or gravel
inside. Because the stone is "pregnant", it facilitates the eagle's
raising its young, a belief transferred as amulet to help women to
give birth.
Hortus Sanitatis (Garden of Health), 1509, from Lüschen 1969, p.
168.

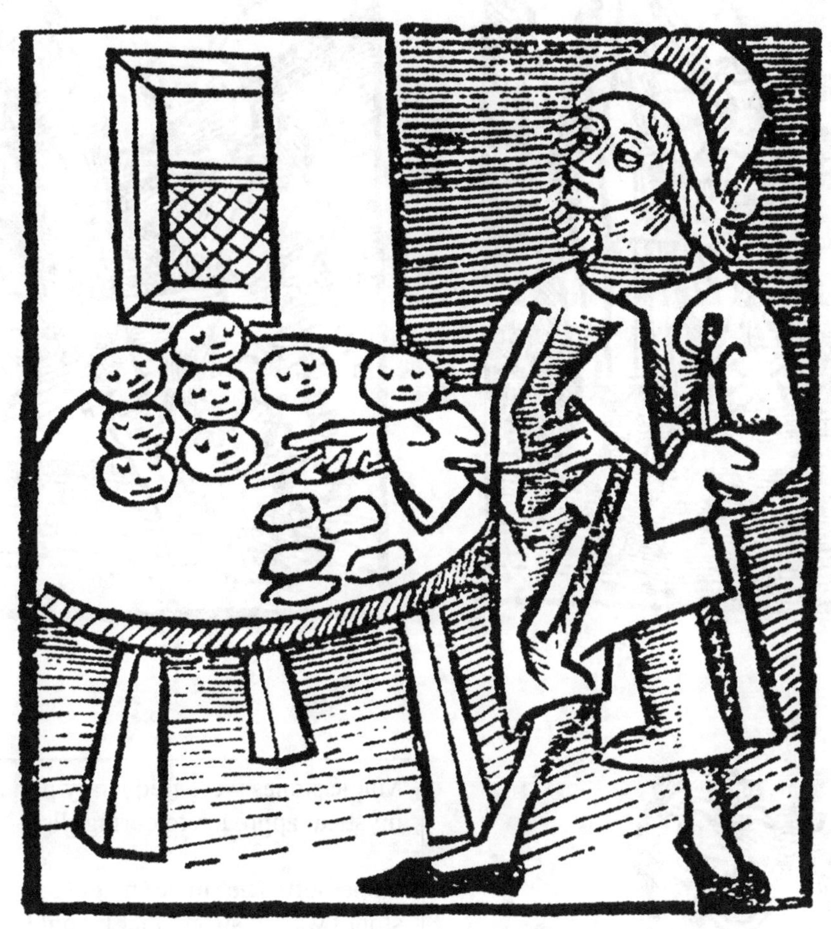

Moon stone (Selenit) was also known as Mary's ice or women's ice, a stone that shone pale like the waxing moon, mostly worn as amulet.
Hortus Sanitatis (Garden of Health) 1509, from Lüschen 1969, p.279

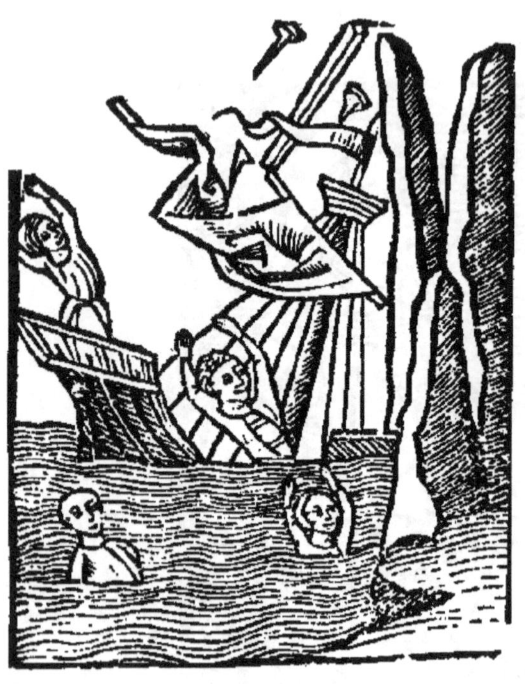

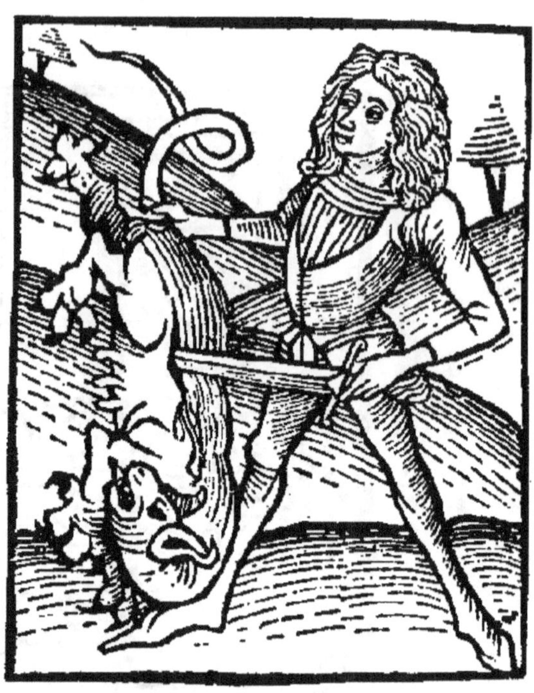

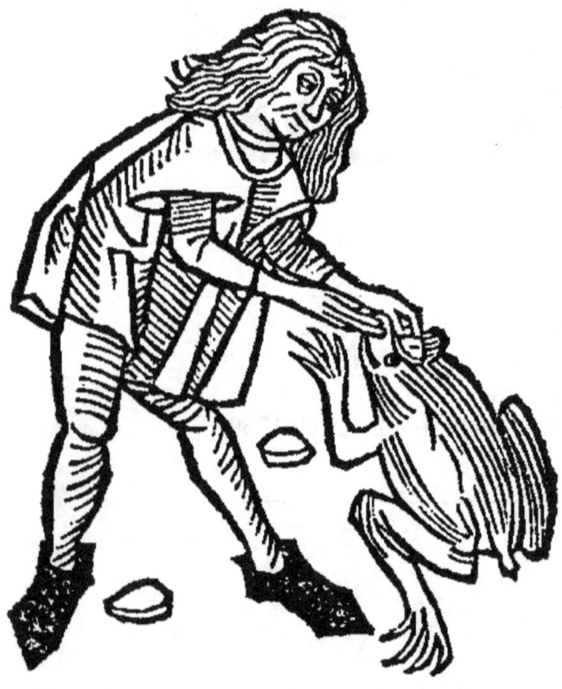

Magic stones were frequently part of the mystical approach to curing ills.

Upper left: The (male) magnet stone (lode stone) was so strong that it could pull iron nails out of ships' planks and sink them. It implied great curative powers when worn as an amulet.

Upper right: The dragon stone was universally considered a panacea to all illnesses, if you could find a dragon, could capture and kill it and remove the stone in its head.

Lower left: The toad would disgorge the stone in its head during the night when the toad was placed on a red cloth. As a child the 16th century physician tried it but the toad was not cooperative.

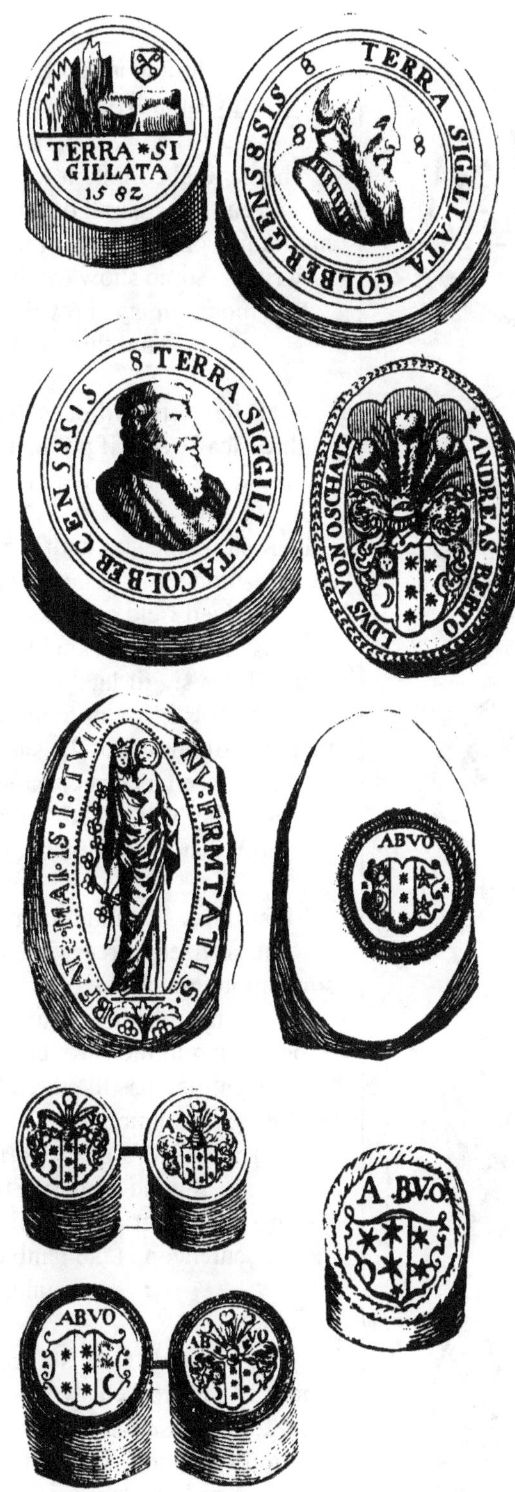

Illustration 400.1
Earth Coins from Germany

This collection of earth coins is from the University of Dresden (C. G. Ludwig, 1748.)

The top left coin has the oldest stamped date, 1582, in this assembly of Silesian coins.
Top right is a coin with the head-and-shoulder portrait of one well known promoter of Silesian coins (Silesia, once eastern Germany, now Polish), Johann Scultetus Montanus. The suffix Montanus or Trimontanus is a location identifier since "his" healing earth came from a region with three distinguishing mountains. The earth origin was spelled as Goldberg/Colberg.

The second promoter, created a fancy coat of arms for himself (2R). He was not a noble, but with the name Andreas Bertholdus von Oschatz (ABVO) gave that appearance. (Oschatz is a small town halfway between Leipzig and Dresden in Saxony.)

The ABVO escutcheon was above a shield with 2 stars, 3 stars, sun and halfmoon, in three vertical strips. One cannot but consider these coins as advertising samples.

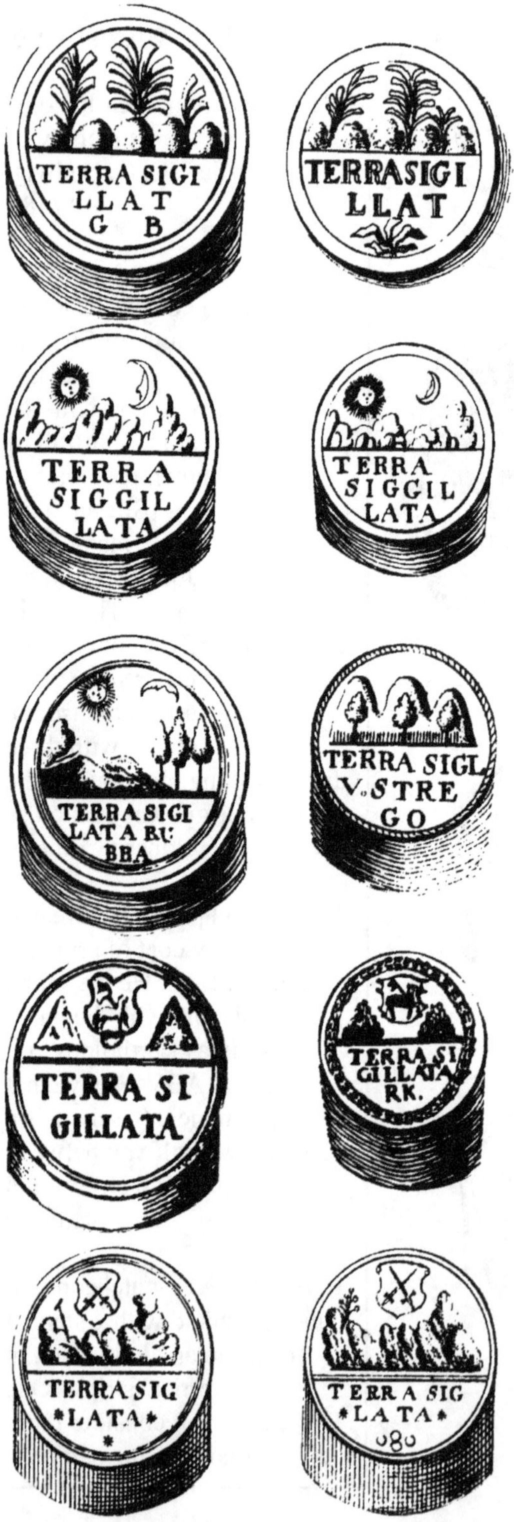

Illustration 400.2
<u>Earth Coins from Germany</u>

The general comment for Strigian earth is that all of them show mountains or hills, all of them show writing, some show the sun and a half moon, many show three trees and three mountains.

1L+R have five hillocks, basically three leaf-trees (if not palm trees) and the unusual hyphenation Terra sigi-llat.
2L+R show the sun with a face and the half-moon with a face, both over a stylized field of rocks or rocky hills. This coin maker spelled the earth Terra siggil-lata, the double g is error. It is difficult to understand that the coinmaker of 2R should not have seen a correct sample, but probably was asked to make the coin just from somebody else's memory.
3L still has sun and moon, first of the stylized 3 trees. The left has some mountain in the back but also the adjective "rubra" (red) pertaining to the earth color. The right one has the three hills of Striegau, a fence, and the legend Terra sigl. V(on) Strego(nien) = minted earth of Striegau.
4L+R have 2 triangular hills. The rarer escutcheon is the lamb of God and a flag.

Row 5L+R, aside from stylized hills and tree has crossed swords in the coat of arms, said to represent the sword of St. Paul. The words lack an i and an l in Terra sig(i)l(l)ata.

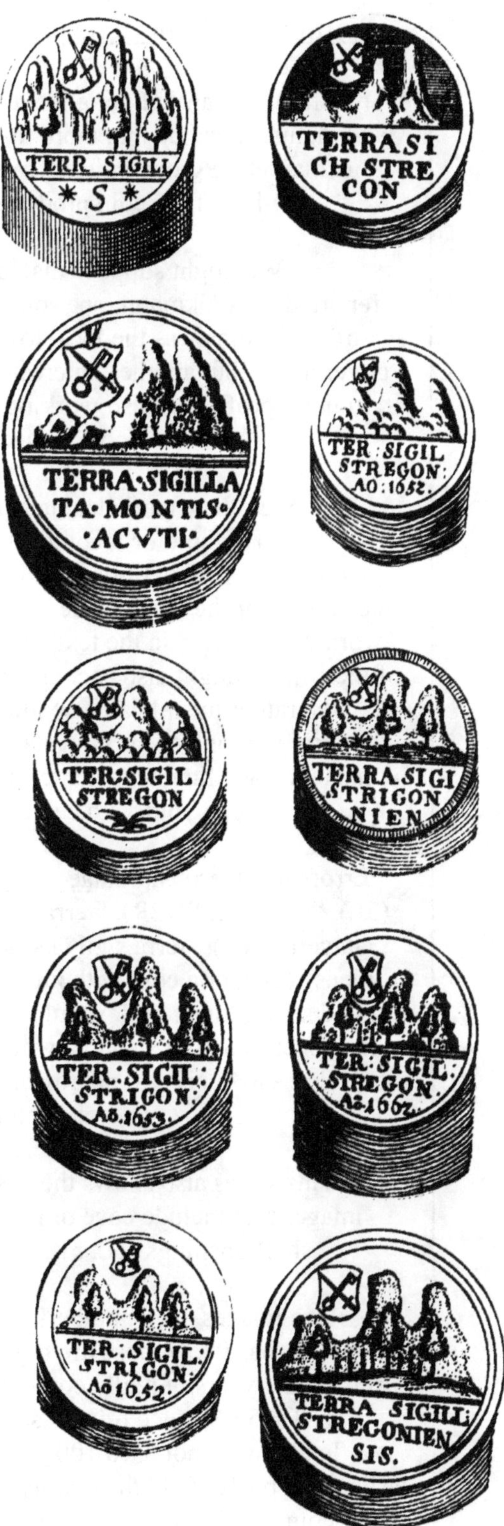

Illustration 401
Earth Coins from Germany

This continuation of Striegau earth coins bewilders with its varying back ground pictures, even though all have three mountains, all but 1R have three trees, and all have the coat of arms of key crossed with sword.

2L with the inscription Terra Sigillata Montis acuti refers to a peaked mountain, Volkmann claims it to be near Groß-Plusnitz, a hamlet not far away from Strigau. The area of the majority of Silesian earths is an uneven trapezoid from Liegnitz SW 20 km to Goldberg, E 20 km to Jauer, 15 km to Striegau, 40 km to Breslau and 60 km back to Liegnitz.

Dates in the coins go from 1652 (2R and 5L) to 1653 (4L) and 1662 (4R). More than one person or entity must have made coins, they surely never intended to make enough for 200 years at one time. It is also possible that since the lettering is so uneven that a printer was not involved setting type, but that the seal was carved by hand. Yet it appears that the lettering was done from an impression of a print font. The image impressed would make coins more durable and easier to handle. In the literature I was able to find out that the clay was flattened to the desired thickness (it varies between coins sizes, which may be a "price" concession), but I have not seen a reference on the making of the mint seal. It could have been made of lead.

151

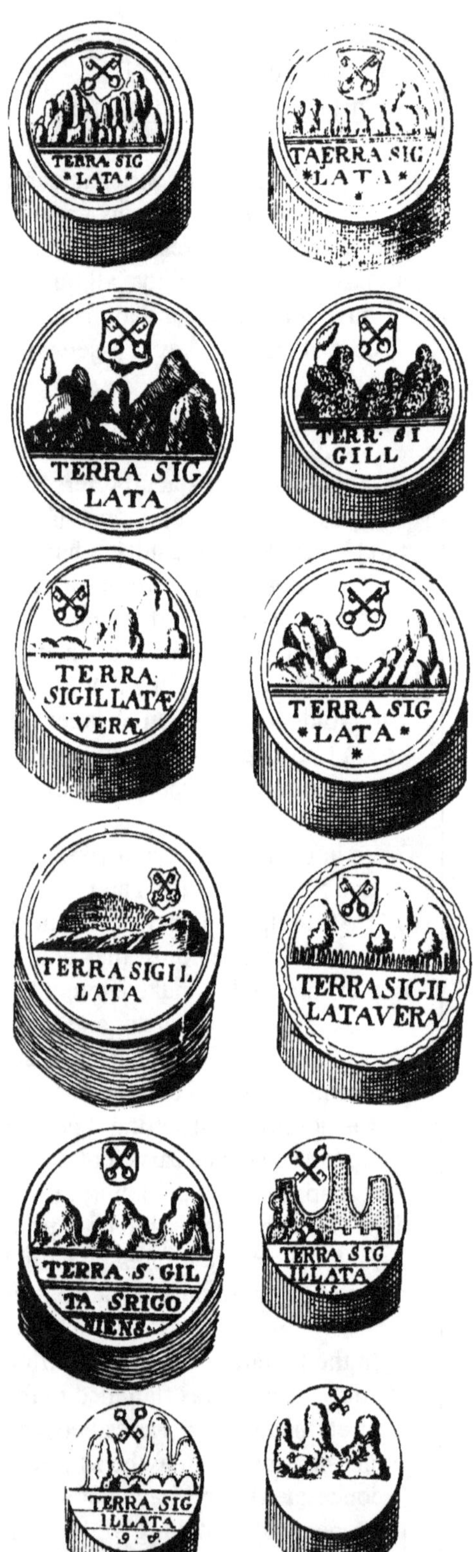

Illustration 402
<u>Earth Coins from Germany</u>

The often similar, but not alike text and picture, must be that more than one marketing group existed over the life of the coin products.

We might suppose that, as reported by Volkmann, one source of earth coins was the local town government, but another, interested in more profit was also working a coin project.

It could be a marketer such as Berthold or it could be a pharmacists. Competition could be the reason for the appearance of the word "vera", true, in the text space of the coin, it might also account for the rather inexplicable spelling errors, if one of the coin stamp makers was illiterate, a matter not rare in 16th/17th century.

Errors like "terra sigillatae verae" (3L) "terr. si gill" (2R), "terra sigil latavera" (4R), "terra s.gil ta srigo niens" (5L), or a coin without any text and a bare lower half, should not have occurred with a source which had access to a printer, pharmacist, or doctor.

This series also shows the first images that include cave or mine shaft openings (1L, 5R, 6L).

Two images have numbers: 5R has 95, 6L has 98. If those are digits of calendar years, it really could be only 1595/98, since printed style letters were not used 100 years earlier, and by 1695/98 the quality of coin minting was much better.

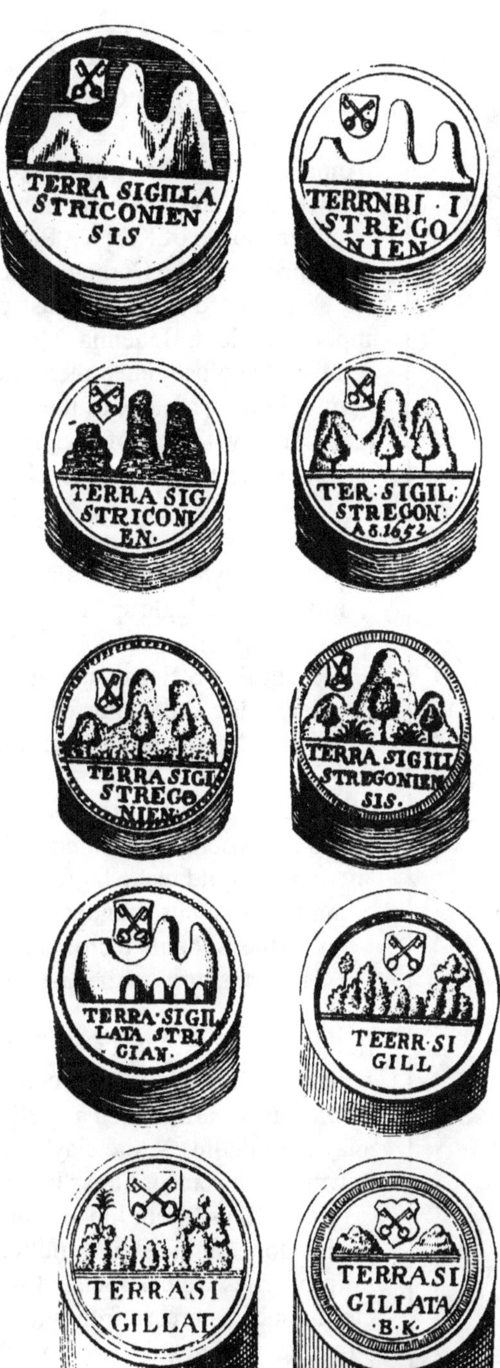

Illustration 403
Earth Coins from Germany

Only very few earth coins were published as photographs from collections. The reason is that many of the coins, as those in the German National Museum in Nürnberg, studied and published by Heller (1964) are in poor condition, some are 400 years old. The ikons we have here are all drawn.

Seven of the images on this page have the crossed flags in the shield, three the crossed sword-and-key. Both styles seem to have co-existed.

1L spells Strigonian with a c, same as Colberg on an earlier page. One rather bland one, 1R, reads "terrnbi I strego nien". 2R has the standard three hills and three cone-shaped trees and a 1652 date. 4L is very stylized and either shows four mine shaft entrances or one entrance and three bushes/trees.

4R spells "teerr si gill", only faintly expressing the basic product mark *Terra sigillata* which must have been the best quality selling point.

I have found no reference how these coins were taken as medicine: Were they hardened or only dried clay, were they broken and then chewed or were they dissolved in water? Volkmann reports that putting clay pieces in water causes an almost explosive reaction, not a gentle fizz.

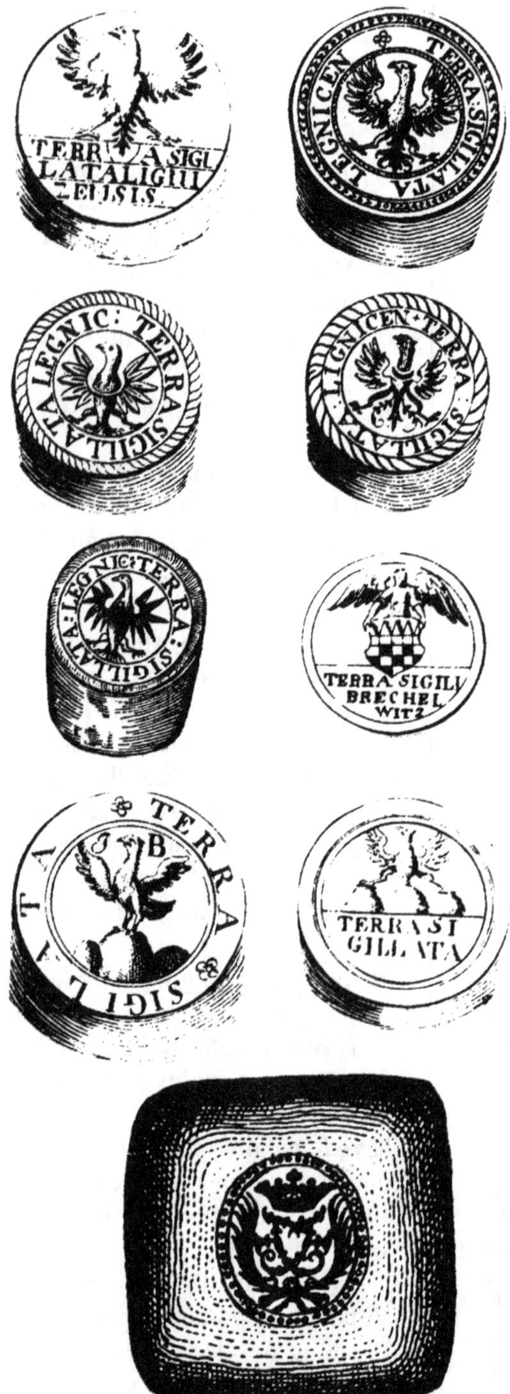

Illustration 404
Earth Coins from Germany

Anna, the daughter of the Duke of Schweidnitz and Jauer (in Silesia), later spouse of Karl V., Roman emperor of the German nation, inherited the right to use the imperial eagle in Bohemia. Most of the earth coins minted thereafter, would have the image of the eagle and the town name of Liegnitz in various spellings (1L+R, 2L+R, 3L.)

Even where the locality was missing, the eagle spread its feet over three hills (4L+R) and thus identified Striegau and the the region of the Dukedoms of Jauer and Schweidnitz.

When competition to sell the earth coins increased, some enterprising merchant would make larger coins or amulets like this rounded square with the Bohemian crown from Hubertusburg in the last coin.

Metals were born, lived and died in the fire of the earth. They created planetary earths, such as yellow clay (from gold), white clay (from silver) for instance. Thus "healing clays" were looked for in abandoned mine shafts and their properties were associated with terms such as grease from the sun (axungia solis, gold) or from the moon (axungia lunae, silver). The living metals were seen as proof of the continuity of creation where God had delegated creative functions to planets and angels.

154

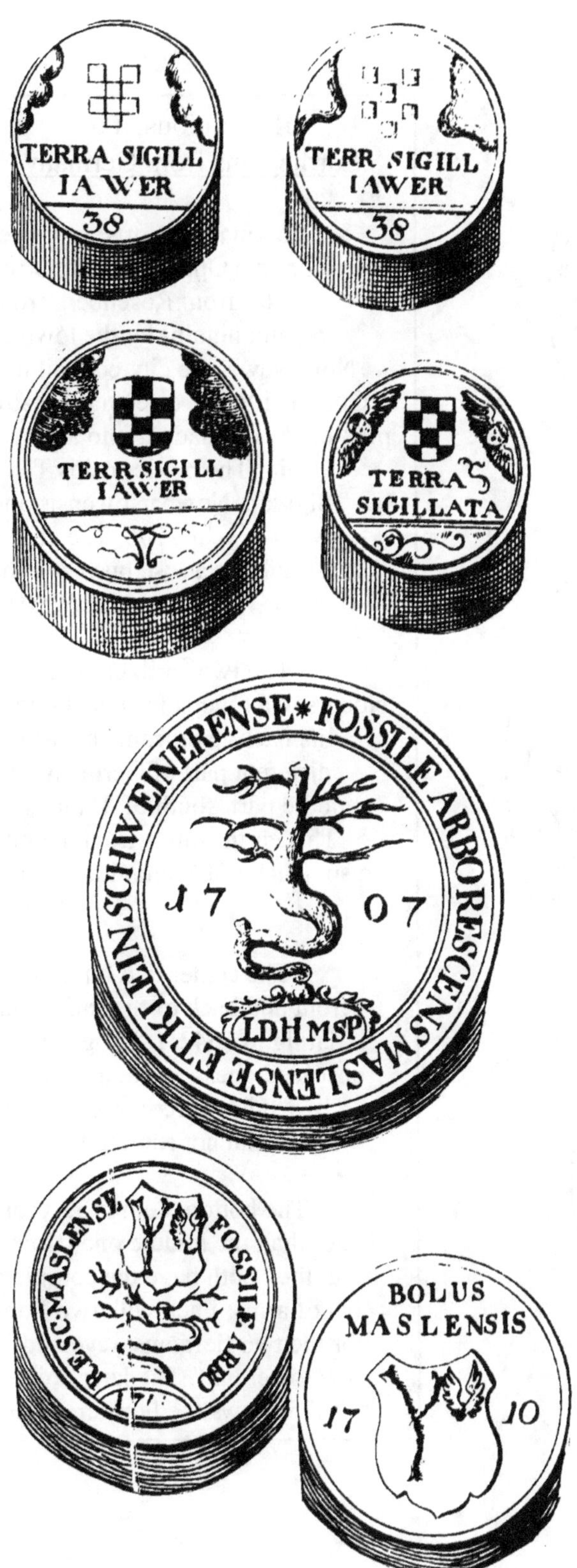

Illustration 405
Earth Coins from Germany

The top four illustrations pertain to the Dukedom of Jauer (here spelled to Iawer). The area with the little squares is depicted in various ways, as engraved interconnected lines, as separate squares (which in reality would be the white squares in the Jauer checkerboard flag.

1L has clouds as part of the frame, 2R has two "flights", heads and wings. The top two have the numeral 38; it might be a calendar year.

The following three ikons refer to clay from Massel (Maslense), a clay find near the mini-village of Klein-Schweinerense (little pig village) at a place where there is an old, dead tree. The specific location is the water trench in the church garden. All three are dated early 18th century. The initials in the large disk refer to the earth's finder Leonhard David Hermann, the parish parson or priest (religion in a fiefdom varied with the belief of the feudal lord).

The escutcheon of the bottom two coins has three fishes nose to nose and a pair of angel wings, the seal of Kreck Witzisch nobility.

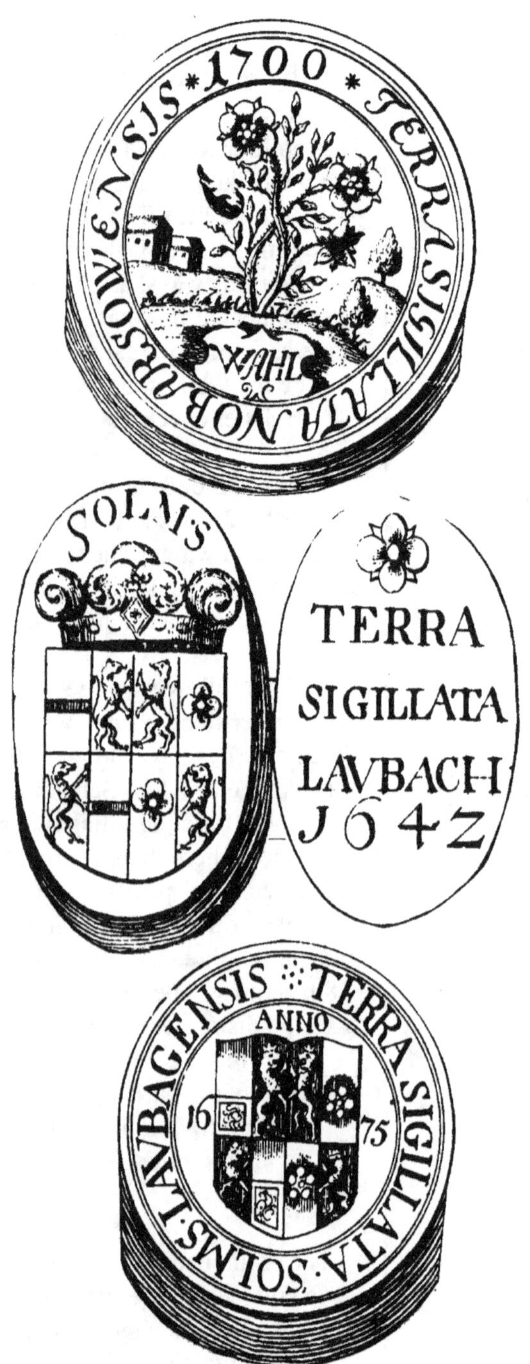

Illustrations 406
<u>Earth Coins from Germany</u>

Volkmann reports: In Upper Silesia, at the Oppelisch border not far from Rosenberg (rose mountain) by the town of Nobarsowa, the city councilman Gottfried Wahl, discovered a soft pink earth. He made it into an earth coin: The border reads Terra Sigillata Nowbarsowensis and gives the year 1700. The center illustration is a rose bush and the name WAHL

The two earth coins below Nobarsowa (one is front and one is its back) are from an entirely different part of Germany, the middle part south of Hannover. This earth comes from the city resp. Duchy of Solms-Laubach in Hesse.

The center two images are front and back of the same coin dating to 1642. It brings up the unsolved question about how the two sides were impressed, the second not ruining the first.

The bottom coin is 33 years later than the middle one (front), but they both have the complete coat of arms: Each with two lions for the two fiefdoms, reversed in the lower half. The later coin of 1675 shows the lions crowned.

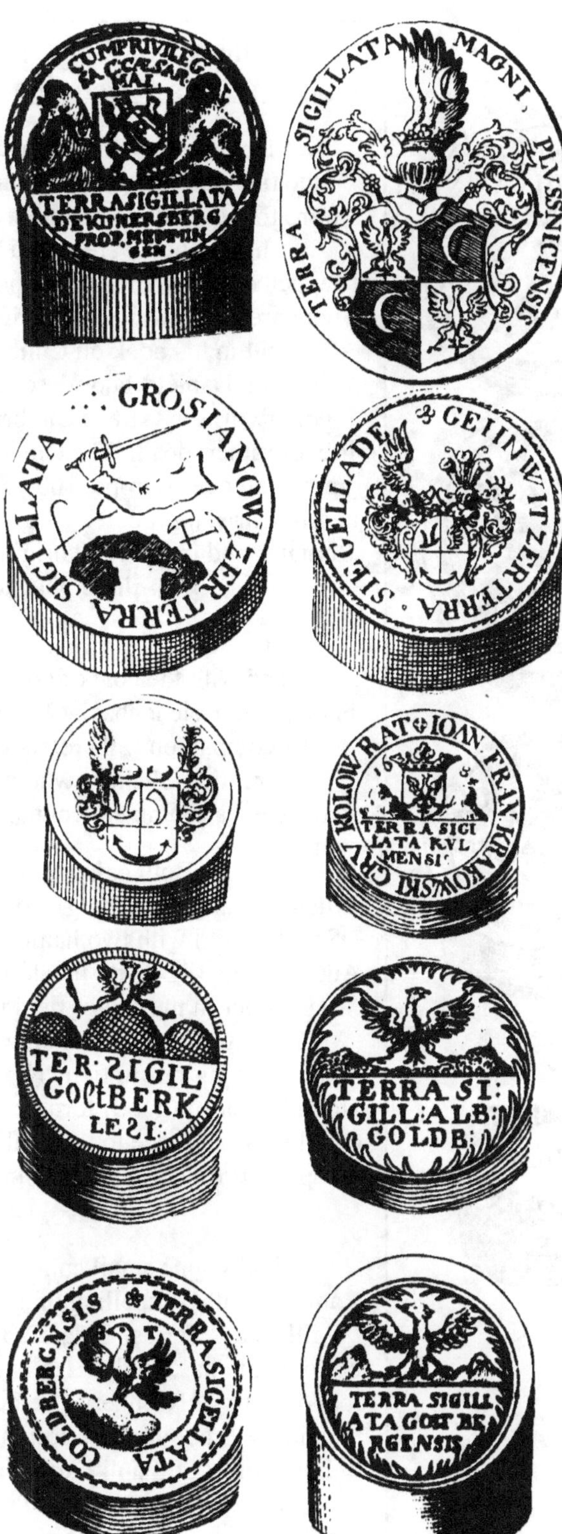

Illustration 407
Earth Coins from
Germany

1L Kümmersberg and 1R Gross-Plußnitz show the diversity of style, details and appeal that can be built into a seal for the earth from a specific location

No town wanted to be left behind in the marketing of "their" earth. Groß Janowitz (2L) combined tools, a strong arm and sword and what may be an anvil in their seal. Gehnwitz (2R. 3L) had not only one, but two elaborate seals.

The Kulmenser Terra Sigil-lata (3R)has a circular inscription that bears witness to the closeness of Silesia, then Germany, and Poland.

The last four earth coins on this page all contain symbols previously seen in Striegau earths, but incredible errors in writing, spelling, and the grace of the hill-perched eagle. 4L probably has the wildest attempt at spelling Terra sigillata from the gold mountain, and (4R) the eagle has not landed on the hills.

157

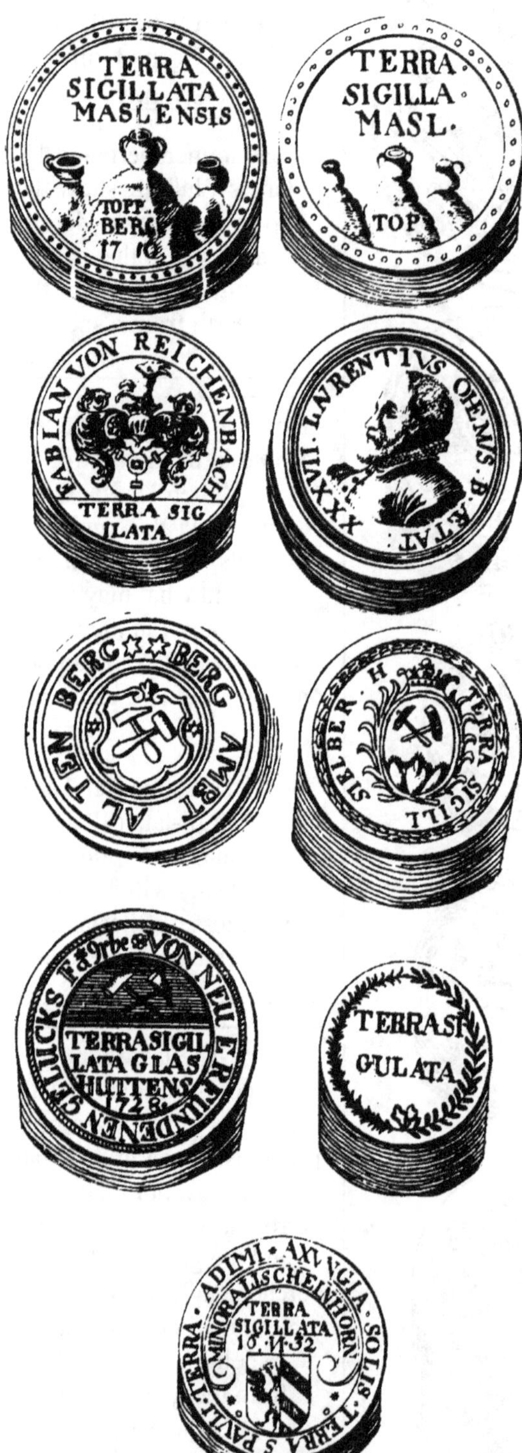

Illustration 408
Earth Coins of Germany

Not far from the church yard in the tiny hamlet of Massel, urns were found on three neighboring hills. They were called the Toeppelberge, the hills of the pots. There are no indications of origin, but in his book on Cimbria, Johann Daniel Major describes pottery urns as part of Cimbrian life, or rather: death. The Cimbers spread all over Europe 100 years before Christ until defeated by the Romans, and may be the origin of these pots, too.

A gray earth from Hanau was sealed with the coat of arms of Fabian von Reichenbach (2L) and its companion (2R) refers to a Laurentius Oheimb, who may have been a prominent councilor.

Both coins in row 3 (Altenberg and Silberberg) have a Saxon shield with two hammers. Another coin (4L) with the double hammer in the center field is a 1728 coin from Glashütten with the intriguing inscription "Newly found color of (good) fortune". It could be a reference to the healing properties associated with this earth.

Finally, one small coin (4R) amuses with its spelling of Terra sigillata as "Terrasi Gulata". The bottom coin has the date 1632, the coat of arms of Nürnberg (Velden) and the bragging description of being like "St. Pauli Earth, pain removing grease of the sun, healing earth equal to mineral unicorn (horn"). Indeed that promises everything.

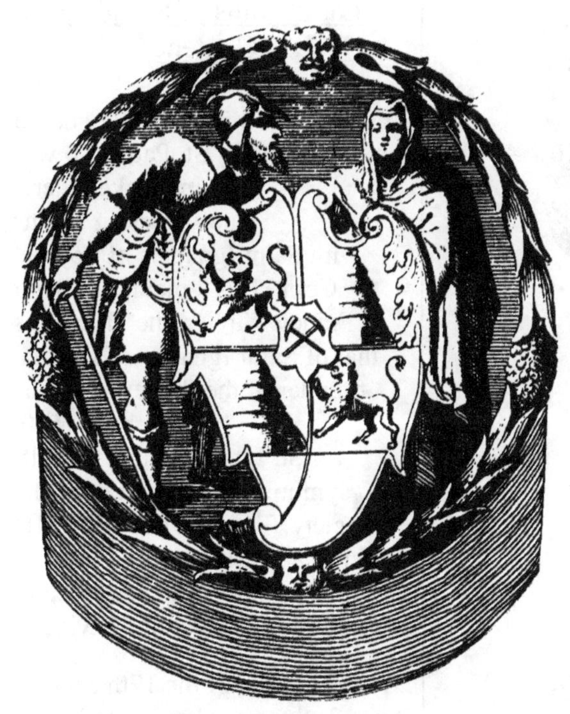

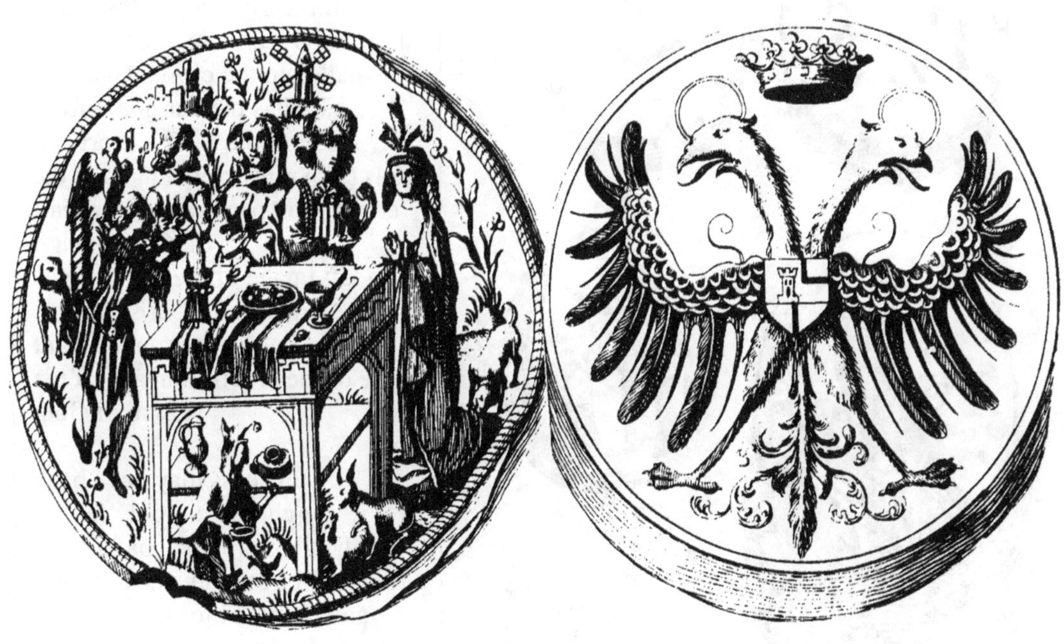

Illustration 409
Earth Coins from Germany

Elaborate large earth coins could have been precious gifts as   had been coin tablets of the ancient earths. At left is a coat of arms design from Saxony with the hammers of the miner in the shield.

The lower images are the front and back of a large earth coin from Bohemia, at least the double eagle is the imperial eagle used in Bohemia. The front picture may be a scene of making and distributing or selling earth coins. As in many old engravings, their dogs and other domesticated animals included with the people in a given scene.

159

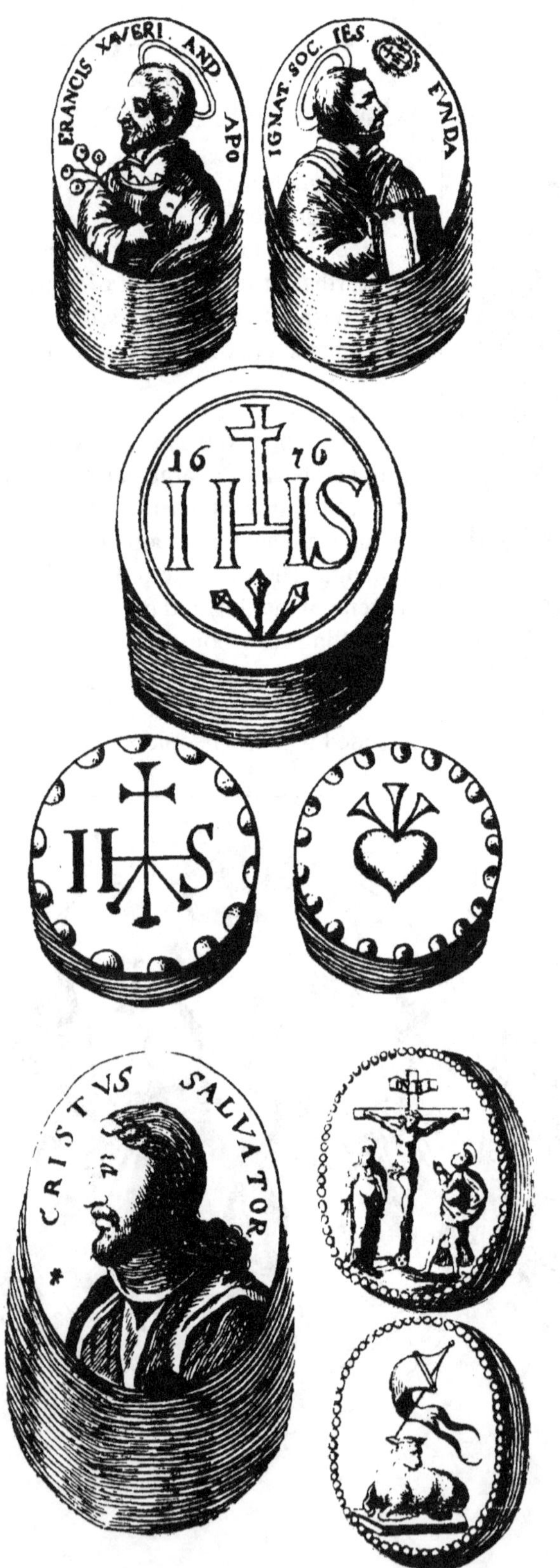

Earth coins from Malta are based on the legend of St. Paul who was shipwrecked there.
Known dating begins with Saint Ignacius of Loyola. Coin 1L is a picture of Saint Francis Xavier, the 1R coin is that of Saint Ignatius of Loyola, founder of the Society of Jesus about 1540.
St. Ignatius liked the HIS symbol and adopted it for the Society. The first two letters IH refer to an early Greek version of Jesus Christ, the S is a later Latin designation "Salvator" (Saviour).

By the middle of the 17th century (row 2) the cross bar of the H was base for a cross and below it are three nails with which Christ was nailed to the cross. A later(?) version has the bar going from the H to the S. The heart and nails (3R) must be the nails of the crucifixion penetrating the heart of Christianity.
The left image of the 4th row is a representation of Christ Savior, the two engravings on the right are of the crucifixion and of the Lamb of God.

Such coins may have been purchased not only for the healing promise, but also as amulets or as evidence of a sum paid to plead for shortening a sinner's period in purgatory or as plea for help from a saint.

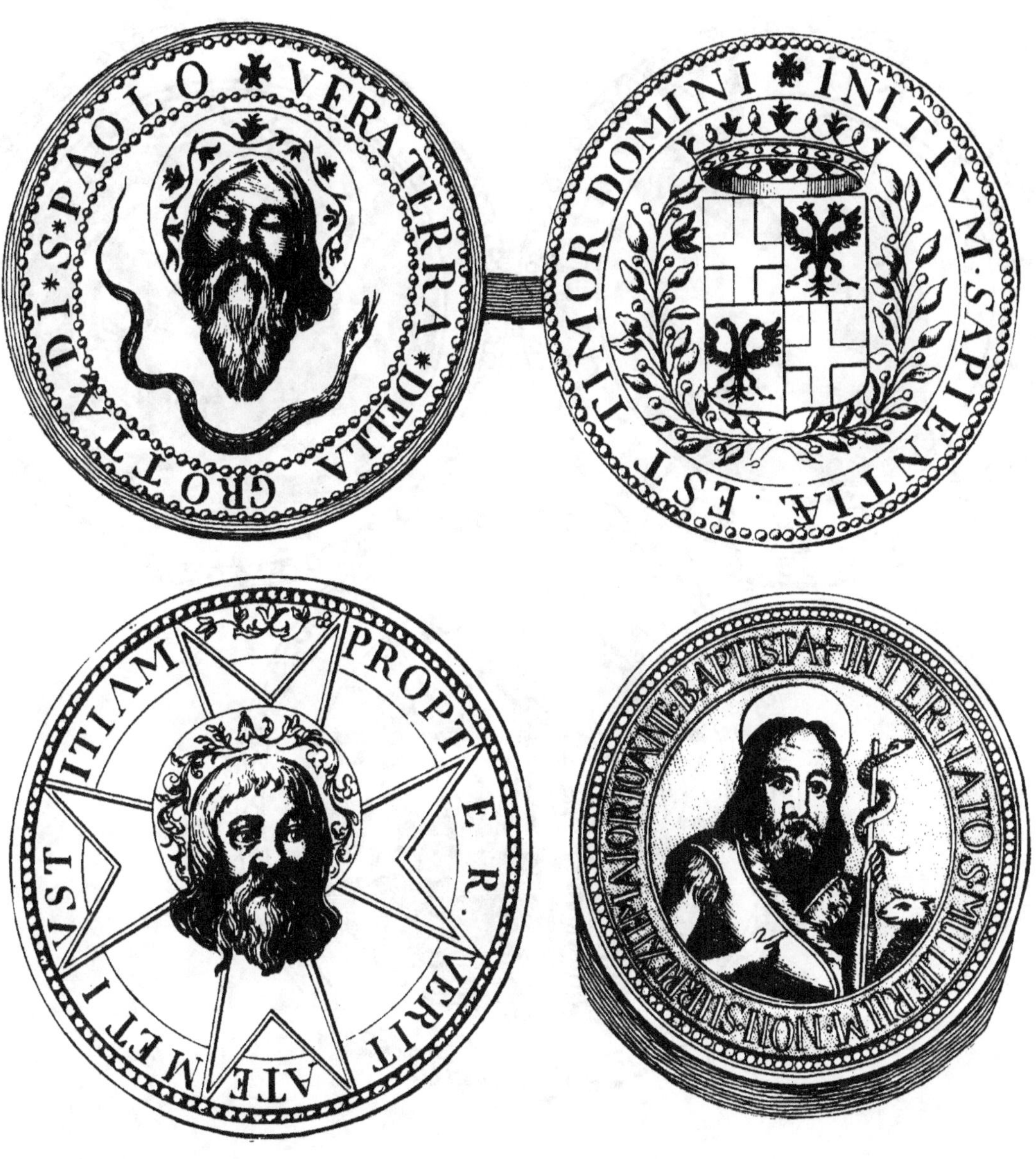

The top two earth-coin images are the front and back of a St. Paul coin. The front has the text "The true earth from the cave (grotto) of Saint Paul" and with his image one of the serpents that St. Paul banished from Malta after one bit him. The lower left represents a likeness of Jesus and the words imply that the beginning of wisdom is the fear of the Lord. The lower right is an image of St. Paul(?) with staff and lamb. The inscription by John the Baptist says that the Lord was born of, but not resurrected, by a woman. The lamb is watching in the corner.

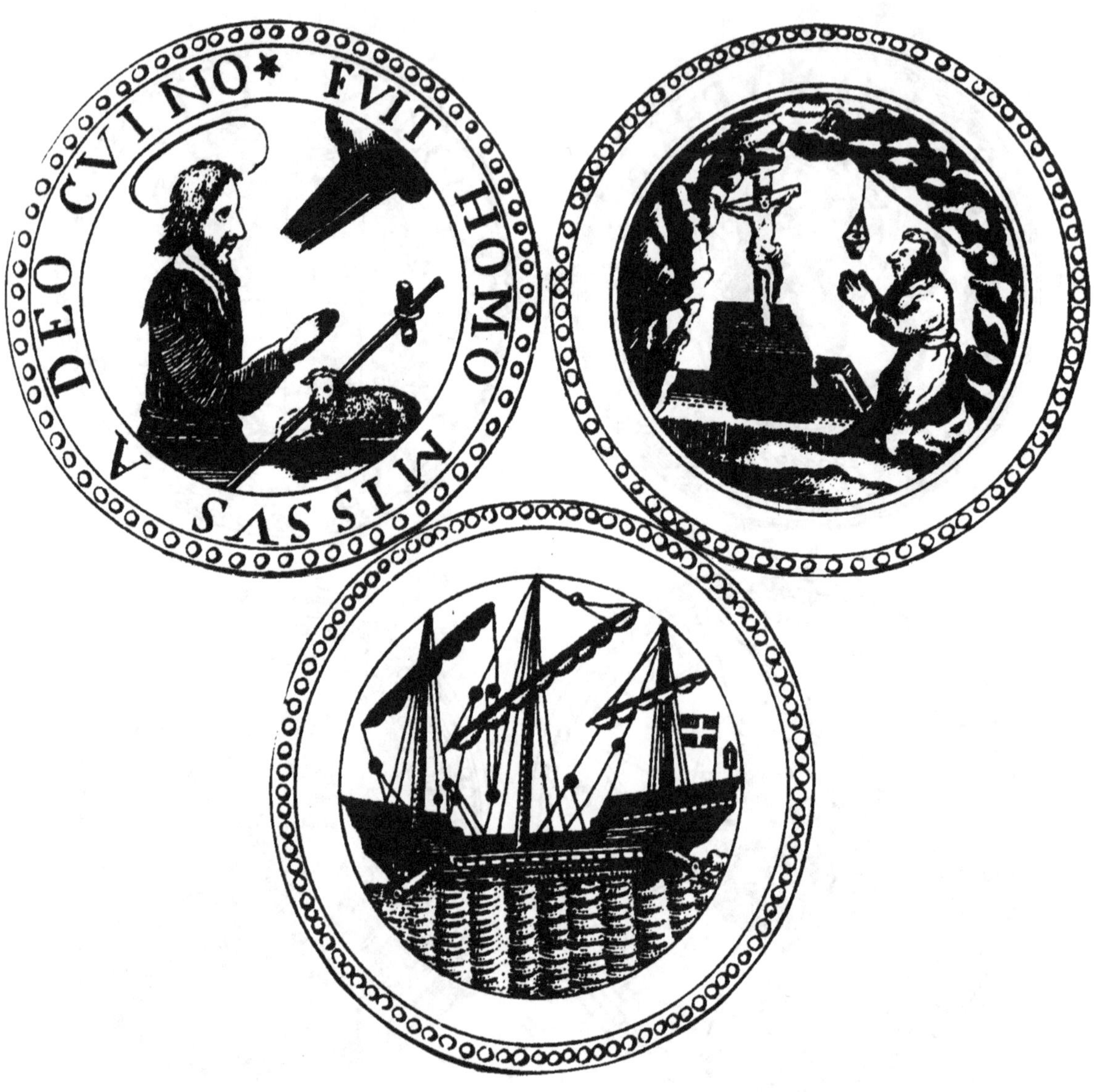

Except for the bottom illustration, the ship which carried St. Paul to an involuntary rest in Malta, these earth coins were described by personal interpretations of G. Spanudis (1945). The Johanniter Knights of Malta, (in English usually called "the Knight Hospitallers) founded 1530, may have taken St. John as a surrogate for the St. Paul legend of banishing the serpents and making their teeth to stone. Concerning the right image, Spanudis saw a supplicant praying and a bag with healing earth hung up to dry. I would think one needed a light in a cave to pray at an altar and cross in a dark cave. If it were a bag of earth, it would have had to be re-wetted for internal use. This earth was popular with Christians, Moslem and Jews alike, who scraped it off the wall of the cave to use as medication. It miraculously always grew

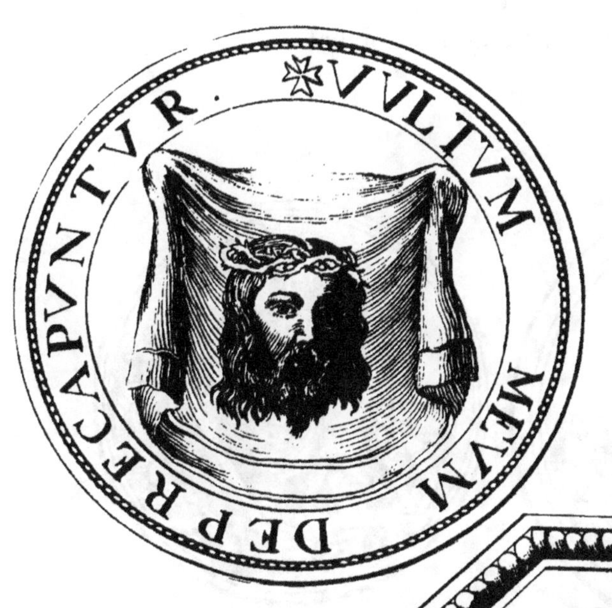

Illustration 413
Earth Coins of Religious Content

Top: Face cloth of Christ (but with crown of thorns, legend: "Pray for my sadness"

Middle: Holy Mary, Mother of Jesus.

Bottom: St. Francis praying at the crucifixion of Christ.

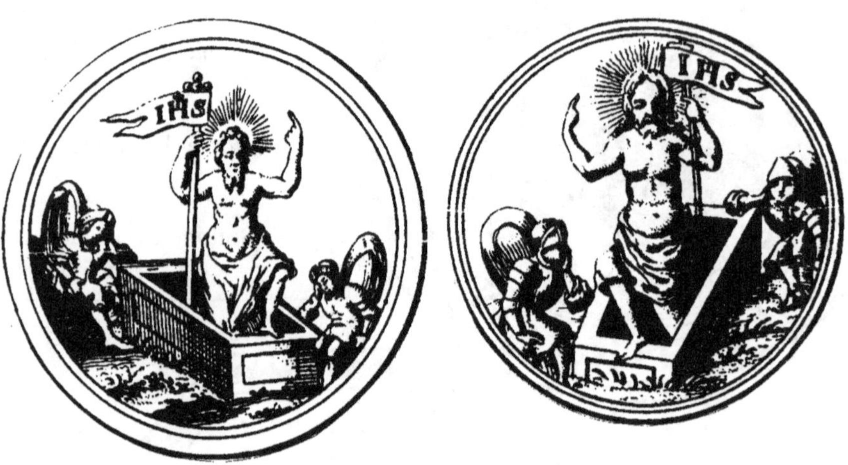

The graphics of these earth coins are very unusual for several reasons: They appear as mirror images, but are not. They appear as front and back, but they are not the same coin. Viewed carefully, they are separate different drawings which merely resemble each other.

Obviously, in both coins the scene depicts the moment of the resurrection of Christ.

I found the description in Aldrovandi's "Museum Metallici", Lib. II. P. 243 under the headline "Syriac chalk in circle with the effigy of the Lord's resurrection." They are supposed to be coins from an order of nuns, who also had coins of the Milk of Mary and here represent that the coins are made from the earth in the sepulcher of the Lord. The coin material, when taken with wine, becomes milk from the breasts of Mary to help women to lactate normally after having given birth. Lack of lactation was often the result of overwork, undernourishment and pregnancy in ancient times.

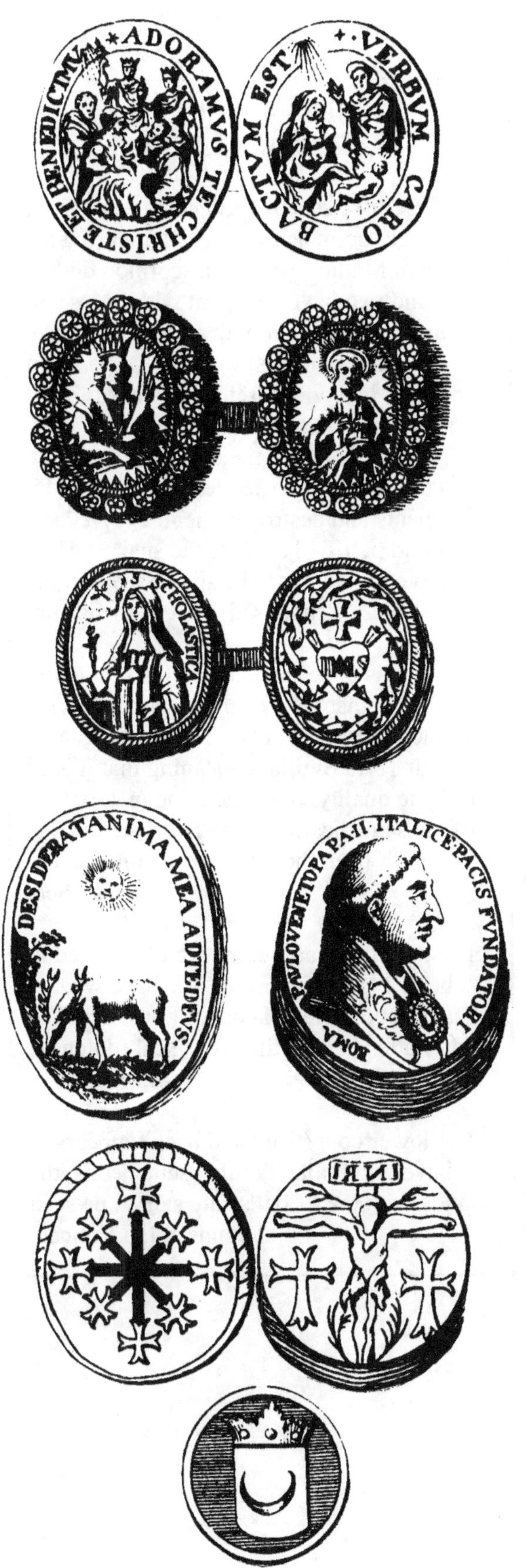

Illustration 415
Earth coins of Italy

The adoration coin (front and back) was probably sold to visitors to the Vatican
(2R&L) Heavily decorated earth coins with the images of crowned women may have originated in the Medici family.
(3L+R) shows a nun and the word "scholastica". St. Scholastica (the biological sister of St. Benedict) was the Saint of Nuns. The cross of crucifixion in the front and on the back the letters IHS previously were identified as "Jesus Christ Savior".
"I wish my soul to be with you" is a coin of unknown source. The right coin is a dedication of Paulo, the Venetian as pope of Italy, exhorting fundamental peace in Italy. There is no date, but the subscript "Rome".

The next two images may have been stamped on an earth called "Milk of the Holy Mary". In a cave she brushed against the wall, spilled some of her milk. From then on the solidified white milk (Calcium carbonate) grew and was scraped from the walls to help women and female animals. The reversed inscription of INRI is an error by the seal maker

The lowest coin is a of a half-round shield with a half moon and crown that could be a Turkish design.

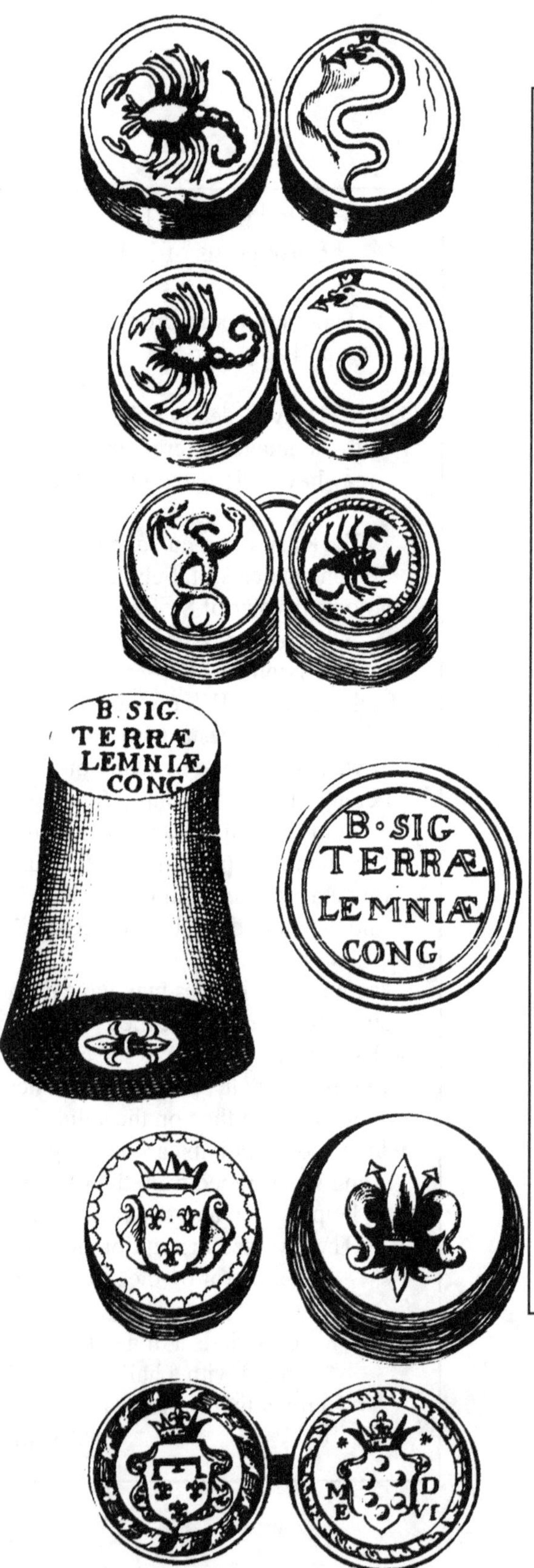

Illustration 416
Earth Coins from Italy

The first three sets of earth coins, each front and back, point again to St. Paul during his stay on Malta: Each has a scorpion on one side and two have a serpent with horns and an arrow in the mouth on the other side. The third coin has two fable serpents on one side, one with forelegs and horns. Paul was bitten by a scorpion, but flung it away and did not die from the bite because he ate of the white earth. He was bothered by serpents and destroyed them. People later found petrified teeth of the snakes. They have turned out to be sharks teeth in the chalk sediment of the island.

This cone shaped creation on the top says that the B(olus), or the B(lois), a French location of clay, is "congenerated" with Terra Sigillata, meaning that it is of the same quality, or of the same material, or of the same healing efficacy as the famous earth from the Island of Lemnos in the Aegean Sea.

The next four earth coins are considered to be of Florentine origin. We have what is said to be a Medici coat of arms, a ball of clay flattened with the "lily" seal (defender of the faith?).

The lower coin (front and back) appears to have two Italian family escutcheons, the side with the 6 "balls" are said to be seen on columns at the Vatican.

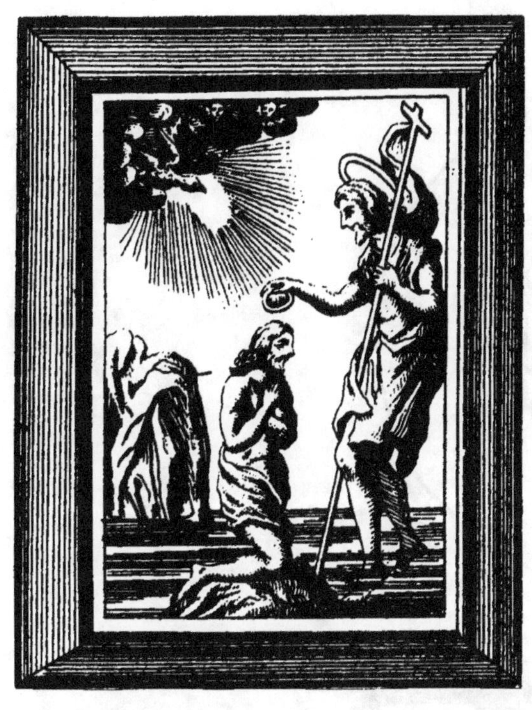

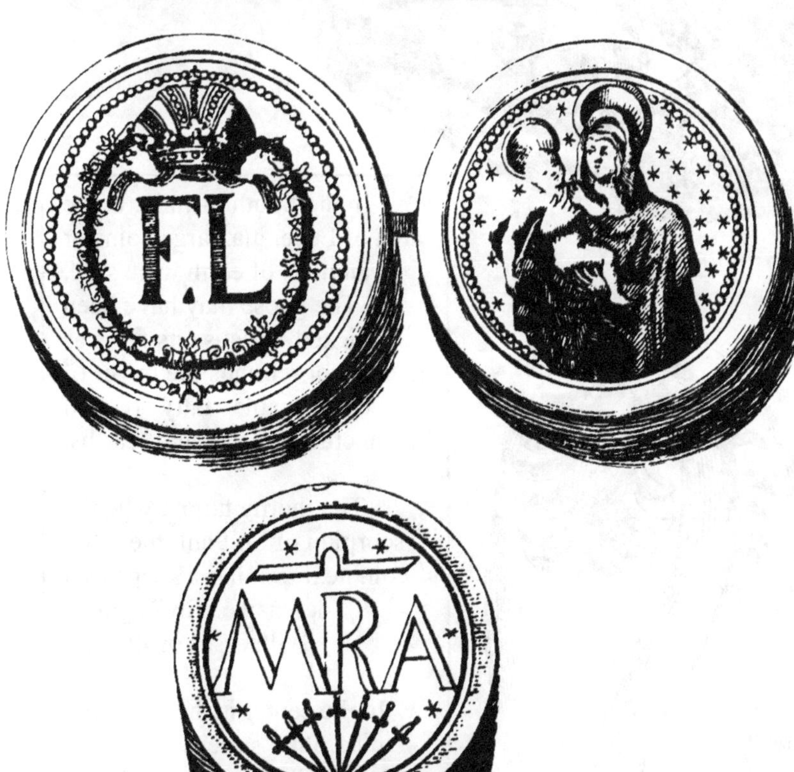

167

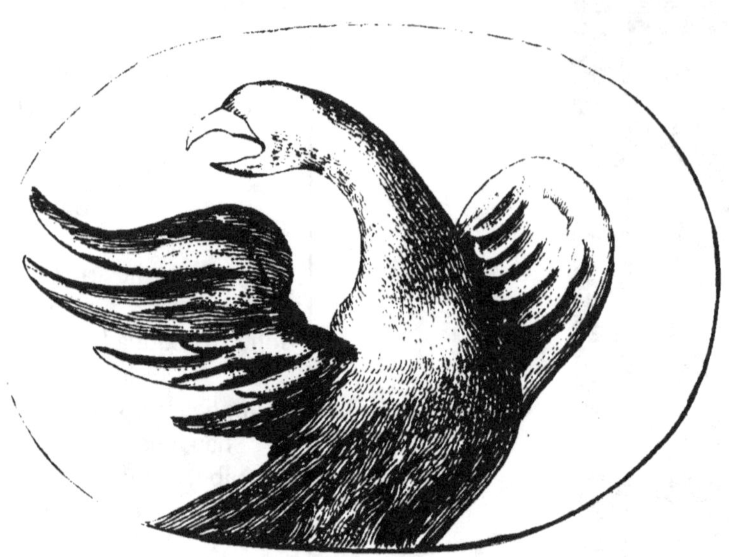

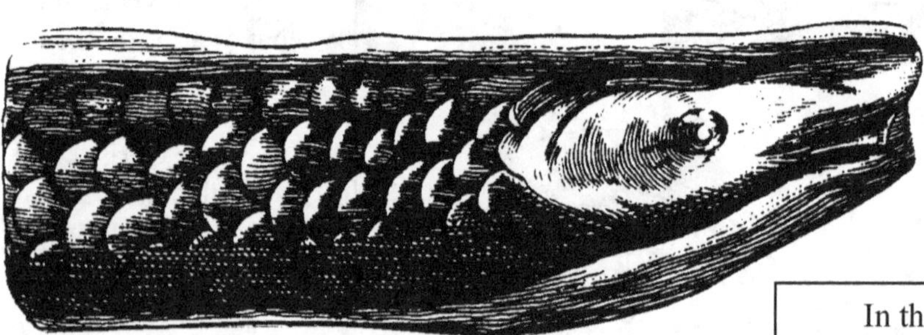

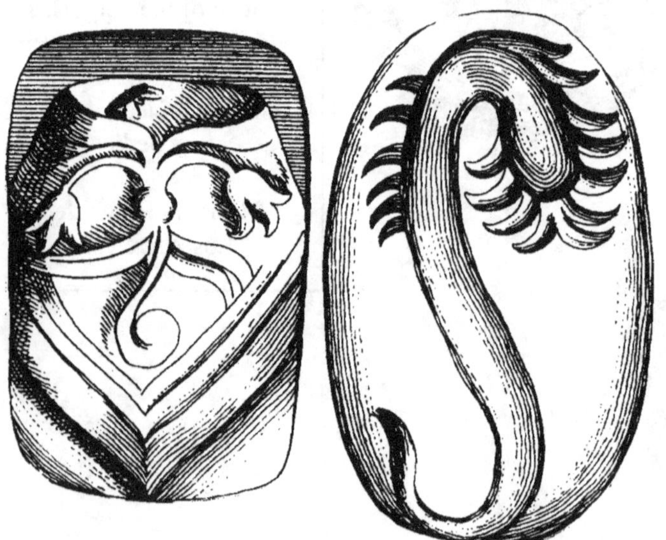

In the South of Italy, in the area of Lucerana, large coins or amulets of earth were sold. The goose may have been picked, because its fat is as good as or reminds the buyer of the valuable "fatty" (called unctuous or pinguid) earths.

The thorny tail may be the scorpion of St. Paul; the other coin next to it has a shape as a defensive "lily" against illnesses or ill luck.

In the center is the head of a pike. Pike's grease, *axungia lucii*, was comparable to unctuous earth as medicine.

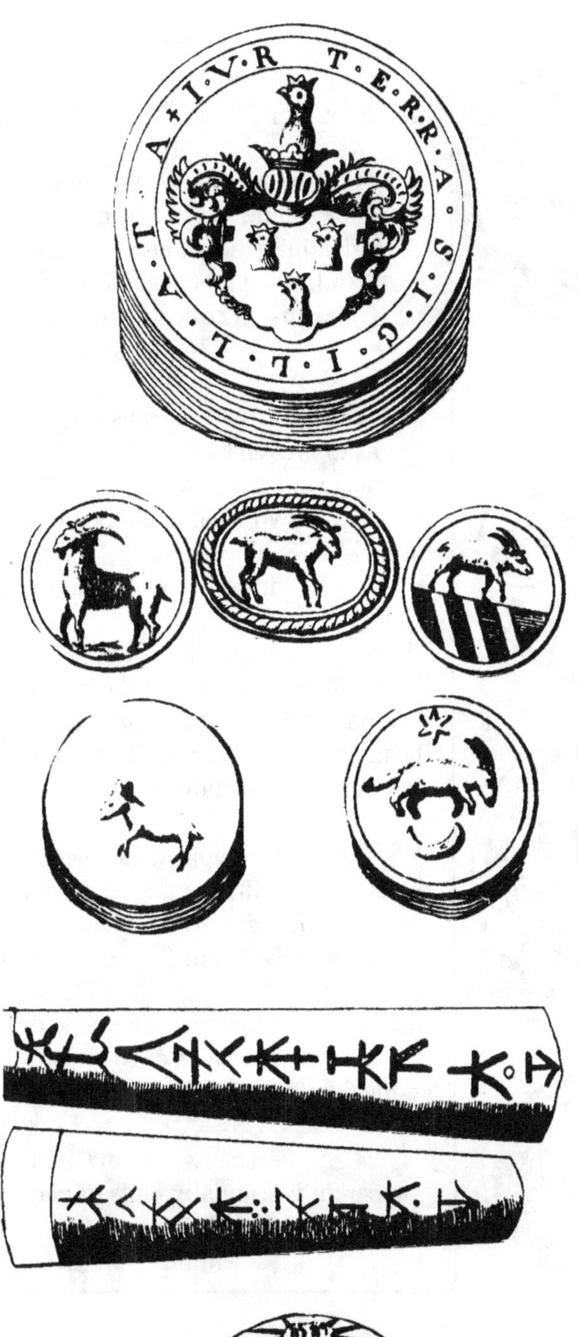

Illustration 419
Miscellaneous Earth Coins

Referring to the first coin, Volkmann sees a brown sigillated earth from the Duchy of Jauer, found near Brechelshof. Ludwig calls it the Praußnitz (Brusnicensis) earth.

The five coins in a cluster of images are supposed to represent the famous healing earth of the Greek island of Lemnos, sealed with the goat mascot of the Goddess Artemis (Greek) or Diana (Roman). There is no doubt that these are copies or memorial coins simulating the value of the Greek earth.

The two conical "coins" are from China and were reported in Athanasius Kircher's Book on China. They were worn on strings and rubbed on to whiten the faces of the noble ladies.

The final coin looks like a preacher's podium and farming or mining tools. The exhortation "ora et labora" should be translated as "pray and work".

Cosmetic use of white earths, such as calcium carbonate, or its use as cleansing agent is also known from Mexico, from the white earth Thicatlalli.

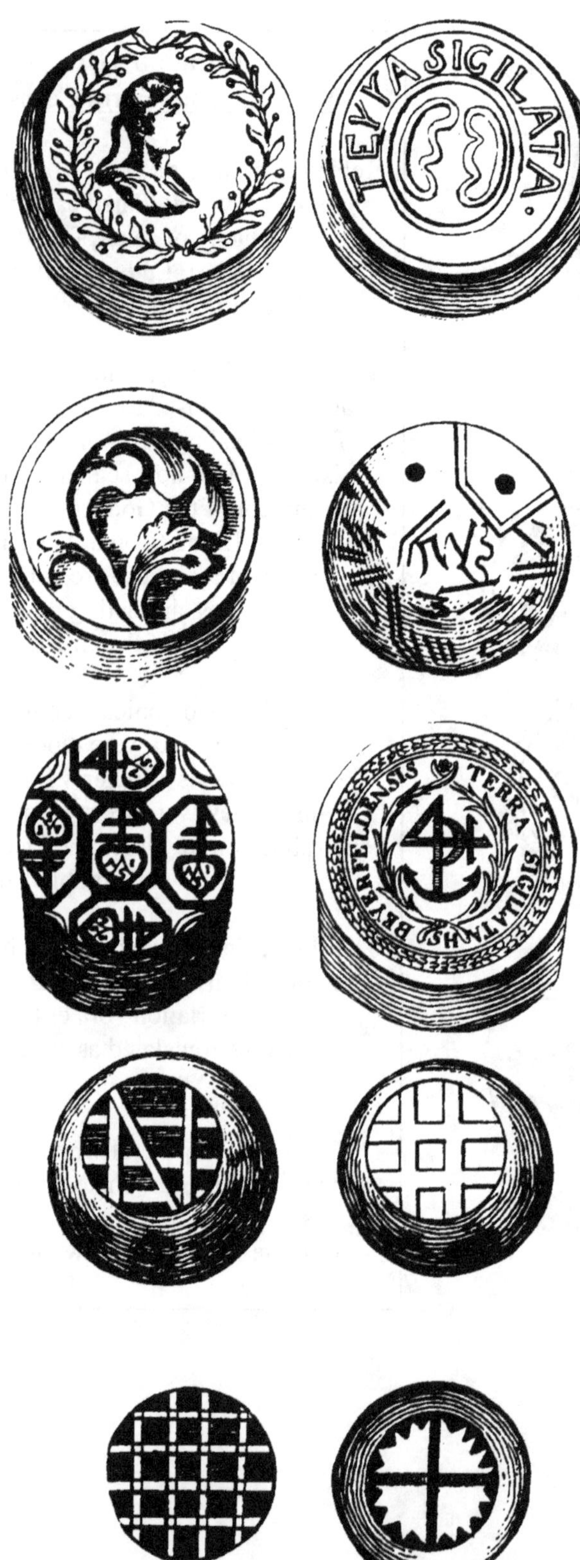

Illustration 420
Earth Coins of Unknown Origin

Of the mineral history authors Aldrovandi, Worm, Volkmann, Valentini, Rivino, and Christian Gottlieb Ludwig, the last has by far the largest collection of coin illustrations.

The first row leaves us no clue as to provenance, neither of the image nor the Terra with small r and two what could be brass knuckles: Schläger, yes, they were in some coats of arms.

The second row left in its execution gives southern Italian flavor and reminds of the "lily", the iron spear heads often buried in the bottom of castle moats or pitfalls as a defense.

Row three appears to show a relationship of the geometric design with the right, so both could be from the hamlet of Beyersfeld in Silesia.
Many earth coins with geometric designs exist and are copied in texts on the coin subject.

The two in row 4 are apparently originally balls of clay (not disks) and flattened by the minting pressure.

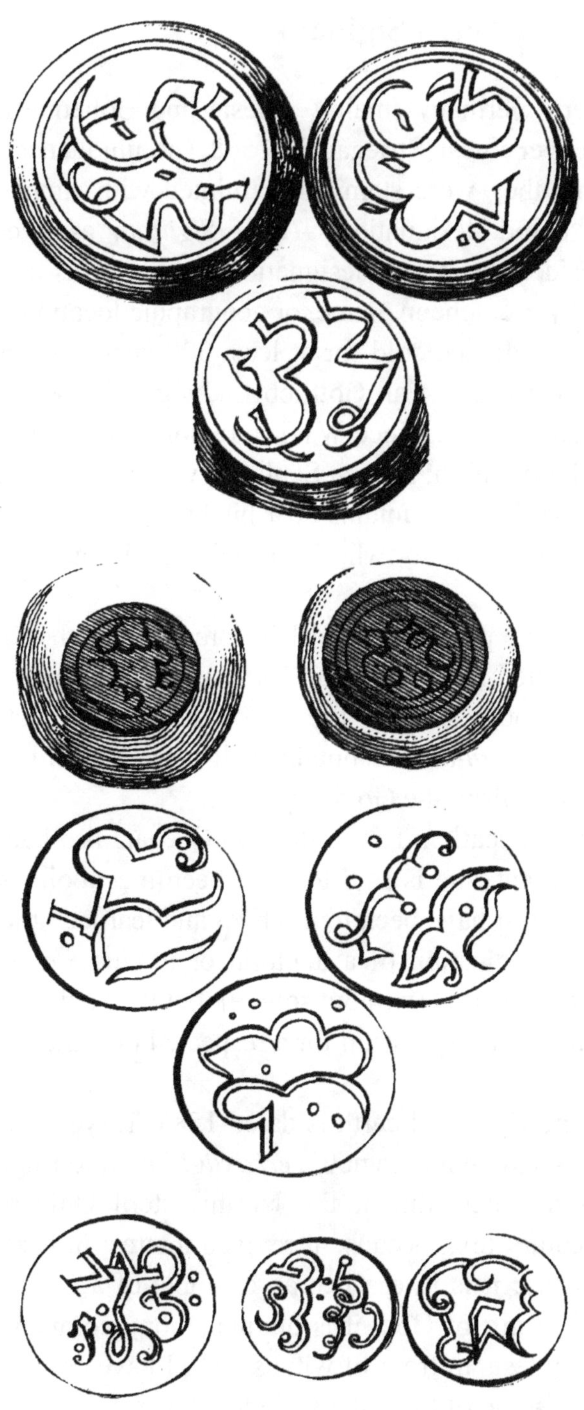

Illustration 421
Earth Coins with Arabic Writing

After Turkey occupied the Greek
Island of Lemnos, the earth coins
made there were stamped with
Arabic characters.

There has been frequent
guessing as to the meaning of these
ikons. Some believe that at least a
few were called "THIN", meaning
from moist, flexible clay. Others had
"BARR" as prefix meaning hard or
friable clay.

Second names attached to either
kind were MACHTUM or
MOHABB, but the meaning is not
resolved. Robertson (1989) thought
Tinmachtum was an alliterated
Greek tini ma chthon "from your
mother earth" expressed in Arabic
writing.

Many earth coins scribed with
supposedly Arabic letters were
European fakes, local clay and
counterfeit images.

Chapter 18 Part 1: Introduction to Andreas Berthold and his Treatise on Terra Sigillata

"Healing earth" coins from then Eastern Germany (mainly Silesia and Bohemia and Saxony) have been known since their discovery near Striegau in 1568.The uniqueness of these earth (clay) trochisks or tablets is that they were stamped or minted with simple to elaborate designs usually including the "brand designation" *Terra Sigillata* as overall symbol of quality since ancient times. Besides the brand designation the seal was also a specific trademark or provenance identifier by escutcheon, name, or geographic location.

German and other European coins were made and sold for at least 300 years. A major collection of these earth coins was described by Christian Gottlieb Ludwig in 1748. As it pertains to coins from Silesia (once a German province, since WWII a region of Poland) two names are associated with the discovery and promotion: Johann Scultetus with the additional name "Montanus" or "Trimontanus", from the three mountains near his birthplace Striegau, and Andreas Berthold (Bertold) from Oschatz in Saxony who later claimed discovery of a new earth inside a gold mine.

Johann (Schulz) Trimontanus was a graduate physician who later practiced in the town of Hirschberg. I believe it was he who identified the new found earth as pliable, unctuous and drying-out to the point where a piece would stick to the tip of the tongue, just as classical descriptions of healing earths, *terrae sigillatae* maintained. It was Berthold who took on the promotion of this new Striegau earth from the Goldberg mine.

Little is known about Andreas Berthold's education. His birth town Oschatz is a hamlet between Leipzig and Dresden in Saxony. Because he is said to have been a schoolmaster and writing teacher in Stettin about 1570, he must have been to a school and learned at least rudimentary Latin, but there is no record or indication of a doctoral or graduate degree. Dannenfeldt (1984) in one place calls him Dr. Berthold (without source), but the "evidence", a capital D before a male name was "Dominus", an expression for a respected man, never an indication of any doctorate.

The first publication in Latin about the newly found earth is dated 1583, 15 years after discovery. The 1587 translation of Berthold's text about the new *Terra Sigillata* into English by an unknown apothecary (B.G.) exists as microfilm at the Northwestern University Library. Because it is a rare printed 16th century text, because it revived interest in healing earth coins when it was published, and because it is in essence an example of a medieval advertising brochure ("it does wonders, it is a gift of God, it is unique among competitors who are misleading the reader, it is proven by tests in front of witnesses"), I have converted it to modern English words, but tried to retain some of the older style for flavor.

The first 20th century writer to cite Berthold's report of a successful trial of his *Terra Sigillata* from Silesia versus deadly poison on a prisoner who had been sentenced to death is D.A. K. Black in 1956, and from a scientific point of view, Black did not think that the test was improbable. Berthold also claimed he had done a series of tests on dogs.

During the 16th and 17th century a number of feudal lords, pressed with the expenditures for court and for standing armies, attempted to improve their financial situation by supporting alchemical experts, especially those who promised to make gold. (A few found it laughable, among them Georgius Agricola, who stated that since everybody believed one can make gold out of a base metal, he cannot say it is impossible, but since none of the gold makers ever got rich, Agricola, tongue in cheek, says that he can't believe it after all).

The court of Hesse was one of those courts known for its alchemical-Paracelsian circle, and that makes it credible that Berthold with his *Terra Sigillata* was received at court. Indeed, in the Archives of the State of Hesse, in personal records of Landgrave Wilhelm IV "the Wise" of Hesse-Kassel (1567-1592) there is a record of the tests, which Andreas Berthold of Oschatz describes as having taken place in the presence of the court. This record is in the archives of the State of Hesse in the town of Marburg (Hessisches Staatsarchiv Marburg, Fürstliche Personalien, Wilhelm IV., Bestand 4a 31 Nr. 77). The English misspellings and errors of the name of the personality and the court of Hesse in the English translation made it more difficult to find the pertinent record.

An archive of the Hohenlohes zu Langenburg (there were many of them) could not confirm that the experiment with a human prisoner did take place as ascribed to Graf Wolfgang II. The reported details of the test make it probable that it took place and was successful.

At first, the subjective promotion of Berthold's terra sigillata, the typical medieval argument sequence "my product is better, the competitors are godless people" and his exaggerations ("I am leaving with an apothecary precious stones for medical treatment for colleagues who may need them") raised a suspicion that the tests were not quite as described, but the reading of the following text gives an insight into the desperate need for medical knowledge and help in the 16th century.

Berthold used "von" in his name, made elaborate coin stamp escutcheons to simulate nobility, maybe to help gain access to courts and credibility. The leading authority on nobility in Germany (Der Herold, Berlin) is certain that Berthold was never ennobled. I also found very disconcerting that the description in his text of where he claims to live in Silesia is a geophysical impossibility, and that he claims he left precious and semi-precious stones available to physicians with a book printer (!) in Frankfurt on the wrong river, may be par for a medieval exuberance in semi-medical writing.

From a Tübingen (Württemberg) diary by a Martin Crusius we learn that in 1608 a Dr. Schopff from Kirchheim unter Teck was permitted a similar experiment giving the prisoner poison and then an antidote, promising freedom if the prisoner survived it. The text says "the prisoner was given a poison (not identified) and after a few hours when the poison started to give effect, an antidote (not identified, but believed to be *terra sigillata*). Within a few days (?) the prisoner was cured and was released". I question the length of time it took to cure the prisoner, it is atypical from other reported tests.

Chapter 18 Part 2: Andreas Berthold von Oschatz Discourse on Terra Sigillata

---

The wonderful and strange effects and virtues

of a new *Terra Sigillata*

lately found out in

Germany

With the right order of
applying and administering it
as oftentimes tried and experienced by
Andreas Bertholdus of Oschatz in Misnia[1]

<u>At London</u>

Printed by ***Robert Robinson***
For ***Richard Watkins***

1587

Introductory letter:

To the right worshipful,
My especially good friends
M.D. Maister and ***M.D. Baylie.*** **Doctors in Physicke**
Attendant upon Her Majesty.

"Well known is it unto you both, Right Reverend and learned doctors, how carefully our good friend **M. Hugh Morgan,** her Majesty's Apothecary, has evermore employed himself and his purse to furnish this realm with the rarest, most perfect and best sorts of all manner of plants, fruits, juices, gums, metals, minerals, boles, stones and whatever else needful for either preserving or restoring of health. Whereby he has not only well served his country but has also become famous for sundry compounds, especially for his exact composition of his *Mithridat*[2] and his *Treacle of Andromachus*[3] for which he had searched throughout France and Italy. It pleased him (and I thank him) of late to send me a new *Terra Sigillata*[4] which lately had been found in Germany. This has not only been tried by physicians of that part of the world and was found most reliable as cure for all poisons and most deadly diseases, it has been experimented with by my good and learned friend *M. Doctor Hector of Nunnes* as well as others of your learned college in London, who also found it most effective against many dreadful and dangerous diseases.

He sent me withall a little book in Latin, written by *Andreas Bertholdus* touching on the benefits and correct use of it.

I thought it good for the benefit of such persons as are ignorant of that language to put it into English and to publish it under the protection of your learning and I ask you to bestow the favor of your support to this translation."

Almingham, this 14th of August, 1587.

Your assuredly loving friend[5],

B.G.[6]

Of the Virtues, Force, and Use
Of the right and approved
Terra Sigillata of Germany

The first and in nature most wonderful and to be revered is that it resists all manners of poisons or venoms which have been ingested, be they ever so furious and deadly, and it expels them by vomit, if either before or presently after the poisons were taken, or if even later, it drives them out by sweating.

Secondly, with the like wonderful quality of nature, it resists the most cruel and horrible infection of the pestilence, not only by preserving of the illness, but by speedy curing and calling to life those infected and half dead [2][7].

Thirdly, it cures the bites or stings of all manner of venomous beasts, or worms, or any wound made by a poisoned dart or weapon.

Fourthly, it is found to have a singular and sweet agreement and wonderful sympathy with the vital parts of man's body, so that it greatly comforts the heart, refreshes the brain, and keeps diseases away from all the inner parts. It assuages all manner of headache, pain, and trembling of the heart. It helps wounded, inflamed, bleary, and watering eyes. It has been found by experience that in [the case of] wounds and inflammations of the brain and the stones[8], this excellent earth has done more good than any other medicine could promise or perform.

Fifthly, against all immeasurable bleeding, either by vein, or artery, or any other part of the body, there cannot be found a more assured remedy.

Sixthly, it dries all manner of rheumes[9], [3] distillations, and murrs.

Seventhly it stops the laske[10], lyentery, bloody flux, and all other too much looseness of the belly.

Eighthly, it thoroughly heals all burns or scaldings by fire, water or metal, keeping them from blistering and speedily restoring the hurt parts.

Ninthly, it soundly and perfectly heals all green[11] wounds, rankled and rotten sores.

Tenthly, it is against quinsy[12] and inner inflammations a most present remedy.

The eleventh, against itch and scabs that are barely cured, this earth is used with very good success.

The twelfth, it is a most effective medicine against all such illnesses as can be avoided by sweating.

The thirteenth, against consumption of the lungs by drying up the sore, staying the spitting of blood, it is a most profitable medicine.

A more full and plainer declaration
of the manner and order
In the using the said earth against
The diseases before named.

First, to speak in general of the use of this earth and the manner of taking it: It is given with the most happy success. Of similar kind as, and against the same unnatural diseases as, the earth of **Lemnos**, which of olden time was so famous and is at this day so highly accounted of by the **Turkish** emperor and his **Bassa** as they esteem it to be far more precious than gold, nay, which is more, in curing of many diseases, it far exceeds the said **Lemnian** earth, which for the most part now is counterfeit and is yet with such difficulties brought out of **Turkey** to us (for that, which is commonly sold at the apothecaries, is in comparison hereof not worthy to be named). [5] And therefore the great good reason is that we confess, and with thankful mind acknowledge, the singularly liberal and generous majesty which extends to our countrymen of **Germany**: That where by reason of Turkish barbarousness so godly and blessed gifts of God, as likewise all learning, arts, and liberal sciences, have been defaced and corrupted, yet it has pleased him this day to so beautify this poor country of **Germany**, not only with all kinds of good learning and arts, and with the profound knowledge of divinity, but has likewise sent unto us such most rare and excellent gifts, whereby we are sufficiently provided of whatsoever concerns the health of either soul or body. And because I would not have men be persuaded by my bare words (who upon a charitable affection have willingly published to the world this worthy benefit of God) I do unto all learned men commit the efficacy for me, and virtuosities of this blessed and never sufficiently commended earth, to be weighed and examined with sound judgment and consideration, which has been proven by good trial and experience. The virtues whereof for their furtherance that have not been much acquainted with physicks, I will here briefly set down.

First, if poison be given to any man in meat or drink or otherwise, or if any have unawares, as many time it chances, tasted deadly or venomous medicine, as soon as he perceives himself diseased, let him take a dram[13] of this earth or more or less according to the strength of the poison, and the age and force of the sick man, and in some convenient liquor let him drink it up, and if the poison has been but newly received, he shall presently bring it up by vomit: But if it be a longer time the venom has been dispersed and carried to the inward veins [even though] yet being well covered in his bed, he shall happily drive it out by sweating. The liquors that are meetest to take it with are these: the water of Cardus benedictus[14,] devil's bit[15], swallow wort[16]. The water of the roots of the greatbroad clott[17], Angelica[18], Pimpernell[19], and such like: If you have not these waters at hand, this sovereign preservative may be taken very well in white wine.

Secondly, against the plague it may be used in the like manner, especially when it is to be given unto such as are already infected. But if you mean to take it but as a preservative, you need not take a whole dram, for half a dram taken in the morning in a little wine or vinegar of marygolds, or any other convenient liquid, will very well serve.

I myself have always used this earth with very good success, in manner as follows, as soon as a man feels any pain of his heart or his head, or perceives any anguish, grudging, loathsomeness, giddiness, or other signs of the pestilence, I do straight [8] dissolve in wine, water or other liquid, a dram of this earth and give it to the sick man in his bed, casting him in a sweat, wherewith the venom is in a very few hours driven out, without any outward sore or swelling: But if it so fall out as it be not taken in time, the blood being for the greatest part infected, there comes out in the sweating either sore or carbuncle. In this case you must open the vein as near the sore as may be: As if it be under the arm, if the botch[20] be in the flank or groin, the great vein on the inside of the leg is to be opened, if the sore be under the knee, open the vein in the sole of the foot. In the meantime be not negligent in qualifying evil humors, least the poison gathering force should strike to the heart, the heart being relieved, will forthwith drive the venom into a sore, which sore being ripe, must by an expert surgeon out of hand be lanced and well healed up, [9] neither must you omit to take a little portion of this earth, and steeping it in vinegar with powder of cinnamon, make it into a plaster, and lay it upon the heart, you shall perceive a great quantity of poison drawn out by the plaster.

Herewithall must you remember after the receipt of the medicine to take a taste wet in very good vinegar, and cause the patient to hold it to his nose to keep him from casting it up again. And if he fortunes to cast it up you must give it again and again till his stomach does keep it. This manner of using it a man of great authority and calling in the **Turkes** Court did send to a noble man, his friend, as a great secret, with the protestation that a principal physician of the **Turkes** did leave his order written in the **Arabyck** tongue, which the experiences of a great number has since confirmed.

Thirdly, against the biting of a mad dog, the stinging of serpents, scorpions, spiders or any [10] other venomous worms, as also against wounds made by poisoned weapons, this earth may in this sort be most commodiously used. Take as much thereof as shall suffice for the bigness of the wound, and with fasting spittle[21] make it into a paste spread upon linen, and lay it to the sore, or being made more thinner anoint the sore with it, whereby the venom shall not only be drawn back, but the force thereof quite abated, so as in this case it is not possible to have a better medicine. And if it were to happen that the plaster be applied too late, then must you of necessity drive out the poison by receiving inwardly a dram of the earth infused in wine or other medicinable liquor.

Fourthly, it does wonderfully assuage the pains and raging of the head, whether it come of heat, wind, labor, watching, care, or trouble of mind, and restores the consumed spirits if it be taken with good **Aqua vitae**, the waters of betony[22], rosemary, marjoram, pennyroyal or such like [11], or in great heat a dram of it taken in the morning with rosewater. The pains and trembling of the heart itself being dumpish it greatly rejoices, if a dram of it be taken with the waters of balm[23], salendine[24] mother-wort[25], buglasse[26], borage or Gelineri?

flowers, or drunk in like sort with good white wine. For the burning heat of the eyes, bleariness, rheumes[27], or any flux, this earth is specially good, applied either with rosewater, the waters of plantain, eyebright[28], valerian[29], fennel, or any such and dropped into the eye with the feather of a black hen, or linnen cloth dipped in the water and laid to it for any stripe in the eye it heals it if it is belayed to with a white of an egg and any convenient water as shall seem good to the physician or surgeon. It helps the wounds of the head or the stones, it being dissolved in rosewater, a linen cloth dipped therein be laid to the hurt place for thereby shall the spare be kept from [12] any inflammation, flux or evil humor or hurtful accident.

Fifthly, you may quickly stanch blood breaking out from any part of the body, if you beat a trochisk of this earth into powder and mingling it with spittle or any other liquid, apply it to the place; you shall soon restrain bleeding at the nose if mingling this earth with vinegar, and white of an egg, and the water of tormentil[30], you spread it upon linen cloth and lay it to the temples to the part of the head, and put it onto the nose, you shall easily also dissolve cluttered blood congealed within the body by any casualty, if you take either this earth alone in warm wine, or if you cause the patient to drink a dram of that bole, which they dig in quarries and find it in the midst of the stones, and name it in Dutch[31] of the color of liverstone, and of the place Steinmarle[32] dissolved in the white of two eggs and warm vinegar with a scruple of saffron. [13]

Sixtly, to cure the rheum use often to drink this earth morning and evening, either in white wine or other liquid, whereby you shall immediately sweat and find great ease.

Seventhly, you shall stop any looseness of the body if you give a dram of this earth in the morning and at night in the water of tormentil, of oak leaves or of the flowers of our **Acacia**.

Eighthly, to keep any part of the body that it blister not after burning and scalding, and to skin it very speedily, powder upon this earth clear fountain water wherein unquenched lime has soaked the night before, and herewithall with the feather of a black hen anoint often times very tenderly the sore place.

Ninthly, if this earth be put in any plaster steeped in any liquid or received any ways into the body, it perfectly cures all pains, inflammations or evil accidents of any wounds or ulcers, especially wounds of the kidneys, stones, or inward parts. [14]

Tenthly, it heals itches, scabs, rubes, skurviness, mange, or other such filthy diseases of the skin and makes the skin smooth and white, if so be it dissolved in spring water or plantain water, if the foul and leprous skin be often washed therewith and not dried after it.

Lastly, this earth of ours doth help quinsy, inward inflammations, ulcered lungs, and such other inward diseases, if a dram of it be taken in any water proper to the disease, as likewise cures all colics and iliac[33] passions. These are in effect the virtues of this excellent earth, as far as I have hitherto had experience. Other virtues of this blessed earth, doubtlessly there are many, which I leave to the experiences of the learned physicians. Only this I will tell them, that this earth is in the nature of the sun, or of gold, for it grows in no place but in the gold mines in the midst of the rocks, as does the precious stone (I mean the yellow earths, for [15] the white is in the silver mines, and likely it is that every metal has his proper bole or earth as I guess, for as yet I have not fully understood it). Whereupon it is called by **Paracelsus** in the first part of his great surgery and in other places, the grease of the sun, because it has in it some show of fatness. Moreover, I have had of some skilful alchymists two sorts of earth, the one drawn from gold, the other from silver very like unto these of ours, which so being, out of all doubt that earth of ours being as it ought to be prepared and applied, will cure all those grievous diseases that gold itself being prepared according to Art[34] will cure, which I leave to the search of the wise and learned physicians: For myself it suffices to have shown the way to others, whereby they may garnish and advance the glory of God and our country.

In time, these and many other remedies sundry doctors have daily found out, especially in the falling [16] sickness, wherein they have found by good trial and experience that divers infected with that disease, by taking of this earth gotten in the golden mine, have been thoroughly delivered, so as they have not any time after been touched with it.

And therefore I heartily desire such to whose hands this earth has come, and who have had any experience of it, that if so be they happen to have any other experience of it either by themselves or others, than a number of learned men have tried (whose witness of great credit, yea, even of magistrates and princes before whom it has been tried I have set down) that for the comfort of the diseased, brotherly charity, and commodity of the universal members of Christ, they would vouchsafe to send me word of it hither into **Silesia**, where I remain in a town called **Kupferberg**, or to advertise the famous and most learned philosopher D. John **Montanus** Doctor in Physick, now dwelling at **Striga**. [17]

Touching the names of both the white and the yellow earth, to speak something thereof, I trust there is no man that can justly be offended with me, in that I have termed the white earth dug out of the silver mines, by the name of mineral unicorn[35], wherein I have not so much here followed mine own fancy (though it may be permitted to the inventors to give names to such things as they have found out) as the counsel and advice of the best miners, and doctors of physick, who commonly give names according to the effect (and quality) of the medicine, and not according to the outward shape or show only, as the unlearned used to do: Or because I have called the yellow earth the grease of the sun, being got out of gold mines, and afterwards with great diligence prepared. For I have found by experience, that the yellow earth has the same force and virtues in curing diseases that gold itself has: as the white has the virtues of silver. So [18] as good reason to me it seems, to name them according to the things whereof they take their force. If these names displease any man, the party may come hither to the mines where they grow, and consider the place, circumstance, form, and property of the thing, before he as unskilful in minerals matters, does maliciously blaze abroad his foolish writings against secret works of God, or upon a covetous conceit, fearing that his kitchen will be the colder, if out of **Germany** that may be had at a small price, which is hunted for out of **Araby**, **Turquy**, and the barbarous places thereabouts, with so great sums of money and with greater gain retailed, although not half as good as this which we may have at less cost by much at home: yet must they in the meantime be accounted great doctors, because they can skill [understand, comprehend] of such things as are far fetched, though they never saw the place where they grew, nor ever have seen [19] them grow or new gathered, as has hitherto happened of that excellent herb **Scordium**[36], which being brought by the merchant out of far countries and sold at a very high price, yet it is now lately found to have grown continually in **Germany**, both as fancy as that which comes from beyond seas, and of better use for the bodies of our **Germans** than the other. In like sort fall out which minerals, metals, and precious stones, which as the learned story writer **Sebastian Munster** affirms, are now found all to grow at home with us, and are sent abroad into other countries in great abundance, which a hundred and fifty years ago were sought for at strangers' hands, and so distributed about.

We that do daily with infinite toil and excessive charges hunt for these hidden treasures in the bowels of our old mother the earth, do every day find new kinds both of metals and minerals, that the old writers never knew of, nor those that at [20] this day inhabit those countries are yet acquainted with, besides the unskilful doctors, and dwellers at home, is it possible that these fellows should have better knowledge of such things, as at home they were never acquainted with; neither know what kind, sort, or nature they be of: than those to whom they be most familiar and who daily gather them where they grow: yet cease they not with their eloquent pens, impudently to lie and to deface the truth, attributing everything most foolishly and feigned names both in Greek and Latin, not weighing the properties and qualities of everything, according to which the Lord God did by **Adam** from the beginning name them: but as seems best to their foolish brain, which fancy of theirs is as foolishly still maintained, and shamelessly defended by their followers, alleging only this slender reason, such and such a philosopher has said it: which for blindness sake and untrustiness of the [21] parties they might rather have deemed to have been most false. And thus not only to God and his gifts but to their own Country of **Germany**, these doctors and philosphers of **Germany** are found to be most injurious, who despise the rare blessings of God that are proper to them and their country: Only commending and desiring such things as are got abroad, suppressing with a vile kind of mind such things as they have at home, nay, which is a fouler thing, they neither have desire to benefit their country nor their brethren, neither will they suffer others that would do it, but study continually how they may with all sorts of railings and slanders stop and deface the good and laudable attempts of such as they know to be studiously and honestly given. Where it had been a great deal more meet for them first to have given thanks to God that in the latter days has so abundantly blessed our country of **Germany** [22] in bringing to light such infinite treasures as having long lain hidden, are now through his mercy found out, to the end that by continual beholding of them we may be called from the dungeon of darkness to light, and to the amendment of our lives. And even of the very bounty and goodness of their disposition, you may easily (good reader) perceive them whom God will have partakers of his hidden treasures, when as they do not with injustice keep to themselves the secret knowledge which they have received from God, but seek by all the means they may to make them common to all men, especially to those that be good and godly: and for the others, his good will is they should continually apply their studies to their private contention, and never attain to the knowledge of the truth: And these good fellows use always to keep in their own custody such things as they themselves have no skill of, neither will [23] they suffer such as are of understanding to handle the use of them. But let us leave this kind of people as withered and rotten stokers, neither profitable to themselves nor others: and according to that which God has given uns, let us be fruitful, always giving praise and thanks to God our merciful father, not seeking our own honor or private commodity, who shall also make us profitable and fit for his kingdom: with which he hath promised to give to us whatsoever we shall have need of, so that we seek for that kingdom before all other things. To this only God who is and has been from everlasting, be everlasting honor and glory.

The testimonials of the Princes & Magistrates, who have seen before them the experience and miraculous force of the *Silesian Terra Sigillata*: and thereupon for the acknowledging of such genuine benefits, and extolling the [24] glory of God, have under their great seals confirmed the truth in order as follows:

First an exemplification, that is an abstract out of the German original faithfully translated into Latin, that the most noble prince William Landgrave of Hesse in Cassel Court[37] in Catzenelnbogen, Ditz, Ziegenheim and Nidda, of his great clemency, did grant to Andreas Bertoldus of Oschatz by his doctors of physik and Chancelor.

Be it known unto all persons, that an honest man called Bertold of Oschatz came into the presence of the most noble prince and lord, the Lord William Langrave of Hesse, Court of Catzenelnbogen, Dietz, Ziegenheim and Nidda &c. our gracious lord and prince, and in humble manner declared unto him, that he had [25] found in an old mine of gold within the dominion of Schweidnitz a new kind of earth which is a present help and most notable remedy against all manners of poisons and sundry diseases, which earth having a stamp upon it he offered to sell unto his excellency: who not trusting the man upon his bare word, committed the matter to his physicians, Maurice, Thaurern and Laurence Hyper: Commanding them to make a perfect trial of said earth, whereupon the said Doctors in Physick to satisfy their prince, did make a double proof of this earth, in this manner. They took four sundry sortes of the deadliest poisons that might be, which were, Mercury sublimate, Aconitum[38], Nereum[39] and Apocinum[40]; and of some one of these they gave half a dram apiece to eight dogs, and to four of them the gave the earth after the poison, and to the other four the poison alone. Of these four that took it alone, the first that took [26]

Apocinum died within half an hour; the second that had taken **Nereum**, died within four hours; the third that swallowed **Mercury**, died within nine hours after: and although they did cast up some part of the poison, yet after most cruel torments with cramps and trembling died: the fourth dog that ate **Aconitum** sustained thirteen great pangs of the cramp, so as everyman thought he would have died with his fellows, yet lived the first day, and having half the dose of this medicine given him, he thoroughly recovered. The other four dogs to whom the poisons before named with the like quantity of this **Terra sigillata** was given, for three hours after the receiving of it, were very sick and feeble, expecially one of them to whom the double quantity of **Aconitum** was given, vomited thrice; the next day they were all well and did eat their meat greedily, so as there appeared scarce any token of [27] poison. When this His Highness had seen the experience of this earth be so present a remedy against such deadly poisons, and the said **Andrew Bertold** had humbly craved his letter of credit, both in your favour of the man and advancement of the truth, that others might have knowledge, he denied not to grant them: but commanded that his letters testimonial sealed with His Highness' privy seal, and subscribed with the hands of the forsaid doctors in whose presence this trial was made, should be given unto him. Which we the abovenamed doctors upon our allegiance to His Highness, and for the furtherance of the truth, because we found it has been declared to be true and unfeigned, most willingly have done. Given the 28th of July, the year of our Lord, **1580**.

Mauritius Thaurer D.
Lawrencius Hyperius MD
Iohan Krug.

[28] In the year of our Lord 1580, the day of St. James: In the presence of the most noble and worth Prince **William Landgrave of Hesse** there was made of the *Terra sigillata* brought unto him by **Andreas Berthold** of **Oschatz** this proof upon certain dogs.

A red dog with a white ring about the neck had given unto him between eight and nine in the morning a scruple of *Mercury* sublimed, and a scruple of *Terra sigillata* therewith: within half an hour after the second hour he vomited extremely, the third hour again he cast up certain colicky matter, so did he in the fourth hour, and without any great harm he escaped.

A yellow cur with a white brest had given unto him a scruple of *Mercury* sublimed and nothing after it, within half an hour after he made water and presently he scummered[41], within half an hour [29] afterwards he was taken with a cramp and fell to the ground, after this cramp he stood up a while panting and grinning[42], and presently afterwards was again taken with the cramp, and withall swelled in the belly: at one of the clock he was taken with a more grievous cramp and lay as though he had been dead for a quarter of an hour, within half an hour after two he began again to go and for an hour and a half afterwards he stood still without moving, between four and five he was again extremely taken with the cramp and sundry times after that, at last he died in the night.

A black little hound with a white tail, had given unto him a great dram of *Aconitum*, and therewith a dram of this earth, within half an hour afterward, he cast up certain frothy matter, after the first hour he vomited the third time and so escaped.

A branded shaghaired dog with a white tail had half a dram of *Aconitum* given him and nothing therewith, within an hour he was [30] taken with a great cramp and that lasting(?) one hour after that about one of the clock he was taken likewise after one, and a half hour after two he fell into the cramp again, so did he at three o'clock, after that he was extremely pulled by the cramp, and by and by after had the like fit wherewith he made a great quantity of water that stank horribly, then was again touched with the cramp, when there was given him at the commandment of our gracious Lord the **Landgrave** of **Hesse** half the dose of this sovereign medicine whereby he recovered and escaped.

A black cur with a white neck had given unto him half a dram of *Nerium* or *Oleander* and half a dram of this earth, within one hour after the taking of it, he vomited extremely, and within a little after he vomited green baggage, within half an hour he vomited he frothed and foamed at the mouth, this was the faintest and [31] weakest amongst them all, yet did he presently recover and escape.

A brown cur with a white neck had given to him half a dram of **Merium**[43] and nothing of the medicine. First he vomited a thin matter about ten of the clock he vomited again, after twelve he was taken with a great quaking and a terrible cramp, which fit was very long and extreme: afterward he was pulled with the cramp til almost three he was terribly raked with cramp, and between three and four he died.

A gray little beagle had given unto him a dram of *Apocynum*[44] half leaves and half roots and withall a dram of this **Terra Sigillata**. This dog as far as we could discern was not all the day long anywise vexed, but escaped very well.

A branded dog had given unto him a dram of *Apocynum* half root and half herb and nothing of the medicine, within half an hour after the receipt of the poison, he was [32] taken with an extreme cramp and quavering, and within a very small while after he fell suddenly dead to the great wondering of those that stood by.

Mauritius Thaurer D.
Laurencious Hyperius D

A copy of the Letters Patents which the noble earl *Wolfgang* Earl of *Hohenlohe*, Lord of *Langenburg &c* had granted to *Andrew Berthold* of *Oschatz,* in witness of the wonderful virtues of the *terra sigillata* found lately in *Germany* which has been tried to be an approved medicine against the strongest poisons, and sundry other grieves: faithfully translated out of the German original.

WE, *Wolfgangus* Earl of *Hohenlohe*, Lord of *Langenburg &c* do openly make known by these my Letters [33] Testimonial, that there came lately before me at

Langenburg, my well-beloved friend **Andreas Bertholdus** of **Oschatz**, and declared unto me that he had a most excellent kind of *Terra Sigillata,* which was not alonely of great force against sundry diseases: but also a most undoubted remedy against all manner of venomous poisons, as had been proved by sundry witnesses upon a great number of dogs, which made me also desirous to see the trial of it. It happened at the same time, that one called W*endell Thumblardt* was by our lieutenant of **Langenburg** for certain felonies imprisoned, who being examined by our justices, confessed himself guilty of a great number of robberies: and therefore brought to the bar was condemned to be hanged. Being yet detained in prison, it came to his ear that there was such a medicine, so souverain against sundry sicknesses, and the most deadly poisons, he made humble request as well by his parents, as by other [34] his friends, of which there were present no small number, desiring for the mercy of God and respect of his poor life, that being thus condemned, he might have given onto him the most deadly poison that might be devised, whereby a perfect trial might be had of the worthiness of this medicinable earth. And in this respect, not only for this pitiful request of his: but also for the accommodation and benefit of all Christendom, (if so be the medicine prove answerable to the report) pardoning the offender, we granted his life upon that condition. Therefore the day of the date of these presents, in the presence of ourself, and our well-beloved Cousin the Count *Georg Friderik* of *Hohenlohe*, and Lord in **Langenburg**, and in the presence of all our nobility and Commoners, the said patient received a dram and a half of **Mercury Sublimate**, mingled with conserve of roses[45], and immediately after it he drank a dram of the *Terra Sigillata* in old wine, and albeit the poison did in the [35a[46]] judgment of our learned physician *Georg Pister* doctor of physick, and *John Lutzen* our apothecary, who were both with him all the while, extremely tormented and vexed him: yet in the end the medicine prevailing overcame it, whereby the poor wretch was delivered, and being restored to his health was committed to his parents. Whereas therefore **Andrew Berthold** has humbly required to have our Letters Testimonial for his farther credit, we have thought good for the furtherance and advancement of the truth, to grant him these our Letters, signed with our manual seal. Given at **Langenburg**, the 25th of January in the year of our Lord, 1581.

The copy of the Letters Testimonial granted by the Magistrate of the City of Juliers[47] unto Master *Crisantus a Cronenburg*, Citizen of Coleine, in the name and behalf of *Andreas Bertholdus* of *Oschatz,* touching the force and virtues of the [35b] sealed earth lately found in *Germany*. Truly drawn out of the dutch original.

We the Mayor and Aldermen of the Town of Juliers do signify unto all to whom this present writing shall come, that there presented himself before us one *Crisant* of *Cronenburg*, a substantial man, and citizen of **Coleine**, declaring unto us that he had an assured remedy against all poisons, called by the name of *Terra Sigillata Axungia Solis, St. Pauls* earth, or *Adams*[48] earth, being made up in diverse trochisks, some of them reddish in color, some greyish, sealed with an escutcheon wherein is portrayed the sun, the half moon, and five stars. In place of the helmet[49] these letters **A.B.** and on the other side **V.O.**, who beseeched us to give him leave to make trial in our sight of the said earth upon certain dogs and beasts, Which when we had [36] granted, the said *Crisant* did will to be brought before him two great dogs, of like color and bigness and therewithal two crowns weight of **Mercury Sublimate** which he divided in our presence and in the sight of *John Ostweiler*, our town surgeon, into two equal portions, whereof the one he gave alone in a piece of lard to the one dog, the other part of the poison he gave to the other in a piece of lard being mingled with the quantity of the trochisks of the *Terra Sigillata*. Both the dogs devoured the portions that were thrown unto them, and both vomited and grew to be feeble, six hours after the receiving of the poison the first dog that had taken the poison pure without any of the earth died. The other which had received the *Terra Sigillata* with the poison, remained safe and alive, and being shut up for a day, after was suffered to go at large. Since these things we saw to be true as they were reported, we thought good [37] to grant to the named *Crisant* of *Cronenburg* these our Letters of Credence, sealed with our common seal. Given at Juliers in the year of our Lord 1580, the 12th of February.

Subsigned Paulus Herle(s?)

This copy was drawn out in the presence of the honorable Henrie Wendelen, & Theodork a Bruck, both the Scauins (?) in Düsseldorf, was by me Antony Burker chief Notarie there, conferred with the true original, sealed and subscribed, neither razed nor cancelled, nor to be suspected, which original remains in keeping of the said Crisantus, wherewith I confess it agrees word for word, which I the aforesaid Anthony Burker do witness with mine own hand. Dated the ninth of March, the year 1582.

Andrewe Berthold to
The loving Reader

[38] Be it known unto all and singular the studious, the searchers out of the treasures of nature, that for their own necessity or their friends, desired to be partakers of the wonderful & medicinable force of the *Terra Sigillata* of *Silesia*: as well for recovering & keeping of their health, as to be preserved from all deadly poison: That I, **Andrew Berthold** of **Oschatz** upon the mountain called **Kupferberg**, dwelling near onto the Golden river named in the German tongue the **Bober** about seven miles from the head of the river called **Elbe**[50], have been earnestly required by sundry doctors of physick and other men of name, to leave some quantity of this precious earth in some place near unto the **Rheyn** specially at **Franckfort**[51], where in my absence, as oft as occasion served, it might be had.

When as therefore I caused these books to be printed by that virtuous man **Christopher Corvin** a printer & citizen of **Franckfort**: I thought it good not anywhere [39] better leave it, than with him who might utter it at a reasonable price to all such as have need of it: which I could hardly entreat him to trouble himself withal, but only in respect that he had printed the copies. Wherefore I intend, God sparing me life, to send abroad Marte not only good store of this earth, but also certain precious stones needful in physick: as **Rubies**, **Emeralds**, **Saphires**, **Hyacinths**, **Cornelians**, **Citrins**, **Crystals**, **Serpentines**, **Amethysts**, **Granats**[52], and such like. And whosoever lacks any stones belonging to Physick or otherwise, he shall be sure at the said **Corvin** to have not only them, but also the earth ready prepared, which our merciful God has bestowed upon **Germany**. For the common profit of Christendom. To which almighty Lord be all honor, glory, and praise, for ever and ever.

Andreas Bertholdus

of Oschatz

Finis

Final notes and comments

[1] Misnia (Meissen) was part of Northern Silesia. Oschatz is in Saxony, not Silesia. Again there is suspicion of an attempt to formulate nobility.

[2] A so-called herbal "poison against all poisons", invented by Mithridatus V. of Pontus, also called "Eupator" after the name of the poison he ingested until he believed himself inured against all poisons.

[3] English spelling for "theriak", a Greek nostrum against bites of wild beast and poisonous stings and venoms, still in apothecary lists in 1900.

[4] Healing Earth, a clay formed into little balls and made into flat disks or tablets, impressed with the words *Terra sigillata* and a trademark to imply quality.

[5] This was an ordinary subscription to a letter at that time, like "yours truly".

[6] I have not found a name to fit these initials.

[7] Corner brackets [ ] enclose numbers of the manuscript page at its beginning.

[8] Kidney stones and bladder stones were a curse on humanity then. At times surgery without anesthesia was tried for bladder stones, with 5 men holding the patient, but most succumbed to infections from unclean hands…

[9] Rheum: Medical definition: Mucous discharge from head to lungs: "distillations" and "murrs" are variations of the same "catarrh" or discharge, phlegm or runny nose.

[10] Laske, lyentery, bloody flux, all were names for Diarrhea, dysentery, loose bowels.

[11] I believe that in antiquity, the word "green" appears a frequent synonym for "fresh".

[12] Quinsy: Tonsillitis, sore throat.

[13] Dram= 3.888 grams, 1/16th avoirdupois ounce, 60 grains, 3 scruples. One scruple = 1.295 grams.

[14] A wild growing but edible thistle, cardoon, artichoke.

[15] Any plant of the genus *Succisa pratensis*, most likely *Scabiosa succisa.*

[16] *Vincetoxium officinale* or *Cheledonium majus.*

[17] A burr, burdock, *Anthium* fam. *asteraceae.*

[18] *Angelica officinalis*, angelic water, from the herb angelica.

[19] Great burnett poterius, *Sanguisorba officinalis.*

[20] A boil, ulcer, pimple

[21] Spittle of a fasting man was a recognized specific among human medicines.

[22] Stachy's betonica formerly credited with medicinal and magic virtues.

[23] Balsam an aromatic exudation of trees of the genus *balsamodendron*

[24] Celendine, and eye salve, *Cheledonium majus,* also swallow-wort.

[25] *Leonurus caridaca*, used for diseases of the womb, formerly also called mug-wort, *Artemisia vulgaris.*

[26] Correct: bugloss, a baginaceous plant, cows-lip.

[27] Watery discharge, often with fever.

[28] Prepared from *Euphrasy* as kind of a beer, *Euphatasia officinalis.* Used for treatment of eye diseases.

[29] Many plants of the genus *Valerian* were used medicinally as stimulants and antispasmodics.

[30] A rosaceous herb, *Potentilla tormentilla*; its astringent roots are used in medicine.

[31] Probably meaning deutsch, German

[32] Misprint for Steinmark (stone marrow) a soft (talcum?) filling in cracks of rocks.

[33] Probably intestinal blockages, but could be lumbago, word means flank or entrails.

[34] This term generally refers to the art of alchemy; created by humans, as opposed to nature.

[35] A mineral with the same magic powers of the famous horn of the (land) unicorn.

[36] *Teucrium scordium*, a garlic-like plant

[37] Landgraf Wilhelm IV., "der Weise" (the wise one) of Hessen Kassel (1567-1592).

[38] Oder *Ranunculaceae*, monks-hood, wolf-bane, *Aconited repellens*, poisonous.

[39] *Nerum oleander*, fam. *Apocybaceae*, twice mispelled in the text.

[40] Dog bane family of the order *Gentionales strophantus*, rauwolfia.

[41] To scummer: to throw up, to bring forth scum.

[42] written "grinning", probably should be "grimming", from suffering the grims.

[43] Should be Nerium.

[44] *Apocynum*, dog-bane or dog's bane, reputed poisonous to dogs, A "bane" is that which destroys life, brings ruin, harm, woe.

[45] A conserve: About 1500 a medical confectionary preparation with sugar or honey, jam, or syrup, also called an electuary.

[46] Error by the printer, two sequential pages numbered 35

[47] Juliers is the French name, Jülich in Flemish or German: a town in western Nordrhein-Westphalia, close to the city of Aachen and the Belgian border with Germany.

[48] Adam's earth, *Terra Adamas*, an earth untouched by human hands; the clay god used to make Adam.

[49] In heraldics, the "helmet" is placed above the escutcheon in an "achievement" honor, supporting the crest, being an armorial granted in memory of an "achievement".

[50] The entire "address" and location description of Kupferberg, Bober River and Elbe River is very confusing and not possible according to pre-1945 Prussian maps. Nowhere do the two rivers, or even their springs come together anywhere within seven miles, and Kupferberg is not to be found within 100 km.

[51] Frankfurt is not on the Rhein, but on its tributary, the Main.

[52] This list of precious and semi-precious stones is correct in that these stones are mentioned variously in literature as of medical use, but it is difficult to believe that the promoter Berthold would have deposited "quantities" of such stones with a printer for dispensation to physicians.

Bibliography

<u>Frequently cited journal:</u> Münchener medizinische Wochenschrift cited as MMWS

Abu Mansur Mowafik Ben Ali et Herwi, 1833, Liber fundamentorum pharmacologiae, Vindobonae (Vienna) 2 vols.

Ackerknecht, Erwin H., History and Geography of the most important diseases, Hafner Publishing Co., Inc., New York & London, 1965.

Adam, Patrick, 1967, "Ancient Greece and Rome", in: Diseases in Antiquity, Ch. 18, pp. 238-246,

Aegina, Paul of, (625-690) Seven books of medicine, transl. see Berendes.

Agricola, Georgius, 1546, de natura fossilium, translated as "Textbook of Mineralogy" by Mark Chance Brady and Jean A. Brady, The Geological Society of America, Special issue 63, 1955.

—————, 1655, Bermannus, 1530, A dialogue of mines. I have used the Latin and French edition see Halleux

Albertus Magnus, ~1250, Book of Minerals, transl. Dorothy Wyckhoff, 1967, Clarendon Press, Oxford

—————, de mineralibus, hgg. Erwin Braun: Texte zur Geschichte der Präventivmedizin, Birkhäuser Verlag, Basel.

Albinus, Petrus, 1589, Meisznische Land und Berg Chronica / in welcher ein vollstendige *description* des Landes / so zwischen Elbe und Sala, Dresden.

Aldrovandi, Ulissis, 1602, Musaeum Metallicum in libris IIII, distributum Bartholomaeus Ambrosinus.

American Pharmaceutical Association, the National Formulary, 1908, Chicago.

Amsler, 1852, Das Bad Schinznach in der Schweiz, R. Bertschingers Buchdruckerei, Lenzburg (Aargau, Switzerland).

Anderson, Frank J., 1977, An illustrated history of the herbals, Columbia U. Press, NY, Ch.6: the Circa Instans of Mathaeus Platearius.

Anglicus, Gilbert, ~13th century, Compendium medicinae, see: Getz, Faye M.

Aristotle, The Book of Stones, see: Ruska, Julius (Author not Aristotle), parts which appear to have been written by Luka ben Serapion and/or Costa del Luca.

Arneth, 1916, "Zur Behandlung der Cholera", in: Deutsche medizinische Wochenschrift, # 31, pp. 935-938.

Aschner, Bernard, 1930, Paracelsus sämtliche Werke, Vol. 3, 4, 5, Verlag Gustav Fischer, Jena.

Aufrecht, 1905, "Der Bolusverbandstoff", in: Deutsche medizinische Wochenschrift, Stuttgart, Nr. 38, pp. 1508-1510.

Aufreiter, Susanne, and Mahaney, William C. and others, "Mineralogical and chemical interactions of soils eaten by chimpanzees of the Mahale Mountains and Gombe Stream National Parks, Tanzania", in: Journal of Chemical Ecology, Vol. 27, Number 2, 2001, pp 285 – 311.

Bacon, Roger, Translation of "De erroribus medicorum", in: Essays of the History of Medicine Presented to Karl Sudhoff on occasion of his 70th birthday Nov. 26, 1923, ed.

Charles Singer & Henry E. Sigerist, 1924 Verlag Seldwyla, Zurich. (Translator anonymous).

Badianus Manuscript, Codex Barberini, see: Emmart, E. W.

Bahrliep von der Müllen, Christof Heinrich, 1705, "The variously moving pain of podagra and The use of the medicinal earth of Freyenwald" (Disputatio inauguralis medica de Arthritide Vaga Scorbutica & huius occasione quaedam de Terra Medicinali Freyenwaldensis), Doctoral dissertation under supervision of Conrad Johrenus, Brandenburg, University of Berlin:

Balbinus, Bohuslao Aloysio, 1664, Vita venerabilis Arnesti, Prague, Archiepiscopali Typogr.

Balkema A. A., 1989, "A checklist of wild African bovidae related to montane habitats with expanded notes on geophagic behaviour of buffalo on Mt. Kenya", in: Quaternary And Environmental Research on East African mountains, Rotterdam, pp. 309-324.

Bechhold, H., 1925, "Chlorsilber-Kieselsäure", in: MMWS, 39, pp. 16-25.

—————, H. and L. Keiner, 1927, "Spezifische Adsorptionstherapie", in: MMWS # 15 pp. 613/4

Bech-i-Borràs, 1987, Les terres medicinals, Discurse a la Reial Acad.de Farmàcia de Barcelona.

Beck, Claus H., 1940, Studium über Gestalt und Ursprung des Circa Instans, doctoral dissertation, Berlin, Druckerei wissenschaftlicher Werke Konrad Triltsch, Würzburg-Aumühle.

Belon, Pierre, du Mans, 1554, Les observations de plusieurs singularitées et choses memorables Trouvées en Grece, Asie, Judées, Egypte, Arabie, et autres pays éstrangés, redigée en trois Livres, Paris, chez Guillaume Cauellat.

Benade, W., 1937, "Die Nomenklatur der Heilsedimente und Heilerden", in: Der Balneologe 4/2 15 Feb 1937.

—————, 1938, "Reports on Proceedings of the International Society of Medical Hydrology1938", in: Der Balneologe: 2/1937 pp. 46-58, 9/1938, pp. 434-436, 9/1938, pp. 419-423.

—————, and R. Teichmann, 1944, "Torf in der Wundbehandlung", in: Der Balneologe, 11. Jahrg. Jan-Mar 1944, Heft 1-3, pp. 82-88.

Bent, James Theodore, 1966, Aegean Islands - life among the insular Greeks, Argonaut Publishers, Chicago.

Berendes, J., 1902, transl. & comm., Des Pedanius Dioskurides aus Anazerbos Arzneimittellehre, 5 Vols., Verlag von Ferdinand Enke, Stuttgart.

—————, 1914, transl. & comm., Paulus von Aegina, des besten Arztes sieben Bücher, Verlags buchhandlung vormals E. J. Brill, Leiden.

Berlu, Jacob, 1860, The Treasury of Drugs Unlocked, a full and true description of all drugs, London, printed for John Harris at the Harrow against the Church in the Poultry and Thomas Hawkins in the George Yard in Lombard Street.

Bertholdus, Andreas (von Oschatz), 1587, The wonderfull and strange effect and vertues of a new *Terra Sigillata* lately found out in Germanie:…, London, R. Robinson for R. Watkins. Microfilm 196 from Northwestern University., Evanston ILL. This is a Translation by a "B. G." from Latin(?) into English.

Bingen, Hildegard von, ~1100, Heilkraft der Natur (Physica), translated by Marie-Louise Portmann, published by Verlag Herder, Freiburg (Breisgau) 1993.

Black, D. A. K., 1956, "Evaluation of Terra Sigillata", in: The Lancet, Special articles, Oct. 27, pp. 883-884.

Bloch, Iwan, 1917a, "Ueber austrocknende antiseptische Behandlung venerischer Affektionen mit Boluphen", in: Berliner klinische Wochenschrift, # 44, p. 1058.

————, 1917b, "Ein Fall von schwerem tertiärsyphilitischen Phagedänismus der männlichen Genitale, Heilung durch kleine Dosen Jodkalium und örtliche Behandlung mit Boluphen", in: Berliner klinische Wochenschrift # 52 pp. 1240-1241.

de Boot (de Boodt, de Bôôt), 1609, Gemmarum et lapidum historia, Hanau, (Third ed. 1647 by Tollius, Leiden.

British Pharmacopoeia 1993, Volume I: Kaolin and Morphine, Martindale ed. 31, London.

Brothwell, Don and A. T. Sandison, eds., 1967, Diseases in antiquity, pp. 191-246, Charles C. Thomas, Springfield, IL.

Brouillard, M.-Y. and & J.-G. Rateau, 1989, "Pouvoir d'adsorption de deux argiles, la smectite et le kaolin sur des entérotoxines bactéeriennes", in: Gastroenterol. Clin. Biol. 13, 18-24.

Bruckmann, Franciscus Ernest, 1739, Epistola Itineraria LXXXIII, Museum Metallici, Wolfenbüttel.

Bryan, Cyril P., 1931, The Papyrus Ebers, transl. from German, D. Appleton & Co., New York.

Budge, Wallis E. A., 1913, The Book of Medicines, translated as Syrian anatomy, pathology, and therapeutics, Oxford U. Press.

Burmeister, R., 1912, "Bolus alba im Handschuh", in: Zentralblatt für Chirurgie, Nr. 5, pp. 157/8.

Burk, W., 1912, "Ein neues Verfahren zur Händedesinfektion", in: Med. Klinik # 39 p.1026.

Byk, 1918, "Ueber Geox", in: Allgemeine medizinische Central-Zeitung, # 22, pp. 85-86.

Cabanès, Dr., 1899, "Les anciens traitments de la peste", in: Bulletin générale de Thérapeutique médicale chirurgicale, obstréticale et pharmaceutique, Vol. 138. Pp. 764-781.

Caley, E. R., and John F. C. Richards, Theophrastus on stones, Introduction, Greek text, Engl. Translation and Commentary, Columbus Ohio, Ohio State Univ. 1956

Cantor, Horman F., 1963, Medieval History, The life and death of a civilization, MacMillan, NY

Castiglione, 1940, Arturo, "Aulus Cornelius Celsus as a historian of medicine", a Fielding H. Garrison lecture, in: History of Medicine Volume VIII, No. 7, 1940, Transactions of the 16th Annual Meeting of the American Association of the History of Medicine, ed. H. E. Sigrist.

————, 1941, A history of medicine, transl. E. B. Krumbhaar, Alfred Knopf, New York.

Castle, George, 1667, The Chymical Galenist, printed by Sarah Griffith for Henry Twyford in Vine Court, Middle Temple, and Timothy Twyfors at Inner Temple Gate.

Celsus - see Frieboes

Chambers, J. S., 1938, The conquest of cholera, Macmillan, NY.

Chen, K.K., and Amy S. H. Ling, 1926, "Fragments of Chinese medical history", in: Annals of Medical History, Vol. III, #1.

Chopra, R. N., 1933, Indigenous Drugs of India, The Art Press, 20 British Indian Street, Calcutta.

Clay eating, 1978, Anon. "Clay eating", in: Lancet Sep 16 pp. 614-615.

Cohn, Max, 1907, "Erfahrungen über Xeranatbolusgaze", in: Medizinische Klinik #24, p.707/9

————, 1910, "Zur Frage der Bolusbehandlung", in: MMWS # 46.

Cordus, Valerius, 1540, Dispensatorium sive pharmacorum, Lugduni Batavorum apud Franciscum Raphelengium.

Coe, Sophie D. and Michael D. Coe, 1996, The true history of chocolate, Thames & Hudson, London. I used the German translation "Die wahre Geschichte der Schokolade", 1997, Fischer Verlag GmbH, Frankfurt/M.

Cowan, Savid L. and William N. Helfand, 1988, Pharmacy, an illustrated history, Harry N. Abrams, Inc., New York.

Cumston, Charles G., 1920, Letter to the Editor, Annals of Medical History, Vol. 2. (re: Ancient Egyptian papyri).

Dannenfeldt, Karl H., 1984, "Introduction of a new sixteenth-century drug: Terra Silesiaca", in: Medical History 28: 174-188.

Dawson, Warren R., and Paul B. Hoeber, 1930a, "The Beginnings, Egypt and Assyria", in: Clio medica, Vol 8., NY, p. 357.

Diamond, Jarel, 2001, "Death of Languages", in: Natural History, April 2001, Volume 110 #3 pp. 30-38.

Diepgen, Paul, 1911, Die Summa Medicinalis von Gualteris Agilonies ~ 1300 AD, Leipzig, Ambrosius Barth.

Dirks, Emil, 1916, "Beitrag zur Bolus-alba-Behandlung bei Ruhr", in: MMWS Nr. 12 pp. 441-2.

Drigalski, Wilhelm, 1943, "Erde, ein indifferentes wirkungsvolles Heilmittel" in MMWS Nr. 26/27, pp. 405-406.

Dumezil, Georges, 1924, Le crime des Lemniennes, Librairie Orientaliste Paul Geuthner, Paris.

Ebstein, Erich, 1928, "Zur geschichtlichen Entwicklung der Bolustherapie mit besonderer Berücksichtigung des Bolus", in: Knolls Mitteilungen für Ärzte, pp. 26-29.

Ebbels, 1937, transl., The Papyrus Ebers II, Levin & Munksgaars, Copenhagen.

Emmart, Emily Walcott, 1940, The Badianus Manuscript (Codex Barberini, Latin 241) Vatican Library, An Aztec Herbal of 1552, introduction, translation and annotations by Emmart, E. W., The Johns Hopkins Press.

Erlenmeyer, 1855, "Ueber die Anwendung der Schlackenbäder", in: Balneologische Zeitung, Vol. I, 26 Feb 1855 # 5, pp. 65-67.

Ernstingius, Arthurus Conradus, 1770, Nucleus totius medicinae oder der vollkommene und Allzeit fertige Apotheker, 5 Vols, 2d ed. From Meyersche Buchhandlung.

Exkremente - see Meyer's Konversationslexikon, 4th ed., vol. 5, Leipzig & Vienna. 1890.

Fischer, Hans, 1899, "Gangraen der Weichtheile und des Knochens beider Füsse bei einem Paralytiker, Thonbehandlung, Ausgang in Heilung,", in: MMWS #12 pp. 378/9

Fischer, Herwart, 1932, Obituary of Julius Stumpf, in: Zeitschrift für gerichtliche Medizin, Volume 19, issue 3.

Forbes, R. J., 1936, Bitumen and Petroleum in Antiquity, Leyden.

Frankenberg, Siegmund, 1848, Geschichte der Heilkunst und Heilschwärmerei, Verlag von Christian Ernst Kollmann, Leipzig.

Fredrich, C., 1906, "Lemnos", in: Mitteilungen des Kaiserlich Deutschen archäologischen Instituts, Athenische Abteilung, Athen-Berlin 1906 pp., Part I: pp. 60-86, Part II: P. 241-278.

Frei (Niederzuwil), 1909, "Zur Ehrenrettung des Bolus alba, eines alten, aber seit langer Zeit verkannten Heilmittels: die Bolus alba", in: Korrespondenzblatt für schweizer Ärzte, Nr. 13.

Freind, John, 1744, The history of physick from the time of Galen to the beginning of the 16th century, London 4th ed. printed for J. Walther over against the Royal Exchange in Cornhill.

Frieboes, Walther, 1906, Aulus Cornelius Celsus über die Arzneiwissenschaft in acht Büchern, Transl. & explained Braunschweig Friedrich Viehweg.

Gardiner, K. R., N. H. Anderson, M. D. McCaigue, P. J. Erwin, M. I. Halliday, B. J. Rowlands, 1993, "Adsorbents as anti-endotoxin agents in experimental colitis", in G.U.T 34:31-55

Garrison, Fielding H., 1929, An introduction to the history of medicine, 4th ed., W. B. Saunders & Co., Philadelphia.

Gelfand, M. E., 1998, cited from African Medical Journal 1945, # 212. 1998. Original not found.

Georgii, 1899, "Ueber die Verwendbarkeit des Thons (Bolus alba) bei der Behandlung des Cervicalkatarrhs", in: MWS, #14, p.48.

Gerondoudis, Leonidas N. & Christophorous L. Gerondoudis, "The Island of Lemnos", no date, no publisher shown, copy extant in city library of Myrina, Lemnos (Greece) dated 1971.

Gesner, Conradus, 1555, "Descriptio montis fracti", in: De raris et admirandis herbis.

————, 1565, De rerum fossilium, lapidum et gemmarum maxime, figuris et similitudinibus, Zurich, bound together with Kentmann's book (see Kentmann).

Gesundbrunnen - see Zedler under that word.

Getz, Fay M., 1992, "The pharmaceutical writings of Gilbert Anglicus", in: Pharmacy in History, Vol. 34, pp 1-60, No. 1, Am. Institute of the History of Pharmacy.

Gilardi, James D., Sean S. Duffy, Charles A. Mum, Lisa A.Tell, 1999, "Biochemical function of geophagy in parrots: detoxification of dietary toxins and cytoprotective effects", In: Journal of Chemical Ecology, Vol. 25, No. 4.

Giseler, Lorens (Laurentius Giselerus), 1663, Observationes medicae de peste Brunsvicensi, Brunsvigae, Sumptibus Christoph Friderich Zilliger.

Glorez, Andreas, 1700, Des Mährischen Albertus Magnus Andreas Glorez eröffnetes Wunderbuch..., Regensburg und Stadtamhof.

Görner, Johannes, 1907, "Die Stumpfsche Bolustherapie, ihre Verwendbarkeit bei Diarrhöen und Meteorismus verschiedenen Urpsrungs", in: MMWS # 45, pp. 2383-4.

Graf, 1923, "Über Erfolge mit Eifelfango", in: V. Praktische Winke, Zeitschrift für ärztliche Fortbildung 20, p. 123.

Graepel, Peter Hartwig, 1999, "Tierversuche zum Wirksamkeitsnachweis von Siegelerde am Hofe Wilhelm IV. von Hessen-Kassel (1580), in: Hessische Heimat, 49. Jahrgang Heft 2. 1999

Gräser, 1911, "Bolus alba gegen Darmerkrankungen", in: MMWS # 37, p. 1991.

Groß, Ludwig, 1927, "Geophagie", in: Die medizinische Welt, Stuttgart, 42-2 pp. 1580-1581.

Grube, Karl, 1919, "Ueber Fangobehandlung mit einem neuen Fangopräparat: Polyfango", in: Medizinische Klinik, # 43 p. 1087.

Güterbock, Hans, 1962, "Hittite Medicine", in: Bulletin of the History of Medicine, Volume 36, # 2, pp. 109-113.

Hager, Hermann, 1874, Commentar zur Pharmacopoea Germanica, Julius Springer, Berlin

——————, 1876, Manuale pharmaceuticum seu promtuarium, adjumenta varia chemica et pharmaceutica atque subsidia ad parandas aquas minerales, Ernst Günter, Leipzig.

——————, 1919, Handbuch der Pharmaceutischen Praxis, Vol 1, 8th ed. Berlin, Julius Springer.

Hahn, Martin, 1906, "Ueber Cholera- und Typhusendotoxine, MMWS # 23, pp. 1097-1101.

Halleux, Robert, and Albert Yans, 1990, transl, & commentary on Agricola, Georgius "Bermannus" (Le Mineur), un dialogue sur les mines, Les Belles Lettres, Paris.

Halsted, James A., 1968, "Geophagia in Man: Its Nature and Nutritional Effects, in: American Journal of Clinical Nutrition, Vol. 21, No. 12, pp. 1384-1393.

Handmann, E., 1916, "Zur Diagnose und Therapie der Bazillenruhr", in: Deutsche medizinische Wochenschrift # 30, pp 908-909.

Hariot, Thomas (1560-1621), privately reprinted 1900, A brief and true report of the new found Land of Virginia, Sir Walter Raleigh's colony of MDLXXXV, First part, notes on Alum and terra sigillata "Wapeik", republished by the Fort Raleigh National Historic Site, NPS, Rt 1, Box 675, Manteo NC 27954.

Harvey, Gideon, 1678, The Family Physician and the House apothecares, 2d. ed. printed for M. R. and to be sold by the booksellers of London.

Hasluck, F. W., 1910, "Terra Lemnia", in: Annual of the British School at Athens, Nr. XVI, Session 1909-1910, London, pp. 220-231

Hartston, William, 1963, "Medical Dispensaries in 18th century London", in: Proceedings of the Royal Society of Medicine, Volume 56, Section History of Medicine, p. 753ff.

Hayward, 1917, "Boluphen in der Wundbehandlung", in: Medizinische Klinik,# 21, p. 583.

Heller, Florian, 1961, "Die Nürnberger medizinischen Siegelerden", in: Altnürnberger Landschaft, Mitteilungen, 10. Jahrgang, Heft ½, Mai 1961, pp. 49-57.

——————, 1964, "Medizinische Siegelerden aus den Sammlungen des Germanischen National-Museums Nürnberg", in: Pharmaz.Zeitung Nr. 40, pp. 1461-1471

Hewson, Addinell, 1872, Earth as topical application in surgery, Lindsay & Blakiston, Philadelphia.

Hippokrates sämtliche Werke, transl. Dr. Upmann, Berlin, Albert Nauck & Co, 1847, Annotations are from pages 397 - 435.

Hoffmann, Georg, 1910, "Zur Lehmbehandlung", in: Der Naturarzt, Nr. 9, p. 234ff.

Holland, Bart K., 1977, "The medicines of Greco-Roman Antiquity", in: Prospecting for drugs in Ancient and medieval European texts, Harwood Academic Publishers, p.15.

Höpfel, Rudolf, 1899, "Der Thon als Verbandmittel", in: MMWS, #14, p. 448.

Horn, F., 1899, "Ueber Nabelschnurbehandlung des Neugeborenen", in: MMWS # 12, 377/8

Horst, Johann Daniel, 1651, Pharmacopoeia galeno-chemica, catholica post renodaeum aliusque huius generis celeberrimos utriusque medicinae doctores practicos adornata, Francofurti ad Maenum, Impensis Joannis Godofredi Schönwetteri.

Humboldt, Alexander von, 1859, Ansichten der Natur, Vol. I., Stuttgart, Cotta 1859, p. 163, Transl. of "Sur les peuples qui mangent de la terre", in: Annales des Voyages II, Paris, 1809, pp. 248-254.

Isensee, Emil, 1840, Die Geschichte der Medizin und ihrer Hülfswissenschaften, Teil I: Ältere und mittlere Geschichte, Liebmann & Co., Berlin.

Isidor of Seville, Hispalensis Escopi, "Etymologiarum sive Originum", XX Vol., transl. William Lindsay, Oxonii, 1911.

Joachim, H., 1890, Papyrus Ebers III, das älteste Buch der Heilkunde, Georg Reiner Verlag.

Jones, Claude E., 1957, "A Pharmacopoeia Empirica of 1748", in: Bulletin of the Medical Library Association, Volume 45, Jan.-Oct. Quarterly.

Jung, H., 1939, "Die Eigenschaften des Lößes und dessen Anwendung in der Heilkunde", in: Deutsche medizinische Wochenschrift, annual 65, Nr. 29.

————, 1948, "Zur Geschichte der Heilerden", Museum der Pharmazie, in: Die Pharmazie, Vol.3, Berlin, pp. 278-284.

Just, Rudolf, 1928, "Heilerde in innerer Anwendung", in: Biologische Heilkunst # 34, p. 929-933.

Kamal, Hassan, 1967, A dictionary of pharaonic medicine, National Publication House.

Karfunkel, Hans, 1905, "Ueber die Heilwirkung einer neuen Schlammart", in: Medizinische Klinik #53, pp 1369-1371.

Kegeler, Casparus, 1608, 3d. ed., Ein nützliches und tröstliches Regiment wider die Pestilenz/ und Pestilenzisch Fieber/ die Schweissucht (Suderus anglicus) genannt, und sonst mancherlei gifftige und tödtliche Krankheit.

Kemkes, B., 1942, "Kombinierte Anwendung von Sulfapyridin und Harnstoff in Form von Wundstreupulver", in: Medizinische Klinik #49, pp. 1163-5.

Kenngott, A., ed., 1885, Handwörterbuch der Mineralogie, Geologie und Palaeontologie, Part II, Enzyklopaedie der Naturwissenschaften, hgg. von Förster et al., Breslau, Eduard Trewendt, Vol II, § 51 - clays.

Kentmann, Johann, 1565, "Medici Nomenclaturae rerum fossilium quae in misnia praecipue et in Aliis quoque regionibus inueniuntur", issued and bound jointly with Conrad Gesner De rerum fossilium, lapidum et gemmarum maxime, under the combined title De omnia rerum fossilium genere, gemmis, lapidibus, metallis et huiusmodi…, Zurich, Gesner Fratres.

Kinnier Wilson, J. W, 1967, "Organic Diseases of Ancient Mesopotamia", in: Diseases in Antiquity, ch. 15, pp. 191- 208.

Kircher, Athanasius, 1665, Mundus subterraneus, Amstelodami, Volume 7, Section II, Chapter 4, de usu variarum terrarum, pages 337-338.

Klobius, Fidel, 1644, De ambrae historiam, Leipzig.

Kneipp, Sebastian, 1955, Mein Testament und Codizill, Neue Ausgabe von Dr. Christian Fey, Ehrenwirt Verlag, München 1955; original edition "Mein Testament für Gesunde und Kranke", Verlag der Jos. Köselschen Buchhandlung, Kempten, 1894.

Kneipp, Sebastian, curriculum vitae, in: Catholic Encyclopedia.

König, Roderich, and J. Hopp, 1995, transl. Pliny the Elder "de natura historia", Vol. 37.

Kronacher, 1890, "Über Moosverbände", in: MMWS Feb 11, 1890, pp. 9-10.

Krueger, Haven C., 1963, Avicenna's Poem on Medicine, Charles C. Thomas Publ. Springfield Ill.,

Kugelmeier, Rita, 1980, Vergleichende Untersuchungen über die Adsorption von Makromolekülen und Bakterien an poröse Kieselsäuren, doctoral dissertation at the University of Bonn.

Kunze, R. und M. Vogel, 1936, "Über Wesen und Wirkungen von Heilerden", in: Der Balneologe, 3, pp. 80-98.

Lachmund, Friedrich, 1674, de ave diomedeae, Amsterdam.

Langemak, 1899, "Frage über die Verwendbarkeit des Thons als antiseptisches und aseptisches Verbandsmittel", in: MMWS January 1899., pp. 111-112.

Lasch, R. 1898, "Über Geophagie", Mitteilungen der Anthropologischen Gesellschaft Wien. 28, Pp. 214-222.

Laufer, Berthold, "Geophagy", 1930, Field Museum of Natural History Publication 280, Anthropological Series Volume XVIII No. 2.

Lawson, Alexander, & H. P. Moon, 1938, "A Clay adjunct to Potato Dietary", in Nature, 141/3357, Jan 1, p. 40

Lehman, Dieter, 1985, "Zwei wundärztliche Rezeptbücher des 15. Jahrhunderts vom Oberrhein, In: Würzburger medizinhistorische Forschungen, Band 34, Horst Wellem Verlag.

Leonhard, Andrea, Marie-Thérese Droy-Lefaix & Adrian Allen, 1994, "Pepsin hydrolysis of the inherent mucus barriers and subsequent gastric mucosal damage in the rat", in: Gastroenterological Clinical Biology 18, 609-616.

Levey, Martin, 1966, transl., The medical formulary of Agrabadhin of Al-Kindt (Rhazes), U. of Wisconsin Press, Madison.

Levy, Walter, 1908, Die Bolustherapie, ihre Geschichte und Begründung durch Empirie und Experiment, Doctoral dissertation at the University of Freiburg im Breisgau, Speyer & Kaerner Universitätsbuchhandlung.

Lewis, S. Judd, 1938, "What is a peloid?" in: Archives of medical Hydrology, October, pp. 76-77.

Lindsay, William, 1911, transl. of Isidore of Seville, Hispalensis Escopi, "Etymologiarum sive Originum Vol. XX"

Li Shizhen, Pen Ts'ao Kang Mu (2 Vols), published by the Association of Chinese Medical Documents, the Research Institute of Chinese Medical Culture and the Research Institute of Ancient Chinese Medical Literature, ed. Li Jianzhong, governor of Pengxi County, 1997. Cited translations by Yanfeng Sun, Beijing, and Mrs. Wang, Hoover Institute, Stanford, personal to the author.

Lowe, C. B., 1920, "Clay as medicine", in: American Journal of Pharmacy, April 1920.

Ludwig, Christian Gottlieb, 1749, Terrae Musei Regii Dresdensis quas digessit descripsit Illustravit D.C.G. Ludwig accedunt Terrarum sigillatarum figurae, Leipzig, ex officine Libraria Gleditschii, ADR MDCCXLVIII.

Lu Gwei-Djen & J. Needham, 1967, Records of Diseases in Ancient China, in: Diseases in Antiquity, ch.17, pp. 222-237.

Lüschen, Hans, 1979, Die Namen der Steine, das Mineralreich im Spiegel der Sprache, 2 ed., Ott Verlag Thun, Switzerland.

Lutz, Alfons, 1958, "Die heilige Erde von Lemnos", in: Österreichische Apotheker Zeitung, Wien, after a lecture on April 16, 1958

MacGill, E. R., 1977, "Examples of a primary source: this booke of sovereign medicines", in: Prospecting for drugs in ancient and medieval European texts: A scientific Approach, ed. Bart K. Holland, Harwood academic Publishers.

Magner, Lios N., 1992, A history of medicine, Marcell Dekker, Inc. NY.

Mahaney, William C. and R. G. V. Hancock, 1990, "Geochemical analysis of African buffalo geophagic sites and dung on Mount Kenya, East Africa", in: Mammalia, Revue Trimestrielle publiée avec le concours du Centre National de la Recherche Scientifique, # 54 No.1, 1990.

————, R. G. V. Hancock and M. Inoue, 1993, "Geochemistry and Clay Mineralogy of soils eaten by Japanese Macaques", in: Primates, 34(1): 85-91, January 1993.

————, Anna Stambolic, Mary Knezevich, Kandiah Sanmugadas, M. J. Kessler and M.D. Grynpas, 1995, "Geophaghy amongst rhesus macaques on Cayo Santiago, Puerto Rico", in: Primates (36)3:323-333, July 1995.

————, and R. G. V. Hancock, Susanne Aufreiter and Michael A. Huffman, 1996, "Geochemistry and clay mineralogy of termite mound soil and the role of geophagy in chimpanzees of the Mahale Mountains of Tanzania", in: Primates 37(2): 121-134.

————, and Michael W. Milner, Kandiah Sanmugadas, R. G. V.Hancock, Susanne Aufreiter, Richard Wrangham and Harold W. Pier, 1997, "Analysis of Geophagy Soils in Kibale Forest, Uganda", in: Primates 38(2):159-176, April 1997.

————, and Jessica Zippin, Michael W. Milner, Kandiah Sanmugadas, R. G. V. Hancock, Susanne Aufreiter, Sean Campbell, Michael A. Huffman, Michael Wink, David Malloch, Volli Kalm, 1999, "Chemistry, mineralogy and microbiology of termite mound soil eaten by the chimpanzees of the Mahale mountains, Western Tanzania", in: Journal of tropical Ecology (1999), 15:565-588.

————, M. W. Milner, Hs Mulyono, R.V.G. Hancock, S. Aufreiter, M. Reich and M. Wink, 2000, "Mineral and chemical analysis of soils eaten by humans in Indonesia", in: International Journal of Environmental Health Research, 10:93-109.

Major, Johann Daniel, Dissertatio medica de lacte lunae, Kiel, 1667, as transl. & expl. by W. R. Reinbacher: Leben, Arbeit, und Umwelt des Arztes Johann Daniel Major, Kroeber Verlag, Linsengericht (Germany) 1998, Chapter on Mondmilch (moonmilk).

————, 1674 Vorstellung etlicher Kunst- und Naturalienkammern in America und Asien, Kiel

————, 1675a, Vorstellung etlicher Kunst- und Naturalienkammern in Africa und an den Gräntzen Europas, Kiel.

————, 1675b, Vorstellung etlicher Kunst-und Naturalienkammern in Italien, zu Neapolis und Alt-Rom, Kiel.

Major, Ralph H., 1954, A History of Medicine, Thomas, Springfield Ill, 2 vol.

Majno, Guido, 1973, The Healing Hand, Man and Wound in the Ancient World, Harvard U. Press

Martini and Grothe, 1910, "Ueber eßbare Erden und ihre Verwendung als Heilmittel", in: Deutsche Medizinische Wochenschrift,Nr.19, p. 900.

Megele, 1899, "Ueber die Verwendbarkeit des Thones (Bolus) als antiseptisches und aseptisches Verbandmittel", in: MMWS # 21, pp. 373-377.

Megenberg, Konrad von, 1309-1374 - see Pfeiffer, Franz, ed.

Meige, Dr. Henry, 1899, "Cholera-Preservativ-Mann", in: Janus, Archives Internationales pour L'Histoire de la Médécine et la Géographie Médicale, Amsterdam, 4th, pp. 79-80.

Meigen, W., 1905, "Essbare Erde von Deutsch-Neuguinea", in: Monatsberichte der Deutschen Geologischen Gesellschaft, Berlin, p. 557.

Mendelson, Walter, 1923, "Maimonides, a twelfth century physician", in: Annals of Medical History, ed. F. R. Packard, Volume V, P. B. Hoeber, Publisher, NY.

Mercati, Michele, 1574, Metalloteca Vaticana, Opus posthumum op. J. M. Lancisii, Rom,1719

Meyer's Konversationslexikon, 1890 edition.

Meyer, Theodor, 1909, Theodorus Priscianus und die römische Medizin, Gustav Fischer, Jena.

Meyer, Klaus, 1998, Geheimnisse des Antoni van Leeuwenhook, Pabst Science Publishers, Lengerich (Germany).

Meyer-Schlatter, A., Neues Lehmbuch- Wunderbare Wirkung der Heilerden, 6th ed. Volksgesundheitverlag, Zurich, no publication date given, but based on certain text, it was printed after 1911 at the earliest and 1948 at the latest.

Meyerhof, Max, 1928, "Eine unbekannte arabische Augenheilkunde", in: Archiv der Geschichte der Medizin, ed. Karl Sudhoff und H. Sigrist.

Mez, Lydia, and Michael Kessler, 1999, Womit der Apotheker einst hantierte.

Mielek, W. H. and H. Leisrink, 1882, "Ueber Sphagnum und Torf als Verbandmaterial (Torfmoos contra Moostorf)", in: Berliner klinische Wochenschrift #39, p. 588-590.

Minnich, Virginia, et al: 1968, "Pica in Turkey, II. Effect of clay upon iron absorption", in: American Journal of Clinical Nutrition, Vol. 21, No. 1, pp. 78-86.

Morrison, Rutherford, 1916, "The treatment of infected suppurating wounds", in: Lancet,Vol. II, Pp. 268- 272.

Möser, H., 1909, "Lehm als Heilmittel", in: Der Naturarzt, # 10, pp. 249-252.

Most, Georg Friedrich, Karl Frich und Hans Biedermann, 1973, Encyclopädie der Gesammten Volksmedizin, F. A. Brockhaus 1843, Nachdruck Akademische Druck- und Verlagsanstalt Graz.

Müller, Jo. Rudolph, 1763, Dissertatio Inauguralis Medica de Thermis Schinznacensibus, Basilae, Typis Joan. Henr. Deckeri, Academiae Typog.

Münz, J., 1895, Maimonides als medizinische Autorität, Trier, Verlag von Sigmund Mayer.

Murray, J. L., and Alan D. Lopez, eds.,1992, "Comprehensive assessment of incidence, Prevalence and mortality estimates for diarrheal diseases", in: Statistical analysis by The World Health Organization, Harvard School of Public Health and the World Bank, distributed by Harvard University Press.

Nadeau, Paul H., 1987, "Clay particle engineering: a potential new technology with diverse Applications", in: Applied Clay Science, 2, 83-93.

Nassauer, 1909, Max, "Zur Behandlung des Ausfluß", in: MMWS #15 pp. 753/7.

——————, 1910, "Zur Bolusbehandlung", in: MMWS #2 p. 84/84.

Nunn, John F., 1996, Ancient Medicine, British Museum Press, London, p. 145

Oppenheim, A. Leo, 1962, "Mesopotamian Medicine" in: Bulletin of the History of Medicine, Vol.XXXVI, # 2, pp. 97-108.

Paczensky, Gert von, and Anna Dünnebier, Kulturgeschichte des Essens und Trinkens, 2d ed.

1977, btb Taschenbuch, Goldmann Verlag Div. of Bertelsmann

Pettenkofer, Max von., 1882, Der Boden und sein Zusammenhang mit der Gesundheit des Menschen, 2d ed., Verlag von Gebrüder Paetel, Berlin.

Peyer, W. & W. Röpke, 1927, "Ueber Heilerden", in: Apotheker-Zeitung # 45, pp. 662-664.

Pfeiffer, Franz, editor, 1962, Das Buch der Natur by Konrad von Megenberg, 1309-1364, the first natural history written in German about 1475 with six editions by 1499, reproprinting 1861 by E. Lokay, Reinheim, and 1962 by Georg Ohms,Verlagsbuchhandlung Hildesheim.

Pharmacopoeia collegi regalis medicorum Londinensis 1746, apud T. Longman, T. Shewell et J. Norse, Londini.

Pharmacopoeia of Japan, 4th ed. effective April 1, 1921, published by the Pharmaceutical Society of Japan, Tokyo, 1927.

Pharmacopoeia of the Royal College of Physicians, London 1809, transl. by Richard Powell MD.

Pictorius, Georgius D., Badenfahrtbüchlein, 1979 reprint of 1560, Herder, Freiburg.

Platearius, Matthaeus, ~1350 de simplici medicinae, or: circa instans, related to the Compendium Salernitanum. Now as Manuscript M873 fol. 87 v., Pierpoint Morgan Library NY. As Platearius Iohannis in Collectana medic, leaves 52-99, in Erlangen University catalog of incunabula as # 429, a part of Tractatus Aegidii Carbolinensis, Hermanno de Porta Regio, Iohannis Platearius et alia multa, one of three known surviving copies.

Pliny the Elder (C. Plinius Secundus the Elder), Naturkunde, 37 Vol., ed. & transl. Roderich König & J. Hopp, Artemis & Winkler, 1995, pp. 33-43.

Polette, Lori A., Norma Ugarte, José Miguel Yacamán, and Russell R. Chianelli, 2000, "Maya Blue - Decoding the chemical complexity of a remarkable ancient paint", in: Discovering Archeology, August 2000, pp. 46-53.

Pomet, Lemery, Tournefort, 1712, A complete history of drugs, London, Book IV (Earths).

————, 1717, Der aufrichtige Materialist und Specerey-Händler, Leipzig, Verlag Gleditsch.

Powell, Richard, 1809, Pharmacopoeia of the royal college of Physicians, London, with commentary.

Priakus, Angeliki, 1997, "Limnos, Die Insel des Hephaistos", in Greek and German translation by Gisela Métzias, published in Thessaloniki, Greece.

Priesner, Claus, & Karin Figala, 1999, Alchemie - Lexikon einer Wisenschaft, C. H. Beck, München, pp. 357/8.

Puppel, Ernst, 1914, "Argobol, ein neues Silberboluspräparat", in: MMWS# 51, pp 2406-7.

Puschmann, Theodor, 1878, Transl. of Alexander von Tralles; Original-Text und Übersetzung nebst einer einleitenden Abhandlung, ein Beitrag zur Geschichte der Medicin, 1878 Vienna, reprint Amsterdam 1963 Adolf M. Hakkert.

Rateau, J.- G., G. Morgant, M.-T. Droy-Priot and J. - L. Parier, 1982, "A histological, enzymatic and water-electrolyte study of the action of smectatite, a mucoprotective clay, on experimental infectious diarrhoea in the rabbit", in: Current Medical Research and Opinion, Vol. 8. No. 4.

Read, B. E., and C. Pak, 1936, "Chinese Materia Medica, a compendium of minerals and stones used in Chinese medicine", from: Pen T'sao Kang Mu (Li Shi chen or Zhen), Henry Lester Institute of medical Research, Shanghai 2d. ed.

Reinbacher, W. R., 1994, ""Is it gnome, is it berg, is it mont, is it mond", in: NSS Bulletin 56:1-13, National Speleological Ass. Huntsville AL June 1994.

————, 1998, Leben, Arbeit und Umwelt des Arztes Johann Daniel Major, 1998, Kroeber Verlag Linsengericht (Germany).

Rivinus, Johann August, 1723, Tentamina quaedam physico-medica circa Terras Medicinales, in disputatione pro loco consensu gratiosissimae facult. medicae Lipsensis, exhibita a D. Johanne Augusto Rivino, respondente Gottfried Mieckisch, Med. Candid, Sagan, Sil. D. I. October 1723, Litteris Titianis. (Leipzig).

Robertson, Aitchison W. G., 1926, "the use of unicorn's horn, coral and stones in medicine", in: Annals of History of Medicine, Vol. VIII, pp. 240 ff.

Robertson, Robert, H. S., 1947, "Geophagy, or Earth-eating" in: Discovery, pp. 213-215

————, 1986, Fuller's Earth, a History of calcium montmorillonite, Volturna Press, London.

————, 1996, "Cadavers, cholera, and clays", in: Mineralogical Society Bulletin, 41 Queens Gate, London, SW7 5HR, UK.

Röpke, W., 1928, "Erden als Heilmittel", in: Steinbruch und Sandgruben, Halle, #27, pp. 53-56.

Rösch, K., 1938, translator & commentator, Das Neue Testament, Volume 3 of Die Heilige Schrift des alten und neuen Testaments, Verlag Ferdinand Schöning, Paderborn.

Rose, Valentine, 1875, "Aristoteles de lapidibus und Arnold Saxo", in: Zeitschrift für deutsches Altertum. 18. Band, Berlin. See also Lüschen 1979, p. 355.

Rosen, Nils, 1739, de medicamentibus absorbentibus eorumque perverso uso, Upsala, passim.

Rupprecht, 1856, "Das Schlackenbad bei Hettstedt", in: Balneologische Zeitung Vol III, 5 May 1856, # 5, pp. 103-107.

Ruska, Julius, transl. & ed. 1912, Das Steinbuch des Aristoteles mit literaturgeschichtlichen Untersuchungen, nach der arabischen Handschrift der Bibliothèque Nationale, Paris, Carl Winter's Universitätsbuchhandlung Heidelberg. This is most likely NOT by Aristotle, but rather by the Syriac writer Hunain ibn Ishak.

Said, Sobhi A., Atef M. Shibl and Mohamed E. Abdullah, "Influence of various agents on Adsorption capacity of kaolin for *Pseudomones aeruginosa* toxin, in: Jounal of Pharmaceutical Sciences, Vol. 69, No. 10, 1980, Riyad, Saudi Arabia.

Salmon, William, 1700, Pharmacopoeia Bateana or Bates Dispensatory, 2d ed. printed for S. Smith & B. Walford at the Prince's Arm", in: Biochemische Zeitschrift # 84 pp. 378-381.

Schelenz, Hermann, 1909, "History of the medical earths and of Cataplasma Kaolini", transl. Otto Raubenheimer, in: American Journal of Pharmacy, March 1909.

Bibliography

Scheuchzer, Johann Jacob, 1717, Hydrographia Helvetica - Beschreibung der Seen/ Flüssen/Brünnen/ Warmen und Kalten Bäderen und anderen Mineral-Wassern deß Schweitzerlandes, der Natur-Histori des Schweitzerlandes Zweyter Teil, Zürich, in der Bodmerischen Truckerey.

Scheider, Wolfgang, 1968, Lexikon zur Arzneimittelgeschichte, Bd. 1, Tierische Drogen, Govi-Verlag GmbH, Pharmazeutischer Verlag, Frankfurt/M, Germany, p. 48: Lucius.

Schönenberger, Fr., 1910, "Zur Lehmbehandlung" in: Der Naturarzt # 6 pp. 145-147.

Schröder, Johannes, 1744, (MD, Reip. Moeno-Francfurtanae Physico Ordinario cum Privilegia S. Caesarea Majestatis) Pharmacopoeia Medico-Chymica sive Thesaurus Pharmacologicus, sumptibus Johannis Gerlinus, Bibliopolae, Ulm, 2d ed.

Schultze-Heubach, H., 1934, "Über Wilhelmshavener Heilschlick", in: Der Balneologe, Vol. I, pp. 175-177.

Sealy, F.L. W., 1918/19, "Lemnos", in: The Annual of the British School at Athens, No. XXIII,

Session 1918-1919, MacMillan & Co, London, pp. 148 – 174.

Seligman, S., 1927, Die magischen Heil- und Schutzmittel aus der unbelebten Natur, Stuttgart, Strecker und Schroeder Verlagsbuchhandlung.

Shaw, Trevor R., 1992, History of cave science, the exploration and study of limestone caves to 1900, 2d ed. Sydney Speleological Society, p. 223.

Shipley, Paul G., 1922, "The treatment of convulsions (tetany) with calcium in the 17th century" In: Annals of Medical History Volume IV, pp. 189-191.

Sigrist, Henry, 1951, A history of Medicine, Oxford University Press, 1951.

Sine nomen, 1895, "Clay eating" in: Scientific American March 23, 1895, based on the 9th annual report of the Bureau of Ethnology by J. G. Bourke.

Singer, Charles, 1948, The earliest chemical industry, London, The Folio Society.

Sinh Jeem, Sir Bhagwat, 1981 reprint, A Short History of Aryan Medical Science, New Asian Publishers, Nai Sarak, New Delhi 6, India

Sirasi, Nancy G., 1990, Medieval & early renaissance medicine, U. of Chicago Press.

Sivin, Nathan, 1987, Traditional medicine in contemporary China, Center for Chinese Studies, University of Michigan, Ann Arbor.

Smith, David E., 1920, "Medicine and Mathematics in the 16th century", in: Annals of Medical History, Paul B. Hoeber, Publisher, New York, Vol 2.

Sondhi, S. M. and N. Agarwal, 1955, "Determination of mineral elements in medicinal plants used for the cure of bronchitis, kidney and bladder disorders, skin diseases and ghonorroea etc.", in: Handard Medicus, Quarterly Journal of Science and Medicine. Vol. 38, Jan/Mar. 1995, # 1.

Souci, S. W., 1937, "Eigenschaften und therapeutische Wirkung des Moores, mit besonderer Berücksichtigung seiner Verwendung zu Badezwecken", in: Der Balneologe, Vol. IV. # 1, pp. 1-7.

Spanudis, G., 1945? "Geschichtliches zur Heilerde", two parts, in: Pharmaziewissenschaftlicher Monatsbericht, Heft 15, pp. 302-305, cont'd pp. 322-328, Institut für Geschichte der Medizin, Universität Wien.

Spencer, W. G., 1935, transl. Aulus Cornelius Celsus "de medicina", Harvard U Press, 2 vols.

Sprengel, Kurt, 1821, Versuch einer pragmatischen Geschichte der Arzneykunde, 3d ed. Part I, Gebauersche Buchhandlung, Halle.

Sprenger and Krämer, Malleus Malificarum, 1486. I used the English translation of 1928 (The witches' hammer)

Stamatakis, Michael G. and Ulrich Lutat, Manuel Regueiro and José Calco, "Milos - the mineral Island" in: Industrial Minerals, February 1996, pp. 58-61.

Starkenstein, Emil, 1915, "Ueber die therapeutische Verwendung der Tierkohle", in: MMWS Nr 3, (1915) pp. 27-29, 5 Jan 1915.

Stauder, 1908, Protokoll, Nürnberger medizinische Gesellschaft und Poliklinik, "ueber die Therapeutische Verwendbarkeit des Bolus alba", in: MMWS, #13, p. illegible.

Stahl, Günther, 1931, "Die Geophagie", in: Zeitschrift für Ethnologie, 63 pp. 346-374.

Stahlecker and Staiger, 1958, The diary of Martin Crusius, 1608,

Stoeckel, Walter, 1900, "Bemerkungen zu dem Aufsatz von O. Frankl in der vorigen Nummer", In: Centralblatt für Gynäkologie, hgg. Heinrich Frisch, No 23, June 9, 1900.

Stumpf, Julius, 1898a, "Ein Fall von tödtlicher Vergiftung durch Essigessenz", in: MMWS # 22, May 1898 pp 69-71.

————, 1898b, "Die Verwendbarkeit des Thones als antiseptisches und aseptisches Verbandmittel", in MMWS, 1898, No. 46, pp. 1466-1468.

————, 1905, "Zur Behandlung der Cholera asiatica, Vorläufige Mitteilung", in: Berliner klinische Wochenschrift 11 Sep 1905, pp. 1199.

————, 1906, Über ein zuverlässiges Heilverfahren bei der asiatischen Cholera sowie bei schweren infektiösen Brechdurchfällen und über die Bedeutung des Bolus (Kaolins) bei der Behandlung gewisser Bakterienkrankheiten, A. Stuber's Verlag (Curt Kabitzsch), Würzburg.

————, 1908, "Über Bolusbehandlung bei Diphtherie", in: MMWS, 1908, # 22, pp. 1181-1182.

————, 1914a, "Ueber Cholerabehandlung und Choleraprophylaxe auf Grund meiner Erfahrungen In Nisch und Belgrad", in: MMWS 1914, #14, pp. 759-763.

————, 1914b, "Bolus alba bei Diarrhoe, Ruhr und asiatischer Cholera", in: MMWS 1914, #40, Pp. illegible.

————, Personnel file of the University of Würzburg, Yaka (Feka) 164/23, Folder 214, seen 1999.

————, 1932, Obituary in Würzburger General-Anzeiger, Tuesday, 12 April 1932, p. 88.

Sussmann, Max, 1967, Diseases in the Bible and Talmud, in: Diseases in Antiquity, ch. 16, pp. 209-219.

Thevet, André, 1554, Cosmographie de Levant, translated by Gregor Horst as Cosmographie Orientis, das ist Beschreibung des gantzen Morgenlandes. *Cited by S. J. S. Thompson without reference, listed in National Union Catalog, but not found.*

Thompson, C. J. S., 1914, "Terra sigillata, a famous medicament of ancient times" in: Proceedings of the 17th International Congress of Medicine, London, 1913, pp. 433-444, Henry Frowde, Oxford U. Press.

Thorndike, Lynn, 1923, History of Magic and Experimental Science, 8 Vols, Vol. I., MacMillan, NY. Also Ch. 25, pp. 566-593.

Thorwald, Jürgen, 1962, The science and secrets of early medicine translated from German by Richard and Clara Winston, Harcourt Brace & World, Inc., NY.

Tozer, Henry Fanshawe, 1890, The Islands of the Aegean, Oxford at the Clarendon Press.

Tralles, Alexander von,(c.525-c.605) see Puschmann, Theodor.

Trumpp, 1909, "Zur Behandlung der Rhinitis acuta", in: MMWS #12 pp. 2422-2423.

Upmann, 1847, transl., Hippokrates sämtliche Werke, Albert Nauck & Co, Berlin.

Urbainski, Helmut, 1940, "Über die antibakterielle Wirkung des Elsterer Moors", in: Der Balneologe, 7. Jahrg. Heft 7, 15 July 1940.

Van den Berg, W. S., and E. J. Brill, 1917, Antidotarium Nicolëi, Leiden, (The Antidotarium of Nikolaus Salernitatus (~1100 AD), Latin ed. By Nicolaus Myrepsus (~1280), written 1351, first impressum 1471).

Valerius, Cordus, 1540, Dispensatorium sive pharmacorum, Lugduni Batavorum apud Franciscum Raphelengium. The 1551 edition was entitled: Pharmacorum conficiendorum ratio vulgo vocant Dispensatorium Nerobergae, in officina Ioannis Daubmanni impremabatur. Variously each of these is considered the first "Nürnberg Pharmacopoeia".

Vardanjan, Stella A., 1993, "Galen und die mittelalterliche armenische Medizin", in: Galen und das hellenistische Erbe, Jutta Kollesch und Diethard Nickel, Hgg, Verhandlungen des IV. Galen-Symposiums am Institut für Geschichte der Medizin am Bereich Medizin (Charité) der Humboldt-Universität zu Berlin, 18-20 Sep., Franz Steiner Verlag Stuttgart.

Verhoeven, John D., 2001, "The Mystery of Damascus Blades", in: Scientific American Vol. 284 January 2001, pp. 74-79.

Vogel, Martin, 1915, "Zur Behandlung des akuten Darmkatarrhs", in: Ärztliche Rundschau, # 25 Pp. 193-195.

Vogel, M., 1943, "Was sind Heilerden?" in: Hippokrates 14, pp. 24-27.

Volkheimer, Gerhard, 1933, "Das Phänomen der Perseption - Historie und Fakten", in: Gastroenterologie, pp. 217, 221.

——————, 1999, "Is the mucosal barrier impermeable for dust? Persorption, Dissemination and Elimination of solid foreign microparticles", Referat 30.10. 1999 zum Jubiläums-Symposium der Charité, Berlin.

Volkmann, Georg Anton, 1720, Silesia subterranea or Schlesien mit seinen unterirdischen Schätzen…, Leipzig, Moritz Georg Weidmann.

Wacker, Leonhard, 1935, "Über die Heilwirkung der Erden und das Erdessen der Naturvölker", In: MMWS, 32 (1935), pp. 1279-1280.

Wald, Georg am, 1581, Bericht und Erklärung…von im erfunden terra sigillata…wider die Pestilenz…(very long title).

Walsh, James, J., 1920, Medieval Medicine, A. &. C. Black Ltd, London.

Waring, George E., 1868, Earth closets: How to make them and use them, The Tribune Association, New York.

——————, 1870, Earth closets and earth sewage, Orange Judd & Co., New York.

Webb, John L., 1957, "he oldest Medical document" in: Bulletin of the Medical Library Association, Volume 45, Jan-Oct.

Welcker, Friedrich Gottlieb, 1824, Die Aeschylische Trilogie Prometheus und die Kabirenweihe zu Lemnos, nebst Winken über die Trilogie des Aeschylus überhaupt, Darmstadt, Verlag C.W. Leske.

Wencker-Wildberg, Friedrich, 1953, "Würzburg um die Jahrhundertwende - die Guillotine auf dem Dachboden", in: Mainpost (daily newspaper of Würzburg and environs), June 6, 1953.

Wigand, Albert, 1879, Lehrbuch der Pharmakognosie.

Winter, D., 1909, "Lehm-Esser", in: Deutsche Rundschau für Geographie und Statistik, 31, pp. 123-125.

Wittich, Iohannis, 1601, Bericht von wunderbaren bezoardischen Gesteinen…, Arnstadt, Typ. Voeglinianus.

Wonnecke von Cube, Johannes, 1483, Hortus sanitatis, Mainz, facsimile print 1966 Konrad Köbel Grünwald, München.

Woodall, John, 1617, The Surgeon's Mate, a facsimile new edition by John Kirkup, originally Printed Kingsmeade Press, Rosewell house, Kingsmeade Square, Bath.

Worm, Olau, 1655, Museum Wormianum sive historia rerum rariorum, Lugduni Batavorum (Leiden), apud Ionannem Elsevirum Acad. Typogr.

Wreszinski, Walter, 1909. ed., Der grosse Medizinische Papyrus des Berliner Museums (Pap. Berl. 3038) Leipzig, J. C. Hinrichs'sche Buchhandlung.

————, 1912, ed., Der Londoner medizinische Papyrus und der Papyrus Hearst, J. C. Hinrichs'sche Buchhandlung, Leipzig.

Wurffbain, Joh, Paul, 1689, "Terra sigillata curiosa", in: Ephemerides of the Miscellanea curiosa medica curiosa Academiae Naturae Curiosorum, Decuria II, Vol. 8

Wyckhoff, Dorothy: see Albertus Magnus

Zedler: Gesundbrunnen, see that word in the Universal Lexikon 1702-1750.

Ziegler, Jacob, 1663, Heilbrunnen - das ist Beschreibung deß köstlich warmen Gesund-Bades bey Schinznach, printed by Hans Caspar Hardtmeyer in Zurich.

Zweifel, P., 1910, "Bolus alba als Träger der Infektion", in: MMWS #34 pp. 1787/88.

Glossary and List of Minerals

A note to the reader: (1) Some obviously Germanic names, mostly from former Eastern Germany could not be found on modern maps, since those are in Polish. Old Prussian field maps do not show some of the very small hamlets or lonesome farms or mine shafts after which earths were named. An inquiry to 200,000 former Silesians through their affinity monthly newsletter did not bring a single reply. The adults who fled after 1945 are now septuagenarians or better, the new generation has never been exposed to names, which are at least 300 years old. The Dresden collection of earth coins described by Ludwig in 1748 was destroyed in 1945. The precise origin of some of the earth coins may be lost. Ludwig, though writing his theory of various types of earths was not always consistent and not reliably accurate—one chapter appearing 1½ times with different content—but worst of all, where he cites the author Rivinus, it appears that the cited tables Ludwig believed attached to Rivinus no longer exist; at least the last extant copy of Rivinus does not have them - and maybe never did. Luwig won't tell us if there was an error.

Abiolith: A sediment of mineral substances, minerogene, compare biolith (Benade, 1937).

Aceldema terra: See calx nativa.

Acetate of lead: White crystalline water soluble substance used in ancient medicine $Pb(C_2H_3O_2)_2$.

Achates: See agate.

Adamea terra: A reddisch earth dust from Assyria, believed to be the clay from which God made Adam, also called Terra damascena, Bagdad earth.

Adamas terra: - a hard stone as carving tool (Theophrast).

Adarkes: A salt crust from Galatia, used against eczema, white spots, liver spots, sciatica (Spanudis citing Dioscorides).

Aetites: See eagle stone.

Agaricus mineralis: Appelation for calcium carbonate: Agaricus was a medicinal mushroom, the cave deposit calcium carbonate was deemed the mineral version or equivalent.

Agate: A common semiprecious silica mineral in bands of varying color and transparency. Named by Theophrast after the river Achates (possibly the modern Carabi or the Cannitello in Sicily). Various versions in Pliny and Isidor: The banded stone is described as onyx, agate more as the stone with pictures or drawings after which it is named: Coral agate, cloud Agate, moss agate. Agate is said to have "eight virtues": against thunder, sorcery, fiendish possession, venom, poison, disease, evils of strong drink and outbreak on skin.

Agate, moss (Mocha stone): Agate with dark inclusions resembling ferns and moss. The inclusions are mainly manganese and iron oxide.

Ajale (red, white, black): Agates used in India for eye diseases, in Egypt and Greece for bites of spiders and scorpions.

Akaustabiolith: Biogene, mostly inorganic material with some remnants of living organisms, not combustible when dry, no organic carbon, or only a very little (Benade, 1937).

Alabaster, dust of: see gypsum.

Alabaster lithos: The hardest form of gypsum, named after pots for ointments made of it to keep, ointments fresh. Confusion with onyx, early modern Alabaster, (Lüschen); softer than marble, almost translucent. Alabastrites probably were compact stalagmitic calcium carbonate, in Egypt called onyx marble or oriental alabaster in contrast to the "real" Alabaster: Gypsum, hydrated calcium sulfate.

Alabaster, meal of: Powdered alabaster, used medicinally, very close to gypsum.

Alana terra: An earth from a town in Ethiopia: Pliny, Paul of Aegina, Erstingius (1770), Ludwig (p. 44/45). Syn. Tripoli earth, probably diatomaceous earth.

Alanelos terra: Yellow clay from a city near Pontus in Cappadocia, similar to bolus armenus (Paul of Aegina).

Alba terra: A white earth described by Pliny. Could be any white clay.

Alcalina terra: Alkaline spring water, deposit of oxides of calcium. (Muller, 1763).

Alexandrine earth: Probably dried Nile mud, 4th to 5th century, Aetius of Amida, (Ludwig, p. 101); red bolus, soft, bubbles in acid. It is the rubrica fabrilis Ægyptiacea of Dioscorides (Lib. V, cap. 103).

Allium: See Alum.

Allum: Ancient spelling, see alum.

Alsatica argilla alba: White clay from Alsatia(?) (Ludwig, p. 115).

Alsatica marga: Marl from Alsatia(?) near Bischweiler (Ludwig, p. 135).

Altenbergensis marga: Marl from Altenberg (Ludwig, p. 134).

Altenbergensis terra: Clay from Altenberg (Ludwig, p. 134).

Altenburgensis terra: Clay from Altenburg (Ludwig, p. 168)

Altendorfina argilla: white clay from near Chemitz near Poenigensee (Ludwig, p. 89).

Althea terra:?, syn. terra judaeicus (Zedler); probably an asphaltous earth.

Alumen: Old spelling, see alum.

Alum: A weathering and evaporation product. Found as weathering product of certain lava, Alum slate is a re-crystallization of alum rich water, when it can contain iron vitriol and bituminosa. Dioscorides calls it stypteria, found in pits in Egypt and all over the Levant; best for medical use is the split alum: It stops bleeding, defeats pus-forming ulcers, Tightens loose teeth with vinegar and honey, helps ear infections, eczema. Used as contraceptive and as abortion facilitator, reduces tonsil swellings. It is found as feathered, round and split alum. In ancient times it came from Turkey and Yemen, the latter prized as mouth wash, styptite, pessary for hemorrhagia, itchy scalp, nasal douche, gonorrhea (?), purulent ophthalmicia, and excessive diarrhea; it is astringent, acidic. Also used as gargle water, alum water to wash frost bite, alum ointment for burn blisters. In ancient times distinguished in 5 kinds: split, round, twisted, plakistis (the leafed one), plinthitis (the brick shaped one), phorimon (milky and soft), Liparian (fibrous and hairy). Roasted Egyptian alum was used for obstinate ulcers. The meaning today has expanded to include other double salts of aluminum sulfate.

Alum, feathered: Also called fibrous or hairy, see alum.

Aluminis terra: Aluminous earth, see alum (Horst, 1651).

Aluminium: British and German spelling for aluminum.

Aluminous clay: See clay.

Aluminum acetate: Aluminum sulfate and glacial acetic acid plus $CaCO_3$ + H_2O + tartaric acid., A moist medium for cataplasms against sprains and swellings, the German name alliterated is "vinegar-sour clay" (Essigsaure Tonerde).

Alum, roasted: See alum.

Alum, round: See alum.

Amazon stone: Historic one not identified, could either be jade or morochthus. The one in the Badiani Aztec herbal could be the feldspar mineral amazonite, yellow green to blue green, pale to deep color, in South America, principally in Brazil. Now not named after Amazon river, but after the Amazons, legendary women warrior tribe in Africa (Monomotape). In South America described by Alexander von Humboldt, who considered it a nephrite or jade.

Amber, gray: The ejected intestinal mucus of the sperm whale enclosing indigestible parts, like beaks of squid. Usually it floats on the sea until washed ashore on beaches of East India, China, Madagascar, Somalia. After this salt water soaking, ambergris(e) is gray and smells very good. Made into pills, used as rejuvenating medicine. Gray amber is NOT the result of gallstones in the whale and it turns gray and perfumey only after at least 24 hours in salt water. (Coe &Coe, 1996).

Amber, yellow: Hardened resin from trees (German: Bernstein), 50,000 years old, usually from a Peninsula near the Baltic Sea of Europe; traded as far south as Liguria (Italy). At times confused with copal from the Indian Ocean, also a tree resin, but much younger. The Roman word succinus (juice) applies to yellow amber. It was chemically dissolved and used in bath water; so-called oil of amber was used against podagra.

Ambergris(e): See amber, gray.

Amber tree or American amber: This is a plant, sweet gum, *Liquidamber styraciflua*, from which Amber balm is won; in Asia it was *Liquidamber formosana*.

Ambra grysea: See amber, gray.

Ambra, nigra: Fresh gray amber, black and smelly, before being soaked in salt water.

Amethyst: In ancient times a stone against drunkenness (Lüschen, 1979). It is a colored quartz. Its effectiveness against becoming drunk is that its color never equals white or red wine (Pliny, liber 37).

Amianthus: feather alum (Schroeder, 1634), but also referred to as asbestos and salamander hair because of its fire resistance.

Ammonia, word origin: 1) From camel dung near temple of Jupiter Ammon in Egypt (probably erroneus), 2) called salt of Aman (M. Jastrow: Amanus = Mountain in Syria).

Ampelitis terra: A bituminous earth used to control insects on grape vines (Ernstingius, 1770). Dioscorides says this earth (also called pharmakitis) is found near Seleukia in Syria: "Choose the black one which resembles pine coals, finely splintered and lustrous, not the thin one". It kills insects and worms from grape vines at the time of budding. Theophrast finds it in Cilicia. It becomes sticky when boiled, then the vines are smeared with it instead of with bird lime. It is also used as an eye cosmetic and as hair coloring.

Ancient brick: Unknown whether fired or not, but an Egyptian medication of either brick dust if fired or brick clay if not.

Angalba terra: Listed in Farmacia de la Familia Salvador, 1760.

Angerburg Terra: (Rivinus, 1723).

Angerburgica tripela argillacea: Diatomaceous clay (Ludwig, p. 91).

Angermanica terra: (Ludwig, p. 178)

Anglica terra: White or yellow Tripoli earth (diatomaceous earth), also called Trippel, from England (Ludwig, p. 82). As Anglica argilla alba: White clay from England (. 113)

Animal stones: Pseudo-Aristotle considers crab (lobster) shells and snail shells as stones. Concerning the squid, its "stone" (beak) is pulverized and used to remove white spots from the eye.

Annaberg yellow clay: Silesian clay (Kentmann, 1565).

Annabergensis marga: Marl from Annaberg (Ludwig, p. 135)

Antimony, balsam of: It subdues and expels infinite diseases, all enemies of human life. Good for wound treatment (Basil Valentine, 1678). Take of Hungarian antimony one part, ½ part of salt, six parts of argilla (not burnt), grind all together and distill vehemently until red Powder remains as balsam for wounds, especially badly healing ones.

Antiscorbutica terra: A Norwegian clay mixed with lemon juice. Today we know it should have helped against scurvy (vitamin C deficiency) but the idea never caught on. The question of why not is one of the puzzles of emerging medicine.

Anwaldina terra: (Ludwig, p. 140, Table XII,11)

Arabian earth: A general name, but considered speckstein or talcum to dry hemorrhoids. Als used for earth with real or phony Arabic seals.

Arabian seal: Turkish or Arabic writing, phonetically Tin Machton (claimed to mean sealed earth) but according to Robertson (1986) is Greek for "of/from your mother earth" (Tin-I-Mach-Ton). But see also THIN (as in THIN-MACHTUM) and BARR.

Arabica terra sigillata: Same as terra hierosolymitica, Jerusalem earth (Zedler Vol. 37, col. 1074).

Argentum vivum: Mercury (Hortus Sanitatis 1485), (Badianus Codex 1552), excessively used in the 17th century in "sweat boxes" where people can sweat after ingesting mercury which is a normal reaction of the body to this poison. In 16th century tests, both a human and several dogs survived the poisoning after ingesting *terra sigillata*.

Argila, argilla: The basic Latin term for white clay, potters' clay, white marl (Ludwig, p.53)

Argilla alba cum acidis non evervescent: White clay not bubbling when acid is added (one of Ludwig's categories).

Argilla, others: cinerea (gray), Eversbach, Wermelandia, Mosconia, Suecica, Numburgensis Purpuream, Leucopetrensis, Weidensis, Halensis, Annaburgensis, Zellerfeldensis, Grubenhagensis, Grützingensis, Markwerbonsis, Glaucham, Osterlandia, glebe badensis

Argilla sigulorum also lutum fictile, potters' clay.

Argillacea lipsiensis (Stettritz): Leipzig earth

Argillacea nigra Glashüttensis (Altenbergensis): Glashütten earth, Altenberg earth (Ludwig)

Argillacea terra: White clayey earth, some noted from Halensis (Rivinus, Ludwig)

Armenian bole: A red clay of legendary value found in caves near the present border of Armenia and Turkey. It was exported to all the known world. Its healing properties included pest (if indeed that always meant bubonic plague). Bolus A. is real earth, feels fat and lubricious, is "thirsty and sticks to fingers".When Europe awoke intellectually after the dark ages, there was a wide search for local replacement clays to skirt the high costs of the original clay. Contains about 43% silica, 36,5% alumina, about 5% oxides of iron. Once so expensive it was a gift between monarchs (Kentmann, 1565). It is smooth to the touch, somewhat glossy, pure. It contains iron, magnetite, sulfite. Pills were prescribed for gastric disorders. "Bole armoniaka" (Alexis of Piemont, 1558). "take mastycke, dragon's blood, bole armonike" (Thomas Cogan, 1584). Gervaise Markham describes bole armony (!); bole armoniack is in the Pharmacopoeia of 1718. Surgeon George Smith made a plaster with bole armenic 1799, bolus armenus 1727-1751 against diarrhea (Robertson, 1986). Used for pus-forming ulcers, dysentery, stomach fluxes, short breath and cough (Spanudis, 1945?). Good for repeated fluxes, diarrhea, menstrual fluxes, catarrhs of the nose (Schroeder, 1644). "Thickens thin humors, resists putrefaction, expels poisonous bodies, stops spitting blood and bleeding wounds, consolidates broken bones(?). is astringent, desiccative, stops looseness of teeth, stops dysentery, sweetens acids internally" (Pomet).

Armenian borax: Myrrh and alumboracic powder for the eyes, (Dawson et al. cite a Coptic medical papyrus of the 9-10th century: "works so well that physician should demand advance payment").

Armenian earth: See Armenian bole.

Armenian stone: Most likely a copper carbonate found in Armenia and also used in healing. The ancients called it vitriol - glass-like, not in the sense of modern vitriols, i.e. metals with sulfuric acid.

Armenica terra: See Armenian bole.

Armenis lapis (lithos): See Armenian stone.

Armenus bolus, same as Armenian bole (Ludwig, 101-103)

Armoniac terra: Confused spelling in English writing, see Armenian bole.

Arsenicalis marga: A marl containing arsenic (Ludwig, p. 124)

Arsenicum: Word created by Theophrast, Arabian root denotes "of gold color," in medieval ages the yellow sulfurous arsenic As_2S_3. Arsenicum was very important to Paracelsus' medicine.

Asphaltus, -tum: See bituminosa.

Assian stone: Theophrast believed it came from Assus "in the Troad." Could be a natural earthy sulfate or sulfate in the form of purified crystals. Said to fill wound caverns, to heal ulcers. With honey it cleans ulcers, with wax it stops ulcers from progressing. Cataplasm for Podagra, helpful for the spleen (Theophrast).

Assyrian earth: For sores, ulcerous wounds. Assyrian has only one word for both swelling and ulcer, mostly translated as "sore" (Majno).

Astacus astacus: River crayfish; around 1879/80 a mass extinction of riverine crayfish ocurred in European waters, caused by water fungus (*Aphanomyces astaci*) which had been imported from the American species that are resistant to this fungus and carry it with them during their lifetime. See also cancer fluviatilis and oculi cancri.

Aster: One of the two earths from Samos, sealed with a star, may have had star-like glimmer from inclusions, good for polishing (Dioscorides, Ludwig, p. 187).

Astra terra: Rapta terra, syn. according to Zedler for Armenian bol (Vol IV, Col. 509).

Atacameños: Original inhabitants of the high Chilean desert between the coastal range and the Andes. Related to the Kiwanakos (Tiuhuanacos) of Bolivia.

Axungia lucii: Fat from the fish pike, medically used the same as fat of the bird Diomedea.

Axungia lunae: "White grease from the moon," a soft stone associated with the moon's ability to create a silver adjunct in the earth with dew from the moon as side product (moonmilk, calcium carbonate). Used against headaches, to strengthen brain, to relieve the white flux of women, relieve diarrhea.

Axungia solis: "Red or yellow grease from the sun," a soft stone associated with the sun's ability to create an adjunct to gold in the earth. Used to strengthen the heart, it is best for men, whereas axungia lunae is best for women.

Bactiacarum bolus cinereus: Gray Bolus found near Bern, Switzerland.

Badiani Manuscript: A 1552 illuminated herbal from Mexico, believed to be untainted by Western medical thought. Contains earths and minerals used in Aztec medicine.

Bagdad earth: Mesopotamian earth? River sediment meant for aching joints, wound treatment still observed in 20th century (Majno), see also Adamea terra.

Baira, earth of: Earth from near Palermo (Italy), (Volkmann, p. 276), also called lapis della montagna di Cane belonging to Principe della Catholica, Duke of Miselmeri.

Balearica terra: Clay from Balearic Islands in Mediterranean. Pliny mentions in liber LVII.

BARR: Arabic meaning "hard, friable", adjective for an earth, opposite: THIN

Basilensis rubra: Red clay from Basle, Switzerland (Rivinus, 1723),

Basilensis cinerea gleba: gray earth from Basle. (Ludwig, p. 114)

Bath bricks: (China) a mixture of sand and clay.

Beaver testicles: German Bibergeil, thought to be beaver testicles but were special glands both male and female beaver have between their hind legs. Legend says that when a beaver spotted a hunter, he bit off his testicles, threw them down for the hunter, and ran away. Syn: castorium.

Beierfelder terra sigillata / beyerfeldensis: Actual location Graul near Schneeberg (Heller, 1964).

Belgica terra: Clay from Belgium? From Kila (Belgis) a tributary of the Mosel? (Ludwig, p. 173)

Bergen earth: Earth from Bergen in Norway (Volkmann, p. 276)

Bernstein: See amber, yellow, once thought to be petrified lynx urine.

Bethlehemitica terra: Bethlehem earth, Milk of the Holy Mary, see Hierosolymitica terra. Depending upon which of the Gospel stories are considered, when Mary was lactating she was either in Nazareth, Bethlehem, probably not in Jerusalem, but fleeing Herod and going to Egypt. Hasluck (1909/10 p. 229) mentions a cave refugium where Mary nursed The infant Christ. This cave was known to Mandeville (1361). they sold earth trochisks with several image stamps or sigillations, including that of Mary, the child and the star.

Bezoar: A concretion within the intestines of animals, the type bezoar is a leather like fibrous accretion in stomachs of the mountain sheep, but variously the term has been applied to such concretions or even stones anywhere in an animal. Bezoars unfailingly detected poison and thus were cherished by noble personages. Prices were enormously high. Word origin from Persian Padh-zähr. Bezoars could also be animal gall stones etc. but all stones in humans (kidney, bladder, gall) were not called bezoar, but "calculus,", little stone.Aristotle considers it a precious smooth stone which protects against any kind of poison.This legend lasted into the 19th century and kings and princes had their own expensive bezoar "just in case". Bezoar was long known before the Europeans adopted it (Coe & Coe, 1996, p. 146).Bezoars: Bezoar bovinum - ox bezoar; Bezoar cervinum -

hart bezoar; Bezoar elephantum - elephant bezoar; Bezoar equinum - horse bezoar; Bezoar lunare - Bezoar powder made from (or with?) silver; Bezoar mulinum - mule bezoar; bezoar simiarum - monkey bezoar; (all Ernstingius, 1770).

Bezoar of snakes: Reported only from China, described as metallic nodes vomited up by snakes during their hibernation (Pen Ts'ao Kang Mu).

Bezoardica aqua: A liquid made from bezoar, ingredient in Horst's pharmacopoeia (1651).

Biolith: A sediment of organic materials at least partially made by organisms, organogene (Benade, 1937).

Bismuth subnitrate: Component of a wound dressing material from England, 1916.

Bismuth subsilicilate: An anti-diarrheal over-the-counter medication (Pepto-Bismol®).

Bitumen: Any natural petroleum tar product, pitch, liquid tar etc.(Lüschen).

Bitumen judaeicum: Globs of tar found floating on the Dead Sea.

Bituminosa terra: An earth containing tar, e.g. ampelitis terra.

Bituminosa torfacea terra: A peat earth containing tar (Ernstingius, 1770). Used medically about 1850 - 1900 in wound treatment.

Blanca terra: A white earth or clay from the island of Elba (Cesalpinus)

Blanckenburgica terra: (Ludwig, p. 99)

Blois, terre de: Red clay from Blois in France (Moise, 1670?), replacement for Armenian bole. Blois is the capital of Loire-et-Cher, first mentioned in 6th century. Joan of Arc set out from Blois. Late in 14th century Blois was sold to Louis de France, Duc d'Orleans.

Blosiensis terra: See Blois (Ludwig, p. 212, Table V, 16-18)

Bloodstone: See hematite.

Blue jade: Chinese term for sapphire.

Blue vitriol: See Chalcanthos.

Boëmica friabilis: Bohemian clay with many pebble inclusions (Kentmann, 1565).

Bohemica terra: Clay from Bohemia (Ludwig, p. 109)

Bolaris terra: Clay from Pennsylvania, a "bole-like earth", an oxymoron. (Ludwig, p. 94).

Boleslauensis argilla alba: White clay from Boleslau (Ludwig, p. 113).

Bolus alba: A white Kaolin-type clay, a German pharmaceutical term for a pill constituent. Stumpf tried it because the particle size is smaller than the bacterium, thus the grade of bolus alba he selected was Bolus alba officinalis subtilissime pulverisata.

Bolus armenus levanticus seu orientalis: A red clay from the Levant similar to Bolus armenus (Kentmann).

Bolus Gallica: Generic for a red clay from France.

Bolus Juliers: Bol from the Jülich, in the Aachen (Rheinland-Westfalen) area near Belgium. (Kentmann, Gessner, Berthold).

Bolus pannonicus: An Hungarian red earth (Kentmann, 1565).

Bononiensis terra: Clay from Bologna? Neusatz (Yugoslavia)? Boulogne-sur-mer? (Ludwig, p. 155)

Borax: A soft white crystalline substance (sodium tetraborate decahydrate), medicinally used as disinfectant and mouthwash, against itch and as clyster. Originally mined from Tibetan Lakes and used first as flux for metal processing in the middle ages.

Bornensis marga: Marl from Born near Freiberg (Ludwig, p. 135)

Bourgogne, bole de: French yellow clay (Pomet, 1712).

Brachmanum terra: Zedler says: From India or Malaysia, a fat brown sticky earth, used for chewing only.

Brasiliensis terra:? possibly an earth from Brazil, named by local Jesuits. Could also be a misprint for Basiliensis terra from Basel, Switzerland.

Brechelwicensis terra: Fat clay from Brechelwitz, Germany (Rivinus, 1723).

Brembergensis marga: Marl from Bremberg (also: Brechelwitz) (Ludwig, p. 131)

Brick clay: With vinegar helps against itch, podagra, swollen neck glands (Spanudis).

Brick dust: (Ancient Egypt, also Greece), powdered and mixed with vinegar, helps against itching and eczema, helps sufferers from podagra, mixed with wax ointment reduces swelling of glands. Mentioned in Berendes' translation of Dioscorides.

Brick earth: Qua lateres ducuntur (Kentmann, 1565). Probably either clay or ground brick.

Brundisiaca terra: Earth from Brundusia= Porrentruy (Switzerland) Listed in Pharmacopoeia Galeno-chemica, catholica (J. Daniel Horst, 1651, also Ludwig, p. 206, Table IV, 1,2).

Brusnicensis terra: Earth from Prausnitz (Ludwig p. 99, Table III, 6)

Burkhartsdorf bolus cinereus: Gray bolus from near Chemnitz (Saxony) (Ludwig, p. 94).

Cabochon (en c.): gemstone cut with convex rounded surface, polished but unfaceted

Cadmia: See calaminaris terra.

Calabrian earth: from Italy, Valentini and Pococke cited by Hasluck 1910.

Calaminaris terra: White deposit in flues of zinc smelters, used especially as eye ointment. Also called Galmei, Hüttenrauch, white copper of China, tutsch (Uigur), tutija - known to every place where zinc was smelted. (Ludwig, p. 179)

Calamine: See Calaminaris terra.

Calamus: root of a member of the Araces families (2), 123 genera, 2400 species which are all fertilized by captured insects. Some (such as calamus) are considered aromatic.

Calcarea (calcaria) terra: Chalk, chalky earth, alkaline earth (Mullen, Schinznach Bad. 1763), also found as deposit around thermal springs.

Calciolith (Kalziolith): Chalks such as sea chalk ($CaCO_3$), riff chalk (Island of Rügen), Akaustabiolithic sediment raised above sea floor (Benade).

Calcium: L. calx, raw and slaked lime; often named for any variety of white earths or clays.

Calcium carbonate: $CaCO_3$, as cave deposit called moonmilk. This is still the geologic name and the type location is the moonmilk cave in the Pilatus mountain near Luzerne, Switzerland.

Calcium montmorillonite: See cimolite, earth of Kimolos, Cimolia terra, also Fuller's earth.

Calculus: "little stone," often refers to human stones in kidney, bladder, gall, etc.

Calx: Lime, calcium.

Calx extincta: Slaked lime.

Calx nativa: See calx viva.

Calx viva: Unslaked lime.

Cancer fluviatilis: A riverine crayfish, Astacus astacus from Eastern Europe, prized for its calcium exoskeleton and the calcium "button" the crayfisch assembles when a new skeleton is needed. The name comes from the "eye" appearance, like an "eye" on a soup or an eye like leopard spots. See also oculi cancri and cancrorum lapis.

Cancrorum lapis: Calcium carbonate "button" from crayfish's accumulation for a new exoskeleton. See above, cancer fluviatilis.

Candida arenosa friabilis: White crumbly marl from Hildesheim (Agricola).

Candidus bolus Lignicensis: See Liegnitz terra.

Candida saponaria (sive fullonica): A white clay used for washing or fulling cloth, possible like Cimolian earth. (Kentmann, 1565). Absent soap, people often used white clay for cleansing.

Candida terra: Earth to make cloth very white, used by aspiring politicians in Rome called "the candidates" because of their whiter than white togas.

Cappadocia terra: Dioscorides, (Rivinus, ill. 19).

Carbonate of lead: L. cerussa, cosmetic use, $PbCO_3$, also ointment constituent.

Carduus benedictus (also Cardoonin English), edible part of artichoke.

Casselana terra: Earth from the Hessian region of Germany (Ludwig, p. 93 et al., see index)

Casselanus bolus luteus: light yellow, moist clay from Kassel (Ludwig, p. 11)

Castorium: See beaver testicles.

Cataplasma: A poultice, i.e. cataplasma kaolini, an antiseptic clay paste (Am. Pharm. Ass., 1908).

Chalcantos: A natural, native sulfate of metals, here copper sulfate, blue vitriol, used medically (Dioscorides). The term "vitriol" did not exist in L. then, but is in the Translation by Berendes. Sulfuric acid anhydride dates back only to 1580, so in Dioscorides' time it was called a hardened liquid (glass-like or vitreus when hard). The concept of "hardened liquids" and "congealed juices" persisted until late in the 16th century. Medical uses needed clay to be astringent, to warm, to cause wound scabbing and to kill (intestinal) worms.

Chemnitz (Chemnicensis) terra: Earths from the Chemitz Region of Saxony (Ludwig, see index)

Chernite: Maybe true alabaster or white onyx (Theophrastus).

Chia terra: Earth or clay from the Aegean island of Chios, also called pignitis terra.

Chrysolit: Called golden stone in antiquity (Lüschen), but so were many other stones like yellow corund, citrine, beryl, topaz. Helps against all sorcery and magic, dispels night terrors, cures cowardice, calms anger, gives notice of poison by losing color. Stops wound bleeding, cures asthma when powdered and added to wine.

Chrysocolla: In antiquity a crusty earthy copper mineral of green color, could be copper carbonate as well as malachite (Lüschen).

Cilicia earth: Earth from the region of Cappadocia.

Cimbers: Northern European tribe (Denmark) which spread all over Europe and even threatened the Roman empire. Their burial rituals included placing bones and artifacts into clay pots before burying.

Cimolia terra: Earth from the Aegean island of Kimolos, white calcium montmorillonite. Dioscorides writes: One is white, one is purplish, sort of fatty and cool to the feel. Either one, mixed with vinegar disperses swellings behind the ears and other swellings. Spread onto burns it works well instantly to protect formation of blisters. Ameliorates hardening of the scrotum as well as inflammations all over the body, cures erysipelas and is very useful if the genuine earth is used. Berendes (correctly) mentions Cimolite as a fullers' earth and the other earth as an iron-containing talcum. Soran of Ephesus claimed it hinders conception.

Cimolian earth: See Cimolia terra.

Cimolite: See Cimolia terra.

Cinerea Hibernia: Irish clay (area) guarded by a poisonous dragon (Kentmann, 1556).

Cinerea Hispanica: A Spanish clay from which melting pots were made (Kentmann, 1556, Rivinus, 1723, Ludwig, 1748).

Cinerea Patavina: Gray earth from Padua (Kentmann, 1656).

Cinerea rarissima Giselana: Rare gray earth from Giessen in the Land of Hesse (Kentmann, 1656). This clay is used still today to make dark gray stone ware pitchers with a deep blue glaze designed for purchasing apple wine,cider, or draft beer at the local pub.

Cinnabar: A red sulfide of mercury HgS, also a dragon's blood from tree resin. Distinguish from red lead oxide - minium.

Cizenis argilla alba: White clay from near Waldenburg (Ludwig, p. 114)

Citrina terra: A lemon yellow stone, probably yellow hyacinth.

Clay: Basically an unconsolidated sediment consisting of particles with a diameter of less than two one-thousands of an inch, also one of a group of clay-sized hydrous aluminosilicate minerals that can absorb water and other materials.
1. Clay sediment, an abiolithic deposit (Benade, 1937), e.g. "salty" shale of Ischl.
2. Aluminosilicate.

Clay, houri: A renowned ancient Egyptian or Yemenite medical clay.

Clay from the gate: Earth described in Papyrus Ebers.

Clay from a statue: Earth described in Papyrus Ebers.

Clay from the wall: Earth described in Papyrus Ebers.

Clay of Ani: Avicenna's name for bolus armenus. Ani was the capital of the ancient kingdom of Baghratuni in Cappadocia.

Clay, red: Clays were often designated simply by their color. Dioscorides: for ulcerated wounds.

Clay, yellow: Clays in antiquity were often designated simply by their color.

Clunea terra:?Pliny, liber LVII, Cluny, Dep. Saône-et-Loire, France

Colcothar (crocus): Reddish oxide of iron obtained by heating ferrous sulfate.

Coldicensis argilla alba: White clay from? (Ludwig, p. 113)

Cöllnische Kreide: Black or dark chalk or earth from Cologne (Rivinus, ill. 5)

Collyris:? Term used by Kircher 1665 for collyra (a piece of bread for soup) or collyrium.

Collyrium - 1) L. a mass shaped like a suppository as medicine, 2) L. a liquid eye ointment 3) one of the clays from the island of Samos. Retains urine, cures haemoptem (Abu Mansur) (Ludwig, p. 187).

Coloniensis terra: Earth from the vicinity of Cologne; Rivinus (1723) says: creta umbra, dark brown chalk (Ludwig, p. 111).

Color gris, terra sigillata de: Farmacia de la Familia Salvador, 1760 (Bech-I-Borràs).

Concretum vegetabile (compacted plant material): Earth mud of 10% to 100% organic material by dry weight. Benade (1937) divides this into a) natural thermal concretion or compaction, b) natural but "thermalized," c) natural, simplex and d) artefactum commune. See also "Lutum," the inorganic counterpart to concretum vegetabile. Term belongs into medical hydrology.

Confectio: One way of preparing prescriptions in palatable form (German: Konfekt – cookies, chocolates). A drug preparation with fruits, spices. sugar, similar to a conserve or anelectuary.

Conserve: See Confectio.

Coral: Underwater plant with calcitic shells - used as diaphoretic and diuretic, often ground as remedy for sour stomach. Red coral was deemed the best, it consists ~ of 83% calcium carbonate, 3.5% Magnesium carbonate and minor quantity of iron oxide. Considered a "stone tree". Black coral (Antipathes) was a specific against witchcraft in India, the Red Sea area. 15 kinds grow in the Mediterranean Sea. Dioscorides: As powerful as the red coral. In many prescriptions by J. Daniel Horst (1651), Ernstingius (1770). Coral as medicine is often powdered and mixed with rose water, lemon juice, guayak juice, spirits of wine (Schroeder). There is a coral salt, a distilled magisterium. Paracelsus calcinated coral with nitrum and added spirits of wine. Cures inflamed eyes, retains urine. Red coral is better for males, white for females. Dioscorides also lauds coral for urinary troubles, to stay menses, detersive of swellings, to stop bleeding piles, for "worm in the tooth", to check vomiting and acidity from dyspepsia and biliousness.

Corallis/Corallium: See Coral.

Crassa terra:? Demokritus.

Creta: Usually translated as chalk, white clay, white earth, and Cretean earth. Origin of word probably from the past principle creta for "has been sifted," rather than from the island of Crete (Kriti in Greek), but often refers to Crete. It is a group name for fine white clay. Aldrovandus, in Museum metallicum lists all white earth as "creta" like cimolia, selunesia, eretria and terra melia.

Creta cimolia candida: Very white earth from Kimolos, probably calcium montmorillonite.

Creta Gallica: A French clay considered equal to bolus armenus.

Creta Hispania: Spanish clay (Rivinus, Ludwig)

Creta nigrita: black chalk, (Ludwig)

Creta terra: Chalk from Crete, Ernstingius: also terra alba, terra alchichi. Doubtful as earth, feels meagre and dense, deposited from filtering into a rare powder. Draw lines with it (Ludwig).

Cretica terra: See Creta terra.

Creta umbrica: Farmacia de la Familia Salvador, 1760. Brown earth? Earth from Umbria?)

Cuenca terra: Against diarrhea, Baumé (1766) "Eléments de Pharmacie Téorique et Pratique", from Cuenca province of Spain?

Cypria terra: Earth from Cyprus, a greenish montmorillonite (R. H. S. Robertson).

Dachselbergensis tripela argillacea: Clay-like diatomaceous earth from Silesia

Dalmatica terra: Earth/clay from the Dalmatian Mountain region (See page 154, Ch. 7)

Damascena terra: See Adamea. (see also Ludwig, p. 160)

Diatomaceous earth: Light colored porous and friable sedimentary rock composed of silicious shells of diatoms. Compare Tripoli earth.

Diphryges: 3 kinds according to Dioscorides: 1) a red clay from Cyprus, twice dried, 2) the red flue residue from copper smelting, 3) Result of roasting pyrites in air. Dioscorides mentions all three in his dispensatory.

Dresdensis argilla: white clay from Dresden (Ludwig, see index)

Dolomite: Calcium-magnesium carbonate $CaCO_3 \cdot MgCO_3$.

Ducis Etruriae, Terra sigillata de: Farmacia de la Familia Salvador (1760), often sealed with the Picture or seal of the Medici, also called Florentine clay (Ludwig).

Eagle stone: A stone that was necessary for eagles to raise young, a "pregnant stone," because a little stone rattles inside it. Amulet for women to ease childbirth.

(Theophrastus). Probably a geode with a clayey or stony nucleus. A persistent legend, selected for medical investigation by Lorenz Bausch, founder of the German first scientific society, Academia Naturae Curiosorum (1660).

Earth dug out of pits: Usually near stables, compare terra nitrosa.

Earth of the Holy Mary: See Hierosolymitic earth, calcium carbonate.

Earths, chinese: See soils, Chinese.

Ebusitanae terra: Pliny, liber LX.

Edulis terra: Edible earth.

Egyptian clays: Tîn Misr generally Egyptian earth, various clays in Papyrus Ebers: clay from the gate, clay from a statue, clay from a wall, masons' clay; curing a series of diarrheal illnesses.

Elba terra: A white earth from the Italian island of Elba, mentioned by Ricarettio Fiorentino and Cesalpino end of 15th century.

Electuary: See Confectio.

Emerald: Aristotle says emerald strengthens the eyes when quietly contemplated; as amulet or signet ring will prevent epileptic attack. 8 grains (8 barley corns) powder taken internally will prevent death from poisoning "so God will."

Eretrian earth: Eretria terra: 1. Clay from the town of Eretria on the island of Euboea. 2. Eretrian cinerea ultramarina: Ashen gray (or blueish) Eretrian earth (Kentmann, 1656). 3. Dioscorides: Best is the ash gray one which shows violet when touched with copper (copper sulfate?). The white one, when washed and cleaned, is astringent, fills wound cavities and glues wound edges together.

Erlachiana terra: Swiss Erlach earth (Ludwig 207, Table IV, 4).

Ethology: Normally the science of ethics, here in its meaning for vertebrate zoology "the study of animal behavior in a natural context".

Eybenstockiensis terra: (Ludwig, p. 87)

Fango (Fanghi): Italian mud, almost a generic term for mud pack in Germany. French: La Fange. Gothic origin: Fani.

Farinacea terra: Flour-like earth from the Mehlberg (Ludwig, p. 94), see also Mehlberg bolus alba

Fechenhusana argilla: Probably a Silesian earth (Ludwig, p. 114)

Ferrifera terra: Mentioned by Ernstingius, but not identified.

Fichtelbergensis argilla: Silesian or Saxonian earth, (Ludwig, p. 114)

Finnlandica terra: Earth from Finland (?) (Ludwig, p. 178)

Florentine earth: Stamped with the seal of the Medici arms, Valentini cited by Hasluck.

Foetida terra: Sulfur, evil smelling earth.

Francabrugensis terra: Zedler: an earth named for or after Franc de Bruges.

Francigena terra: Actually a vegetable: Tragant (dragantum) goat's thorn, rattleweed.

Freybergensis argilla alba: White clay from Freiberg (Ludwig, see index).

Freybergensis bolus: red clay from Freiberg (Ludwig, p. 94).

Freyburgensis terra: (Ludwig, p. 90)

Freyenwaldensis terra: Very oily clay, used for gout (Zedler). Johrenius (1704), Conrad: disputatio inauguralis de arthritide…quaedam de terra medicinali Freyenwaldensis.

Fullers' earth: See calcium montmorillonite, cimolite, cimolian earth

Fullonica terra: See Fullers' earth

Gabel (Jabbel): Earth from Hungaria

Gagates lithos: A hard, polishable coal, today "jet," other meaning possible such as earth from Gagates, a river delta sediment clay.

Galactida lapis: L. galactites, milky color, when rubbed will give a white juice with milky taste, helps lactating women if worn as amulet, increases saliva flow in children, but takes away memory (Dioscorides). Can't be calcium carbonate which does not have any taste. Magnesium containing white clay?

Galactites: Coellnische Kreide is a misnomer, chalk from Cologne, Rivino (1723), (Ludwig P. 41/42)

Galata terra: Pliny, liber LIX.

Gallmey - Galmey: Zinc oxide, residue of zinc smelting.

Geoglyphs - Pictures and designs formed by assembly of small stones on gentle hillsides of the Chilean high desert that form the outline of an image cleared of stones on the "inside". Such images are often mythical, at times represent human figures, in some places they show recognizable llamas or guanacos. Sometimes an assemblage of geoglyphs is in the "negative", the image is filled with stones and at the edges of the image any stones are removed completely to give a black figure on a "white" background. The images are on a roughly 25-40% inclination, but shown so that when viewed from the flat desert over distance the shapes appear geometrically correct.

Geophagy: The habit or custom or practice of eating "earth", usually clayey earths.

Gieshübelensis: (Ludwig, p. 172)

Giessen (Gisela): Gray clay from Hesse (Konrad Gesner, 1565).

Gland terra: A vegetable, the peanut (an earth-nut).

Glashütten earth: Called the "newfound color of fortune", (Ill. in Ludwig, Table IV, 34, dated on the seal 1728). Hammers in shield may be from Saxony).

Glaucham Osterlandiae tripela argillacea: (Ludwig p. 91)

Glauchensis terra: (Ludwig, see index)

Glebis terrae: The lumpy earth as opposed to pulverized earth (Isidor).

Glimmer: Mica.

Goldberg alba terra: Rivinus (1723) - Terra sigillata goldbergiensis from Goldberg near Liegnitz.

Goldbergensis terra sigillata: One of the Silesian boles, also spelled Goltberg, Goldtberg, also called white bolus from Goldberg (Ludwig, p. 94).

Goldberg(i)ensis marga: Marl from Goldberg (Ludwig, p. 131).

Golderde: gold[en] earth, terra solaris, - a clay from Almerod, helps against vomiting, cures lack of appetite, helps with spleen problems, gets rid of intestinal worms. Sounds like a bolus alba. By some reports contains tiny flakes of gold.

Görlicensis marga: Marl from Görtlitz (Ludwig, p. 134)

Goslariensis: Clay from Goslar (Ludwig, p. 97)

Gran, earth of: Hungarian earth (Volkmann, p. 276

Graphium creta: doubtful earth, fat and lubricious, very tenacious in paste form (Ludwig).

Green (fresh) earth: Khespê dhê Sapâ in Papyrus Ebers I.

Green stone, Chinese: Empty green, Evergreen, green green, flat green, white green, application not yet identified.

Greifensteinensis terra: Earth from Greifenstein described by Dr. Geilfas, Darmstadt court Physician, probably like Terra laubacensis from Hesse.

Grimmensis argilla alba: White clay from the Grimmisch Forest near Chemnitz (Ludwig, p. 112)

Großjanowitzensis terra: Earth/clay from Großjanowitz in Silesia, now Poland.

Gross-Plussnitzer Erde: Clay from Silesia, eastern Germany, now Poland, also called terra sigillata montis acuti.

Grunspergensis argilla (Ludwig, p. 114)

Grünhayensis bolus luteus: Soft or yellow clay from Grünhain (Ludwig, p. 100)

Grützingensis gleba: Ludwig, p. 114

Gudensis argilla alba: White clay from Holland (Ludwig. p. 112)

Guinensis aromaticus terra: Rivinus (1723).

Gur: Guhr, silicolith.

Gypsum: Hydrated calcium sulfate named "chalk" (Greek: gypsos) by Theophrastus 300 BC. Also called selenite (moon like) because of its luster. The fine grained massive variety is Alabaster. Gypsum is common in the marls and clays of the Paris basin, therefore the name "Plaster of Paris". Dioscorides lauds it as astringent, it helps form skin over wounds, reduces perspiration and bleeding, but when taking internally, it can kill by Asphyxiation (indeed,, care must be exercised to keep the dust out of the lungs.)

Habsburgica: Collective name for empire including Austria, Hungary, Bohemia, Silesia)

Hainoviensis argilla: white clay from Silesia (Ludwig, p.114)

Halensis argilla alba: White clay from Halle (?) (Ludwig, p. 113)

Halloysite: A form of kaolin type clay but containing water, $Al_2Si_2O_3(0H)_4.2H_2OF$

Haslauiensis argilla: (Ludwig, p. 114)

Healing earth: Transl. of "Heilerde," a term coined about 1925. It denotes an earth used for medical application and includes such as residual weathered stone, clays, marls, loess and Loess clay (Benade, 1937). Benade divides these into 1) naturals: packed in original moist condition, heated and used for treatment, 2) praeparata: prepared by a work process without changing the product (grinding, milling, sifting, washing, drying, and 3) artificial: If altered significantly. Originally the name applied only to externally applied clay.

Healing sediment: Similar to definition of healing earth, but limited to underwater sediments.

Heidelbergensis terra: (Ludwig, p. 91)

Helsingica terra: (Ludwig, p. 86)

Helvetica terra: (Ludwig, see index)

Hematite (haematite): Blood stone, a naturally found iron oxide. Dioscorides: Must be easily pulverize, best color is very dark, even black, clean of dirt or foreign particles. Warms slightly and is astringent, with honey smoothes scars and roughness on the eyes, cures dripping eye when mixed with mothers' milk. With wine drunk to ease urination and to cure female flux. With Pomegranate juice drunk against spitting blood. Makes collyria and other eye medications. Easily faked with alum or cinnabar or the like (Dioscorides); Modern spelling hematite. In Egypt and Ethiopia used for eyes and for burns, as red paste for bilious disorders. At times confused with red clay. The translation of the

Egyptian cuneiform symbol "didi" still not certain - either red clay or hematite. Theophrast also calls it red jasper.

Helvetia "an der Thun" argilla: Clay by the river Thun in Switzerland (Ludwig, p. 116)

Heraclean stone: Lodestone (Theophrast).

Hersbrucker Erde, Terra hersbruccensis: See Veldener earth.

Hibernia cinerea: Gray clay from Ireland (Kentmann, 1565).

Hierosolymitana: see Hierosolymitica, otherwise (Ludwig, p. 222, Table VII, 29 ff)

Hierosolymitica terra: Jerusalem earth, calcium carbonate, in legend milk accidentally sprayed from Mary's breast onto the walls of a cave where the Holy Family was hiding from Herod. Cave continued to produce calcium carbonate. Chronology very much in doubt. Main use of Mary's milk is improving of lactation of human and beast. See also Bethlehemiticum terra, Syriac issue of "earth from the sepulcher (Ill. p. 153, Ch. 17)

Hilbersdorf argilla viridis: Green clay from Hilbersdorf (Ludwig, p. 116)

Hildesiensis terra: (Ludwig, p. 89)

Hirschberg marga candida fissilis (Rivinus, 1723, Ludwig, p. 119)

Hispanica terra (sigillata): Spanish earth (Rivinus, 1723).

Hispanica cinerea: ashen colored earth from Spain (Kentmann, 1565).

Hium Hian Sinensis terra: A sweet soft earth from China (Rivinus, 1723).

Holy Mary earth: see Hierosolymitica terra.

Hortus sanitatis: An illuminated herbal of 1485 from Germany, with earths included.

Houri clay: A fine clay from Egypt.

HTNJ - earth: Frequently mentioned in the Papyrus Hearst and the London Papyrus. Often mixed with dates, antelope tallow, serpent fat, crocodile fat and hippopotamus fat.

Hubertusburg: (Ludwig, p. 241, Table XXII, 26)

Human stone in bladder (China): used medicinally, probably pulverized.

Humolith: See peat.

Hungarica: Hungarian earth (Ludwig, p. 90)

Iablonensis terra: (Ludwig, p. 109, Table IV, 5,6)

Iaspis: A watery green and translucent stone (Theophrast), not today's jasper apparently.

Iauoprensis terra: Earth from Dukedom of Jauer (Ludwig, p. 81, Table II, 40-46)

Ichorous: A wound excretion, watery and serous.

Ienowitzensis bolus: Groß und Klein Gehnowitz, (Ludwig, p. 107).

Ienensis argilla alba: White clay from Jena (Ludwig, p. 113).

Iflebiana candida: White clay with "glittering silver", probably flecks of mica (Kentmann, 1656).

Ilfana terra: Earth/clay from island of Ilfa or Liefland, mixed with lemon juice against evil fevers (Zedler), see also livoniensis terra (Jung). From Livonia (Ludwig).

Iluana terra lutea: (yellow, lemon-colored clay from Iluana (Ludwig, p. 94)

Ilvensem terra: (Rivinus 28).

Imbria terra: Mentioned, no details given. It is either a clay used for roof tiles or a Powdered roof or gutter tile, from Latin imber - hard rain, probably similar to brick dust.

Ioudaikis lithos: Sea urchin spines, helps break bladder stones (?) Sea urchin spines are calcium carbonate

Ipsensis terra:? Ybbs (Tributary of the Donau)? (Ludwig, p. 112)

Italica terra: Italian earths

Iron Pyrite: Bisulfide of iron, Chinese health stone Tzu Jan T'ung, which grows pale when the health of the wearer is about to fail (Pen T'sao Kang Mu).

Iuliacensis bolus candidus ex luteo ad grande rubedinem accedens vero bolo Armenia: A glistening bolus from a clay of such redness that it approaches the Armenian bole, (Kentmann 1656). From Jülich near Aachen.

Iuliacensis pinguis mollis cinerea: Grey soft fatty earth from Jülich (Kentmann, 1656).

Jablonensis terra: From the town of Jablona on the feudal estate of Count Berka of Berkarum in Bohemia.

Jade: Nephrite, Chinese Yü, silicate of magnesia and alumina, also dolomite. In Europe used for edema, calculi (Bartholinus, 1628), in Brazil called "Amazon stone," an amulet against snake bite and difficult parturition.

Jade elixir: Chinese Yü ch'uan, confers immortality.

Japonica terra: A vegetable, once thought to be an earth, but it is a tree sap.

Judaeicus lapis/lithos: Bitumen, asphaltic exudation.

Kaolin: Al $_4$(OH)$_8$ (Si $_4$O$_{10}$), white clay from China. It is the reason fine dishware is called "china" In the US and England; in other countries the dishware designation is "porcelain" because the surface is white and translucent like the shell of the Porcellana snail. Later the term includes other minerals in a group such as halloysite.

Kaustabiolith: Term for sediment of organic, primarily plant, material, combustible when dry, consisting mostly of organic carbon and more or less mineral substance (Benade, 1937)

Kellmünzlicensus tripela argillacea: diatomaceous earth (Ludwig, p. 87).

Kiangnan province: a clay from Kiangnan (Rivinus, 14).

Kieselgur: Diatomaceous earth, Tripoli (triple) earth.

Knee dirt: Soil rubbed off the knee (China).

Kulmensis (Bohemia) bolus ruber: Red clay from Bohemia (Ludwig, p. 100).

Künnersbergensis argilla: a clay (Ludwig, p. 91).

Künnersbergensis tripela: (Ludwig, p. 91)

Kyanos: See Armenian stone.

Lac lunae: Moonmilk: calcium carbonate as cave deposit, Gessner (1555), (J. D. Major, 1667), (Ludwig, 1748).

Lac virginis: 1. An old English mixture of white earth and white of egg dating to Erasmus of Rotterdam and copied down by Isaac Newton. 2. Mary's milk, milk of the holy mother, also called Bethlehem or Jerusalem earth.

Landesleubensis terra: (Ludwig, p. 156)

Langele(u)ben argilla alba: White clay from Langele(u)ben (Ludwig, p. 113)

Lapis: L. a softer, fragile, or smaller stone than "saxum" which refers to harder, rocklike stones. Often the "earths", terrae, are referred to as lapis/lapides.Lapis armenicus: Nicolaus Salernitatus ~1100 AD. It is generally considered a copper vitriol, but could be a mistake for Armenian bole - see Armenian stone.

Lapis lazuli: Occurs in crystalline limestone, the ultramarine pigment comes from sodalite which is a chloride containing aluminosilicate, which, when blue, is called lazurite. Inclusion of Pyrite gives lapis lazuli the gold-like flecks. Papyrus Ebers refers to use together with Malachite milk and Tabasheer (?) for cataract; paste made with ash, astringent mud and caustic earths, used as counter-irritant (Dioscorides). Purges melancholy and strengthens the heart.

Lapis niger - pumice (Abu Mansur).

Lapis qui submergitur in corpore humano: Stones in the human body. Also Latin: calculus.

Laubacensis terra: A fat clay from Laubach, Hesse, Rivinus (1723) "saliva permista"; (Ludwig).

Laubacensis marga: Marl from Laubach, (Ludwig, p.134).

Legnica: Since 1945 Polish name for Liegnitz.

Leisnicensis terra:? Leising (Saxony) (Ludwig, p. 118)

Lehm/Letten: German for a yellow sandy clay (loam?).

Lemnia seu sigillata terra:

1. Clay from the island of Lemnos, with the seal of the goat of the goddess Artemis. The best description is from Galen who was there.

2. Earth from the island of Lemnos was either known as *Terra lemnia* or as *terra sigillata* (sealed, branded earth) which became the synonym for Lemnian earth; later used with other earths, too (Kentmann, 1656, et al.).

3. Red earth from swampy area of Lemnos (but also says: from subterranean shafts) (Dioscorides, who also says the earth is mixed with goat's blood - wrong. Taken with wine will prevent poisoning, good against diarrhea, useful for insect and animal bites. Vitruvius calls it a red clay. Plinius thinks it is cinnabar (Plinius, as usual, is wrong). 4. Pomet says: Good poison antidote, proper for fluxes, hemorraghes, gonorrhoea, vomiting - it is fatty, clayey, soft, dry, friable, astringent. Tozer (1898) says earth is striated and can be white, pink, streaked, or red.

Lemnia sigillata terra: The most famous healing earth in the ancient world from the island of Lemnos. It was sealed (branded) with a seal of a goat, the symbol of the Goddess Artemis (Roman: Diana). Sometimes referred to as *lemnia sphragis* (sealed lemnian earth). Thompson's "safe assumption" analysis (1912) appears to be of a clay other than true Lemnian earth.

Leucopetrensis argilla alba: White clay from? (Ludwig, p. 93).

Levantine bolus: See bolus armenus.

Liegnitz earth: Clay from Liegnitz in Silesia, branded with cross keys, symbol of the city, but many fakes exist - Heller. Now Legnica in Wroclaw district of Poland.

Lignicensis terra: See Liegnitz earth.

Lignicensis marga: Marl from Liegnitz (Ludwig 131)

Lignicensis argilla alba: White clay from Liegnitz (Ludwig 108)

Lignicensis bolus candida: Very white clay from Liegnitz

Lignisch gesiegelt Erd: See Liegnitz earth.

Lignitz, Leignitz: Common misspellings of Liegnitz in English language publications.

Ligurius - see Lyngurion (Ligurius is Albertus Magnus' spelling.)

Limestone in old graves: A Chinese "healing" stone.

Limoges porcelain: fine china earth, found near Montmorillon.

Liparian stone: Obsidian from the island of Lipari (Theophrast); others think pumice. Lipari Islands are west-northwest of the Strait of Messina between Italian mainland and Sicily.

Lipsiensis argilla alba: White clay from Leipzig (Ludwig 113)

Lithomarga: Syn. for rock marl, talcum (magnesium hydrosilicate).

Lithos: Greek for stone, equivalent to L. lapis.

Lithomarga: Filling "earth" in rock crevices, often talc.

Lithuanica terra: (Ludwig, p. 86)

Livoniensis ilfana terra: From Livland, said to have been mixed with lemon juice (Jung).

Livonica terra: Ludwig has earth coin picture (Ludwig, p. 112, Table I # 2).

Loess (Löß): Diluvial wind deposits of very fine sand and calcium particles (Lüschen). Wind sorts the particles by size. Loess primarily shows 65% particles of 0.1-0.02 mm, 25% 0.02-0.002, 7% < 0.002 mm, very porous, high quartz content over 50% (Jung 1939).

Lodestone: Magnetic stone - magnetic iron oxide (Theophrastus).

Lutea terra or bolus: soft, wet clay

Lutea terra Casselana: Soft clay from Kassel (Hessen).

Lutosa terra: Soft yellow clay (Kentmann, 1565).

Lutosa terra candida: White clay, sandy, wherein grow little petrified snail houses (Kentmann, 1565).

Lutum: A moist soft earth such as clay, loam, mud. A predominantly inorganic mineral material with a maximum of 19-15% dry component. See for comparison "concretum vegetabile" (Benade, 1937).

Lutum Apuliae: Soft earth from Apulia (Kircher, 1665).

Lutum artefactum commune: Sediment material being applied in a form which does not exist in nature (Benade, 1937).

Lutum naturale simplex: Natural sediment not connected to a thermal spring (Benade, 1937).

Lutum naturale thermale: Natural thermal mud created by a thermal spring. (Benade, 1937).

Lutum naturale thermalisatum: A mud which is not connected to a thermal springs, but thermal spring water is later mixed in (Benade, 1937).

Lyngurion: Theophrastus apparently was not aware of yellow amber being traded from northern Europe to Liguria (Lynguria) in Italy. It was considered lynx urine dried in earth. Pliny defines it as lynx urine. So does Hildegard von Bingen.

Lyncurium - see Lyngurion.

Lynx stone: See Lyngurion resp. amber, yellow.

Magdeburgensis tripela: Diatomaceous earth from Magdeburg (Ludwig, p. 91)

Magnesite: $MgCO_3$ also called carbonate of magnesia, an anti-diarrheal medicine (milk of magnesia).

Magnet stone: (Lodestone) (Pseudo Aristoteles) When this stone ist softened in garlic and onion water, it loses its power, but sour milk and hot blood strengthens it. A magnetic mountain lies in India which will pull iron nails and locks out of ships. If someone has been injured by poisoned iron, the mountain will cure him. This legend is later repeated in other tales. Aetius of Amida said it cured headaches.

Magnetis lapis: See magnet stone.

Magnetism: According to the Book of Stones wrongly attributed to Aristotle, there is a mountain "in the West" which has a variety of stones which are magnets for gold, silver, copper, flesh, hair, (finger-) nails, wool, cotton, lead and a stone which attracts fish so you can scoop them out of the water.

Magni-Plussnicensis terra: Earth from Great-Plussnitz in Silesia. It was claimed that it resisted the pest (??) when drunk with brandy or beer. Also coined as Montis acuti.

Malachite: Basic copper carbonate $Cu_2CO_3(OH)_2$. Used for cardiac pains and colic, eye trouble.

Malaena: black chalk.

Maslense bolus, in signum Domine de Kreckowitz: Earth from Massel, (Ludwig Table III # 9)

Maslense Fossile arboresense 1711 (Ludwig III #8, in Chapter of Illustrations).

Maslense Fossile arborescense et Kleinschweinerense: (Ludwig Table III # 7), Signum LDH MSP. Illustration Chapter 17 p. 144, Line 3, 4 L.)
Leonhardi David Hermann', Maslensis Silesii Pastoris.

Maldiviensis terra asiatica: Earth from the islands of the Maldives (Ludwig, p. 110).

Maltese earth: From the island of Malta. Usually referred to as St.Paul's earth, but may be dated before Paul involuntarily reached Malta. From comments about "re-growth" of the white earth, it probably was calcium carbonate in St. Paul's cave. Also called Pauladatum after Knights Templar (Knights Hospitallers, Johanniter Knights) arrived ~ 1606.

Majorica terra: Mallorca? From *Mundus subterranous* by Athanasius Kircher 1665.

Mansfeldensis: (Ludwig, p. 93)

Marble: A white stone, a calcium stone. Isidor, who differentiated between stones, classified them as normal stones, excellent stones, marble and precious stones. This could include porphyrites, basalt, alabaster - same as with the definitions of Albertus Magnus.

Marga: Marrow, clay in rock spaces, marl, also marga saxatilis (distinguish medulla saxorum).

Marga candida pinguis mollis Torgana: White liquid marl of Torgau (Kentmann, 1565).

Marga candida lapidosa: White hard marl (Kentmann, 1565).

Marga lemnia: Ludwig, for: terra lemnia.

Margarita: Latin: pearl.

Mariaeburgensis: (Ludwig, p. 172)

Marrisburgensis: (Ludiwg, p. 100)

Markwerkensis pallide rubra argilla: Light red clay from Markwerk (Ludwig, p. 116)

Markwerkensis purpurea argilla: Purple clay from Markwerk (Ludwig, p. 116)

Marl: clayey earth used normally as fertilizer, Agricola (1565).

Marrow stones: Chinese, Wu Se Shih Chih (Read and Pak, 1936). They are very much like kaolin, The blueish one resembles Fuller's or Saxony earth, the yellow variety lithomarge; generally about 47% silica and 40% alumina. Comparable to *Terra sigillata*.

Martialis terra: Iron oxide (iron was the metal of Mars).

Martisburgensis bolus luteus: Yellow or soft clay from Martisburg (Ludwig, p. 100)

Martisburgensis pallide rubra argilla: Pale red clay from Martisburg (Ludwig, p. 116)

Maslensis ochra: (Ludwig, p. 88)

Massel: A small hamlet in Silesia, on coins known as Maslensis.

Masons' clay: Egyptian, from Papyrus Ebers' list.

Medicant: From old Latin medicari something that cures, appeared 1535 in English, modern syn. medicament, medicine.

Medicinalis terra: Non identifying term but classifying those worthwhile having in a chemist's shop as remedy.

Medulla saxorum: Marrow of the rock, usually talcum (talc).

Meerschaum: Sepiolite, sea froth, very famous type of clay for smoking pipe bowls.

Mehlberg bolus albus: White flour-like clay from Mehlberg (syn: Farinacea terra)

Meissen earth: Very well known brand of porcelain clay from Germany.

Melaena terra: Black chalk (Rivinus).

Melanteria terra: A black earth used as shoe polish (Agricola 1546, Bermannus).

Melia terra: Earth or clay from the Aegean island of Melos (Ernstingius, 1770). Dioscorides says it is ash gray like Eretrian, easily rubbed between fingers, but a bit rough. Weak taste, dries the tongue. Cleans body when rubbed on, is a depilatory and removes white spots from the skin. Use it sieved and fresh. Restrains creeping ulcers, stops bloody fluxes, closes moist gums, strengthens wagging teeth. Almost entirely silicon dioxide - 97%.

Melitea (Melitensis) terra - earth (probably calcium carbonate) from the island of Malta, also called sigillated earth of St. Paul (Schroeder, 1634). There were at least four different seals, probably from four different clay digger associations - all had Christian themes of St. Paul who was shipwrecked on the island. See Chapter Seventeen, see pages 150, 151. Melo candissima: The whitest earth (clay) from the island of Melos (Kentmann, 1565)33.

Memmingensis: (Ludwig, p. 94)

Meranensis argilla: From Merano? (Ludwig, p. 114)

Mercurialis terra Beccheri: A quicksilver mixture as medicine by Becher, not an earth

Mercury: Quicksilver, used medically extensively in 16th century (Ingestion of mercury, sweatboxes).

Merita terra: Actually a vegetable - root of curcuma, tumeric.

Mesuè, sigillated earth, mentioned in 1511 Catalan Pharmacopoeia (Bech-I-Borràs), refers to J. Mesuè (1581) "De medicamentorum...Canones...de simplicibus. Grabadin Antidotarium, Venice. Printed by Juntas. Actually Bech-I-Borràs is in error, since there are about 50 different Pseudo-Mesuè. The title which Bech-I-Borràs gives is dated 1513 and the authors as Petrus, Jacque Departs and Nicolaus (the Antidotarium).

Metal stones: In the Book of Stones of Aristotle as translated from an Arabic text, the term stone includes all metals, which is curious because in one place a metal is called a metal. (Probably falsely attributed to Aristotle by a Syriac writer).

Milchheimensis Franconiae argilla alba: White clay from Milchheim in Franconia (Ludwig 113)

Minoralische Einhorn-Erde: Mineral earth effective like [expensive] unicorn horn (Heller 1960)

Miraculosa terra: From Planitz in Saxony (Jung).

Misnensis cinera terra:
1. gray clay from Meissen (Kentmann, 1565).
2. prope Risan - light gray clay from Riß near Meissen.

Mithridat, An antidote for poison named after King Mithridatus of Pontus. He drank Eupatorium until he believed himself inured to all poisons. When he was finally captured by the Romans, they thought it futile to make him take poison and made him fall on his sword instead.

Mitweydensis argilla: (Ludwig, p. 88)

Molaris lapis: Ground mill stone.

Moluccis insulis effossa argilla: Earth dug on the Molukka islands (Ludwig, p. 116)

Mönchensteinensis argilla marmorea; Marbled clay from Mönchenstein (Ludwig, p. 116): gray, violet and variegated.

Montanus: See Trimontanus, Johann Sculterus

Montis acuti terra sigillata: See Groß-Plussnitzer earth.

Montis fracti terra: Moonmilk ($CaCO_3$) from Pilatus mountain near Luzerne, Switzerland

Montmorillonite: Type location Montmorillon in France, basically known as calcium montmorillonite. and sodium montmorillonite (today generally called bentonite).

Moonmilk: Calcium carbonate as cave sediment or drip stone (Gesner 1555, Major J.D., 1667, Dictionary of geology, 1998).

Moor (moor land): Moor is only a location, not an "earth"

Moor: Also fen, bog, swamp(land), marsh(land) - see "peat". Moor is the natural resting place of peat which can count among healing earths.

Moritzburg bolus luteus: Soft or yellow clay from Moritzburg in Hesse. (Ludwig, p. 100)

Morochtus: A leek green and milky sediment stone in thermal springs, used for cleaning cloth. Pliny says it gives a light green juice like leek, Galen and Dioscorides disagree. Claimed efficacious for spitting blood, lower abdominal and bladder problems, also as insert for white flux. With wax ointment helps building of scar tissue. According to Ludwig 1748 The term has variously (wrongly) been appied to moonmilk (calcium carbonate), Maltese earth, Dresden clay and earth from Münchenstein near Basle,

Moskauensis: Ludwig (p. 95) Moscow earth?

Moscovica argilla viridis: Green clay from Moscow (Ludwig, p. 116)

Mud (Schlick): An ocean tideland or river mud flat, silt, ooze, mire; generally a biopelit and Akaustobiolothic sediment MS, Benade (1937).

Mud (Spring): A biopelit, akaustobiolithic sediment occuring near or in thermal springs (Benade 1937) Examples in Europe: Battaglia and Pistyan (mud baths).

Mud of marsh: Mud in the flood area of either Nile or Euphrates

Mud of Nile: 1) "btj", 2) tîr iblîz, syn: crocodile earth.

Mud of Nile, with lemon: For flavor probably, doubtful that it was known as cure for scurvy.

Mumia: In a time period when various body parts and exudations were used in medicine, it is not surprising to have mumia considered dried skin of mummies. However, it is more likely that mumia referred to a type bitumen originating in Armenia, which at times was used as suitable balm for preservation of bodies.

Mumia mineralis: Pitch, tar (Ernstingius, 1770).

Münsterbergensis argilla alba: White clay from Münsterberg (Ludwig, p. 111)

Naphtha: Originating from Babylonian naptu, the burning thing which surfaced spontaneously in Mesopotamia. Liquid petroleum.

Naxius lapis: Powdered marble (Aethius of Amida).

Nericia earth:? Ludwig, see index, but provenance not discussed.

Neosoliensis marga: Marl from? (Ludwig, p. 135)

Nicolstadiensis:? (Ludwig, p. 159)

Niger lapis: See pumex.

Nishapur clay or earth: Rhases in his "treatise on clays" tells of curing people seized by very grave choleric affections with violent fits of vomiting and cramps (cholera?), the clay immediately relieved nausea and indigestion. Also used it to reduce secretion of saliva and to help all people with ravenous appetite (worms?). He prescribed 30 drams of clay twice a day in a decoction of sweet apples, which also cured nausea.

Nitrosa terra: Earth dug from animal stables, rich in urine/ammonia (Ernstingius, 1770).

Nitrosa Thuringia (terra): Clay full of nitrum (soda, ammonia) (Kentmann, 1565).

Nitrum: Natural soda used for bleaching, washing and as mordant for colors.

Nobarsowensis terra: from Upper Silesia (Zedler, Ludwig - see Chapter on Illustrations).

Norimbergensis rubra terra or rubrica: Red clay from Nuremberg.

Noviregni terra: Brandenburg earth.

Norwegica terra: Clay with lemon juice, antiscorbutum alexipharma terra (Rivinus, 1723)

Nubian earth: Egyptians used it for ear aches, tongue inflammations, tooth decay. Also an earth from Shendi in Nubia, gray/brown, mild to the touch, to treat syphilis (?).

Nucerana: various earth coin shapes from southern Italy near Palermo (Chapter 17, p. 157)

Numburgensis pallid rubra argilla: Light red clay from Nuremberg (Ludwig, p. 116)

Numburgensis argilla pallide fusca: Light brown clay from Nuremberg (Ludwig, p. 116)

Oakum - the coarse part of flax separated in hacking, also: a loose fiber obtained by untwisting and picking old rope, used especially in caulking ships' seams. Picking oakum was once a prison occupation (1481)

Oberrabenstein bolus luteus: Soft clay from Oberrabenstein (Ludwig, p. 100)

Ocean animal stones: (Aristotle) When added to eye powder will sharpen the sight and strengthen the nerves, removes the dry eczema and the roughness of skin.

Ocean stone: Curious is the distinction between stones of the "traveled ocean" and the "unknown Ocean" (traveled ocean =Mediterranean, unknown ocean = South Atlantic, then called the Ethiopian ocean well into the 17th century. For instance, the legend of coral involves both oceans.

Ochra (ochre): Take the one yellow through and through, free of stones, easy to disperse by hand, the one from Attika is best. It is astringent, heals infections and swelling… (Dioscorides). From iron pits comes the reddish clay, firing it makes it redder (Pliny). Both red and yellow clay can occur together. Theophrastus: The best red ochre comes from the Cyclades island of Kéa.

Ochre: A mixture of iron oxide hydrate with clay (Berendes).

Ochre, burnt or roasted: Given internally as a pill. Probably little difference to brick dust.

Ockroll red clay: Kentmann (1565).

Oculi cancri: 1) When the river crayfish Astacus astacus needs a new exoskeleton, it collects a button or eye of calcium carbonate near his belly, from which the new skeleton is made. These calcium buttons were collected by the cart full and sold to apothecaries as cure for sour stomach resp. heartburn (Reinbacher, 1998). See also Cancer fluviatilis, Astacus astacus. 2) The gastric teeth or gastroliths from the gizzard of the common crayfish Astacus fluviatilis (Paul G. Shipley).

Oculus - Eye on the skin of a leopard, eye on peacock feather, the bud or bulb of a plant, "the certain thick part in certain places", such as (see above) the oculi cancri.

Officinalis terra: Designation of earth in a pharmacy.

Olsnitiensis earth:? Oels (lower Silesia)? (Ludwig, p. 159)

Oreana earth: From Italy, Worm cited by Hasluck.

Orpiment: A native or natural sulfide of arsenic, As_2S_3.

Osnabrugensis terra: Earth from Westphalia (Ludwig, p. 153)

Ostraca: Fired earth fragments from the oven, finely pulverized, has a drying and cleansing and smoothing power, polishes teeth, mixed with vinegar helps against itch and podagra, with wax ointment disperses hardened glands of the neck (Paul of Aeginas transl. Berendes, 1914). Dioscorides: Prevents pregnancy after taking it with wine for four days.

Ostrea: Fired or burnt oyster shells, cleans teeth, when washed looses the sharp taste and helps to fill wet ulcers (Paul of Aegina).

Ostrobothnica: (Ludwig p. 178 - but may be a sand))

Ostrogothica: Earth from Cimbria? (Ludwig, p. 86)

Oxoniensis terra: (Ludwig, p. 114

Oxymel of Gold: Mixture of vinegar and honey, with gold (flakes or dust) an elixir of life in (China). Danziger Goldwasser: Gold flakes in liqueur as a tonic (Europe).

Pan(n)onicus verus terra or bolus: Genuine Hungarian bole (Kentmann, 1506).

Pappenheimensis argilla marmorea: Marble-like clay from Pappenheim (Ludwig, p. 119).

Paretonian earth: Named after a sea port in Cyrenaica (Ludwig, p. 186).

Paros marble: Marble from Mt. Marpessos on the island of Paros.

Passauensis argilla alba: White clay from Passau (Ludwig, p. 113).

Patnae terra: From India, used geophagically by local pregnant women (Zedler).

Pearl: The Greek myth of the creation of the pearl involves both the traveled ocean and the ocean of darkness forever. A spray from the traveled ocean fertilizes the shell. The pearl is made of an equal amount of heat and cold, dryness and wetness. The pearl helps against a fast beating heart and against fear and panic. The pearl is mixed with medicaments for the eyes and relieves headaches. J. D. Major (1677) had it in his "Potentate tonic" for his Duke of Schleswig-Holstein (Reinbacher, 1998). Sylvaticus prescribed pearls for malignant fevers - pearls to him were celestial dew drops in the ocean. Feeding powdered pearl to leeches made leeches work better for bloodletting.

Peat (humolith): A kaustobiolith that forms mainly in temperate humid climates by the accumulation and partial decomposition of vegetable remnants under conditions of deficient drainage (MS), first exposed to air oxygen and later humified in the absence of oxygen (Benade, 1937). It covers vast areas of moors, such as flat moors, forest moors, high moors, spring moors and hanging moors. Moor earth is mineral rich peat (Benade, 1937).

Pedemontanus (Rochlitz) terra: Bauhinus, Rivinus

Peloid: Created as collective name (Greek: pylos - clay, mud) for all kinds of mud, peat, etc. of natural origin by S. Judd Lewis of the Peloid Committee of the International Medical Hydrology Association (1937). The name was violently objected to by some members, supported by others. Benade preferred his classifications of "lutum". The committee disbanded since no consensus could be reached.

Pennsylvanica: (Ludwig, p. 91)

Pen Ts'ao Kang Mu: The nigh 3,000 year old written collection of medical knowledge of China which was updated continually in every dynasty, first printed in the 16th century, and revised and reprinted in 1997.

Pentelius marble: Found near Athens.

Petersdorf earth: Silesian clay, (Ludwig, p. 203, Table III. 3.).

Petzenstein: (Ludwig, p. 203)

Pharmacognosy: Acquired (by humans and animals) knowledge of minerals, herbs, and animal substances or parts with specific medical benefit.

Pica: The eating of irrational foods (usually by pregnant women) sometimes used as synonum for geophagy, the eating of earths.

Piedmont earth (terra piemonte, now piedmontite): brown or black silicate of aluminum with iron, manganese, and calcium.

Pignite earth: Similar to Eretrian earth or earth from Chios, cooling, sticks very tightly to the tongue. Name comes from Pigneus in Lybia. Very astringent, black, powerful as Cimolian earth (Paul of Aegina). Also called terre étouffée.

Pitch: Cures harmful humors, softens scrofulous tumors, used to treat leprosy and wounds, hemorrhoids, ingredient in salve for boils (Avicenna).

Pix, liquidus: Liquid tar product from pine wood.

Planitz terra sigillata: "iron stone marrow" (Agricola), reddish marl?

Ponderosus terra: Heavy earth, also stibium turcicae - Abu Mansur.

Porcelain clay: White translucent clay like kaolin, named after the almost translucent white shell of the porcellana snail. Therefore German use for fine dish ware is "Porzellan", French "porcelaine", English retained "china" (made from clay from China).

Portugallica terra: Sealed with a rose (source: CJS Thompson, 1913) - name not in Latin dictionary, source not given. Meaning probably "earth from Portugal."

Potters' clay: Any variety of aluminosilicates suitable for fabricating on potter's wheels

Potters' earth: Clay for making pots and other household items.

Pretiosa terra: Common name for all hyped sigillated earths with "healing power" (Zedler).

Primogena terra: From Crete (Erstingius 1770), virginal earth.

Prussica: earth from Prussia

Psoralea bituminosa: A pitch base ointment for head itches (psoriasis, maybe lice) (Mowafik).

Pulvis paretonius: used by Kircher 1665 for an earth from Cyrenaica

Pulvis puteolanis: Volcanic ash from Campana in Italy (Kircher, 1665).

Pumex: See Pumice

Pumice (stone): Rough volcanic stone, lava. Light pumice floating on water, believed formed by the foam of the sea (Theophrast). Abundant on Melos and on Lipari islands.

Pumicum: An African pinguid aluminosilicate clay. Source Ludwig. 3d definition of "lutum".

Purulent: A wound which contains or discharges pus

Puteolana terra, puteolanis pulvus: Cicero: A city in Campagna of Italy, favorite area to relax for rich Romans - volcanic ash and mud for bathing.

Pozzuolana terra: volcanic ash with silica, alumina, lime, earth from near Pompeii.

Quartz: A rock crystal. In Chinese Shui Ching used as "vertigo stone". Olaus Borrichius (1626-1690) made a tincture for dropsy, scrofula and melancholy from quartz.

Quedlinburgensis argilla alba: White clay from Quedlinburg (Ludwig, p. 113)

Radisensis argilla alba: White clay from Radis near Wittenberg (Ludwig p. 113)

Rammelsbergensis argilla: (Ludwig, p. 124)

Realgar: A native or natural red arsenic sulfide As_4S_4, also called sandarac.

Reichenbach earth: Silesian earth (Ludwig)

Reichenbergensis ochra: Ocher from Reichenberg (Ludwig, p. 88)

Reichensteinensis terra: (Ludwig, p. 168)

Reppersdorfiensis bolus luteus: Soft bolus from Reppersdorf (Ludwig, p. 100)

Rock crystal- See quartz.

Rocklitz earth: A soft red stone marrow (Agricola, 1565; Rivinus, 1723), talcum, used as fake Armenian bole.

Röcklicensis bolus alba: A white clay from Rocklitz or Röchlitz.

Rocklicensis bolus luteus: Most clay from Rocklitz (Ludwig, p. 100)

Ronneburgica: (Ronneburg in Hesse?) (Ludwig, p. 153)

Ros. di: Italian:? (Ludwig, p. 157)

Roswinensis: (Ludwig, p. 110)

Rubrica: Syn. for red earth or clay, see also rufus bolus.

Rubrica fabrilis: Red earth from a volcano.

Rubrica sinopia: See Sinopian earth.

Rouen, terre de: An argillaceous (white) diatomaceous earth from Rouen (Ludwig, p. 87)

Rufus bolus: light-red bolus, see also rubrica

Russian earth: (Ludwig, p. 91)

Saarauer Blauton: A blue/black clay dating to Miocene age, from Saarau near Striegau in Silesia, Heller (1964).

Sacra terra: See sancta terra.

Salfeldensis ochra: Ochre from Salfeld (Ludwig, p. 88).

Salmantica terra: In Farmacopoea de Valencia.

Salsburgensis terra:? Salzburg? Salisbury?

Salts in Chinese medicine: Sea salt, pond salt, well salt, stone salt, army salt (?), bright salt (?).

St. Paul's earth: St. Paul was shipwrecked on Malta and lived in a cave near Rabatto by Civitavecchia. The cave contained a self-replenishing white earth (calcium carbonate). The marketing of this earth was done with many variations of allegories from Christian religion in the seals and size of tablets; prices were very competitive. Also Terra sigillata St. Pauli, Vera terra de la grotta di Sao Paolo. Seals were St. Paul, St. Peter, Johannes, thorn-crowed Christ, maltese cross. About 20 different ones. It is possible that marketing of St. Paul's earth is as early as the beginning of the 16th century.

Samia terra: See Samian earth, either collyrium or aster.

Samian earth - Aster: hard as a grinding stone and plate like, when ground as effective as Eretrian earth, reduces blood spitting, effective against female white flux; with water and rose ointment reduces swellings of testicles and breasts. Drunk with water helps against poisonous bites and poisoning. Stamped or sigillated with a six-pointed star (aster) (Dioscorides).

Samian earth - collyrium: Very white and light clay, glues to the tongue, rubs off easily.

Samian stone (Lithos samios): Stone used by goldsmiths to polish. When white it cools, is good for the stomach, dulls the senses (Dioscorides)

Sancta terra:? Could be 1) St. Paul's earth, 2) Mary's milk earth, 3) possibly Lemnian earth.

Sangershusana earth: From Sangershausen, Silesia (Ludwig, p. 148)

Santa Marta, terra de:-From Farmacia de la Familia Salvador, 1760.

Saponaria Elbogiana: Body colored, red and white, Elbogiana soap earth (Kentmann, 1656).

Sapphire: Lüschen says: used for eye diseases (Aldrovandi Museum metallicum 1684 p. 972); in Hindu medicine against phlegm, bite and flatulence, potions for scorpion bites, intestinal ulcers, prevents boils and pustules.

Saprolith: A kaustobolithic (q.v.) mud, Sapropel™ of Bad Bentheim, Liman mud, also Schollener Pelose, Gyttja. Pelose - see peloid. (Benade, 1937).

Saracenica terra: Same as terra lemnia or terra sigillata alba, probably referring to "Saracenes" as eastern heathens, such as the Turks were then considered. Term most likely invented after Turkey took over the island of Lemnos.

Sarda terra: Earth from Sardinia, Rivinus (1723), Pliny liber LVII.

Sardinica terra: Earth from Sardinia

Saumur earth or bole: Red earth/clay from Saumur, France (Pomet, 1712).

Saxonia miraculosa terra: Miracle earth from Saxony, a state of Germany (Ludwig, p. 161)

Schaumburgia terra: (Ludwig, p. 112)

Schlick: gently flowing river mud, coastal mud, see mud of sea.

Schmiedebergensis terra: (Ludwig, p. 164)

Schnabelbergensis (Helvetica) argilla: Clay from Schnabelsberg in Switzerland (Ludwig, p. 116)

Schönauensis marga: Marl from Schönau near Zwickau in Saxony (Ludwig, p. 135)

Schneebergensis ochra: Ochre from Schneeberg.

Schönfeldensis terra: (Ludwig, p. 91 ff)

Schönhübelensis terra: (Ludwig, p. 172)

Schwarzenbergensis: (Ludwig, index)

Schwiednitzensis ochra: Ochre from Siberia (Ludwig, p. 88)

Scrapings from a statue: A clay from Sumer.

Sculterus: latinized name for an appointed mayor or scribe of a town, German Schultheiß, see Trimontanus, Johann Sculterus

Seburgia candida: White clay from Seeburg (Kentmann, 1565).

Seichauer terra sigillata: Seichauensis, bolus from basaltic mountains in Silesia.

Seichauensis marga: Marl from Seichau in Silesia (Ludwig, p. 131, Rivinus, 19).

Selinusia terra: An earth from Selinus on Sicily, smoothes facial skin, rebuilds after ulcers and fills them, especially for burns. (Paul of Aegina).

Sepiolite: Meerschaum used for pipe bowls.

Sepulcher, earth of: Supposedly earth from the sepulcher of Jesus.

Serpents' bezoar: (China) a pisiform iron oxide and nodular pyrites, believed to be a bezoar of snakes which they vomit up during hibernation (Pen T'sao Kang Mu).

Seyferdorffensis terra: (Ludwig, p. 110).

Sessana earth: From Italy, cited by Hasluck (1910).

Sicula terra: From CJS Thompson: Sicilian earth (?).

Siberiense tripela argilla: Diatomaceous white clay?

Siberiensis bolus: Bolaris clay (reddish?) from Siberia.

Siderolith: Metallic akaustabiolithic compound, i.e. ochre in Val Sinestra and Pyrite Sand of Teufelsbad (Benade, 1937).

Sielbergensis: (Ludwig, p. 210, Table IV 35), two hammers in shield: Bohemia? Saxony?

Sienense lac lunae: Mondmilch (calcium carbonate?) from Siena, Italy.

Sigulata terra: Misspelled sealed earth [sigillata] from an unknown source in Germany (Baier, 1708).

Silberberg earth: clay from Silesia, (Rivinus, Ludwig).

Silicolith: Kieselgur, see diatomaceous earth.

Silesia, Silesian earths: A region of former eastern Germany (now Poland) where many earths were found. A strip about 100 km wide extending almost mated to the northeastern border of the Check and the Slowak republics. The border area includes much of the so-called Giant Mountains, here though meaning in lenght, not height.

Silesiaca terra: Generic for any earth from Silesia (now Poland).

Sinopian red (earth, rubrica): Considered the best fine red earth. It is dug in caves in Cappadocia and transported to Sinope on the Black sea. (Dioscorides). It has been reported that the red earth was cinnabar dug near by Sinope, but that appears not likely. It is an iron silicate clay or bolus rubra (Berendes). Theophrastus says it is bolus armenus.

Sinuessa earth: An Italian earth, cited by Hasluck. Cups made from it detect poison.

Sleep bringing stone: Fable stone reported in the so-called Book of Stones by Aristotle. It is a red stone, glowing like fire at night and smoky in the day. Hanging a drachma of this stone around a person's neck will instantly put him to sleep until the stone is removed.

Sleep chasing stone: Same as sleep bringing stone, except gray - he who hangs 10 drachma around his neck will not sleep night or day. Snorting powder from this stone will cure elephantasia.

Smalcaldensis Marga: Marl from Schmalkalden (Ludwig, p. 134)

Smaragdus: In Theophrast's time any green translucent stone from Bactria (Afghanistan).

Smaragdus (false): Probably solid blocks of malachite.

Smectite: Smectite minerals are derived from the alteration of volcanic glass and from the weathering of primary silicates. They are chief constituents of bentonites and fullers' earth. Smectis earth feels fat and lubricius, not thirsty, tenacious and compact, difficult to make into paste (Ludwig)

Soapstone: Syn. Steatite.

Soda, natural: Na_2CO_3.

Sodium montmorillonite: Bentonite, used much the same as calcium montmorillonite.

Soils, Chinese: Soils from: bottom of well, one of Chinese healing earths; bottom of hole of urin, bottom of hole of shit, soil from agricultural field; carriage soil, soil underneath shoe, soil under pillar, soil under bed, soil mixed with dog urine, soil mixed with donkey urine, soil of bird nest, soil of bee nest, soil of rat nest, shit of ghost; soil of white ant, soil of earthworm, soil of snail, soil of white eel, sweet soil, red soil, yellow soil, soil on east wall, sun soil.

Solaris toccavensis terra: Gold flecked earth from the northeast corner of Hungaria (Tokay).

Soliskamskoi tripela: Diatomaceous earth from Russia.

Solms-Laubach: see Laubach, Laubacensis, see also Solmensis terra for illustration.

Solmensis terra: (Ludwig, p. 211, Table V, 5-11)

Sommerfeldensis terra: (Ludwig, p. 90)

Sonneburgensis terra: (Ludwig, p. 90)

Sphragia terra: Same as Lemnia terra or terra sigillata - also meaning stamped or sealed earth.

Spiros lithos: Syn: Thrakian stone, asphalt, bitumen.

Spongiae lapis: Light pumice.

Stag horn: Often roasted and pulverized for calcium content.

Stag's tears: Legend has it that stags ate snakes, but that the ingested poison heated them so that they had to cool off in lakes or ponds where they shed tears which solidified as clear crystals.

Stalactite in China: K'ung Kung Nieh - the middle part of the drip stone with a hole in the center. Considered the stone of immortality.

Stalimene terra: Stalimene is an old name for the island of Lemnos. See Lemnian earth.

Steatite: Soapstone.

Steinauensis: Which Steinau? (Ludwig, p. 119)

Stella terra: Syn: for aster? Star stone, star sealed stone from Samos?

Stetinensis:?Stettin? (Ludwig, p. 150)

Stibnite, also antimony glance: In ancient times often confused with Persian silver, tin and antimony, or tin and lead.

Stockhornius: Stockhorn mountain, Switzerland? If so, Gesner (1565)

Stollbergensis: (Ludwig, p. 117)

Striegauer Siegelerde: See Strigoniensis, named by Johann Schulz called Montanus or Johannes Sculterus Trimontanus after the three clay source hills Breitenberg, Georgenberg and Kreuzberg. Ludwig names 21 kinds of earths (See Illustrations Ch. 17, p. 130-140)

Strigoniensis terra (earth): Rivinus (1723), a fat clay. Colerus (1604) clay against poisoning, bites, insect bites, heart ache, heart palpitation, heart weakness and unconsciousness, eye injuries and inflammations, fluxes and dripping eye, red and white stomach fluxes, fevers, old ulcers.

Strigoniensis marga: Marl from Striegau, Silesia (Ludwig, p. 131)

Stypteria: Syn. for alum (q.v.), later "styptic" as stopping blood flow. (Dioscorides)

Succinus: See amber, yellow.

Suecica argilla: from Orebroam, Sweden.

Suecica argilla: from Wermelandia, Sweden (Ludwig, p. 114)

Suppurating: A wound which gathers pus underneath

Syriac writing: Developed from an Aramaic alphabet. Language and writing of Syriac Christians (1st to 14th century)

Syriaca earth: Earth from the sepulcher of Christ (Chapter 17, p. 133) (Ludwig, p. 122)

Talcosa terra: a bolus from near Jena (Ludwig, p. 94)

Talcum: A fine white powder of low slip, $Mg_6OH_4Si_8O_{20}$, syn: Speckstein, old Lithomarga. The Arabic name is sun phlegm or sun saliva. In antiquity often confused, Aristotle includes in this name mica, asbestos; it falls onto earth like manna or honey dew and hardens. Depending upon surroundings, may be green or even reddish. Fills cracks and recesses between rocks.

Tell(t)anensis bolus: (Ludwig, p. 94)

Termite hill earth: Especially in Australia frequent reference to native consumption for stomach complaints and also for improved lactation.

Terra sigillata: 1) General term for stamped or impressed or "sealed" earths in medical history 2) Not used here, for clarification only: Term for Roman red pottery from 1st to 3d century which had decorations "stamped" by using a negative mold to raise the relief, term of art in ceramic studies.

Theriak: Very old multi-ingredient remedy against poisonous bites and almost all illnesses, usually among 70-100 ingredients, contains at least one earth, much wine or other alcohol. Found in classic medicine well into the 19th century.

THIN: An arabic designation "soft, flexible" as adjective or prefix to a clay name, such as THIN-MACHTUM (Terra Maris), THIN ALBOHERA.

Thrakian stone: Asphalt or bitumen from the district north of the Aegean Sea.

Thuringia nitrosa: An ammonia-rich earth from Thuringia (Kentmann, 1565).

Tin stone, description: Aristotle (?) calls all metals "stones". The tin stone goes into eye ointments. It is a miscegenated silver.

Toccarese earth: Italy?, allegedly sigillated with Medici Coat of Arms. Cited by Hasluck, 1910.

Toccaviensis terra: Rivinus (1723) - like Armenian bol, Hungarian earth, see: solaris toccaviensis terra, (Zedler).

Toccaviensis Marga: Marl from Tokay (Ludwig p. 134) (Volkmann, p. 270)

Tockiensis, tocaensis, toccaiensis, tokaika: Different known spellings.

Tokayensi, terra medicinali: Fischer, Daniel Wratislaviae, 1732.

Töppelberg: The Töppelberg may have been a place where the Cimbrians buried the bones and ashes and artifacts of relatives in clay pots (same as they did in Cimbria, then lower Denmark). A deposit of such pots was found in Silesia on a mountain called Töppelberg.

Torgauiensis earth: Clay from Torgau (Ludwig, p. 158)

Trimontanus: Johann Sculterus Montanus or Trimontanus of Striegau found some of the first Strigian clay earths about 1582. They were soft, pliable, yellowish, fat, stuck to the tongue, disperses when wetted with saliva, a typical healing clay description from old days. Believed to be found in gold mine shafts, where the rising vapors of gold create this.

Tripoli earth: See Trippel earth.

Tripolino Barbariae: See Trippel earth.

Tripolitana terra: See Trippel earth.

Trippel, trippela: diatomaceous earth from Tripoli, German common expression.

Turcica terra sigillata: Most likely Lemnian earth after Turkey annexed Lemnos and took over the marketing of the Lemnian earth (Schroeder, 1644).

Turkish clay: Reddish clay found all over Turkey.

Tutija: Calamine.

Tymphanic earth: A white earth used for [cleaning] clothes, found near Mt. Athos. Theophrast lumps it together with his gypsum which could have been chalk.

Umbra: Earth from Umbria in Italy.

Unicornus ad terras non pertinet: While one promoter called his earth coins "as good as metallic unicorn horn powder", Ludwig disagrees with that. By 1740 Leibniz had published his reconstruction of some fossil bones as a unicorn with two knees per front leg, no hind Legs, but sliding on the tailbone. (Reinbacher, 1998)

Usnea cranii: A moss, probably lichen, grew on the heads of those hanged, after their bodies had been lying in a town's "killing field" unburied for several years. Today usnea are medicinal lichens. Usnea barbata is called the "plant antibiotic" medicine.

Vallis Joachimici terra: Earth from Joachimstal (Rivinus).

Veldener earth, terra sigillata or herspruccensis (also Hersbrucker earth): Chalky clay in the Geisloch caves near Velden (Germany). Also called Veldensis-Norica. Mentioned by Joh. Jacob Maier, 1708, Ludwig, 1748. Volkmann (272) says it was found in the Geisloch cave near the Velden pestilence office near Nürnberg

Vermelandia ochra: Ochre from Vermeland (Ludwig, p. 88).

Veldensis marga: Marl from Velden (Ludwig, p. 135).

Veronensis terra: Green earth from Verona, see also terra viridis.

Virgo terra: A deep underground earth never touched by man.

Viridis terra: Green earth from Verona, also in Farmacia de la Familia Salvador, 1760.

Vitriol: The term vitriol dates to 1580 when sulfuric acid and its relation to metals was discovered.

Waldeckensis: Earth from Waldeck (Ludwig, p. 124)

Waldenburgensis rubra mollis scissilis: Soft, red, friable earth (Kentmann, 1656), (Ludwig, p. 114).

Wartenburgensis: Which Wartburg? (Ludwig, p. 155)

Weapon's salve: An ointment to be applied to the weapon (tool) which caused the injury and the patient would be cured even if he/she was elsewhere. The official prescription from the Berlin dispensatory required moss from the head of a hanged man (usnea cranii),which must be collected when the waning moon stands in Venus, not in Saturn or Mars. Other Ingredients: cleaned earthworms, boar or bear grease, oil, turpentine and Armenian Bole.

Wermelandia: (Ludwig, p. 114)

Weiss sigillata: See Lignitz earth.

Westmannica: (Ludwig, p. 94)

Westrogothica: (Ludwig, p. 153)

Wetterauica terra: Earth from the German region of Wetterau, (Horst, 1651).

Wettinense tripela prope halam Saxorum: Diatomaceous earth near Halle, Saxony (Ludwig, p. 87)

White copper (Chinese): Calamine.

White earth from Elba: See Cesalpino, 1596, see Ricotto Fiorentino, 1498.

Wildenburg clay: One of the favored post-classic clays found in Germany.

Winkelhaydensis argilla: (Ludwig, p. 114)

Woldorpensis tripela argillacea: White diatomaceous earth from Woldorp (Ludwig 91)

Wounds: In the times when infections were still common, an ichorous wound had a watery, serous discharge, a suppurating wound gathered pus underneath, a purulent wound contained or discharged pus. Wound still do this, but aspsis and antibiotics treat it.

Zinc bloom: Calamine.

Zwickauer argilla marmorea: Marbled red and white clay from Zwickau. (Ludwig, Table XII, 5)

INDEX

<u>INDEX</u>

<u>About the Author</u>

Rudy Reinbacher was born and educated in Germany. He graduated as a diplomate in economics and in business administration. He speaks and reads several languages and has traveled worldwide for research.

This book about minerals for healing since the dawn of humankind is a unique effort. Because of the quality of research, several private, public, and university libraries consented to his use of rare illustrations from the twelfth, sixteenth, and eighteenth century for this book dealing exclusively with healing earths.

Rudy and his wife live in Northern California since 1964. The proximity to Stanford University facilitates his research. His first book was a biography, in German, about a professor of medicine near Hamburg who wrote about the cave medicine "moonmilk".

www.ingramcontent.com/pod-product-compliance
Lightning Source LLC
Chambersburg PA
CBHW080253030726
47593CB00009B/2468